Policy Analysi

In *Policy Analysis as Problem Solving*, authors Rachel Meltzer and Alex Schwartz provide a pragmatic yet fresh and original approach to the field. Emphasizing the importance of evidence and sound logic and drawing upon multiple perspectives and methods, the book guides readers through the process of making evidence-based decisions about policies. It offers a series of clear and comprehensive discussions about the key elements of the analytical process, beginning with steps to define the problem all the way until analysts arrive at a recommendation.

The authors break from traditional approaches in their embrace of analytical flexibility and illustrate a broader framework for thinking about policy, both empowering and equipping readers to marshal a diverse array of evidence, techniques, and evaluative criteria in their analyses. Case studies threaded throughout the book illustrate the different ways in which problems can be framed and the kinds of policies and criteria that may flow from these alternative framings. Focusing on child support, voter turnout, water shortage, and short-term rental platforms, they also reveal the challenges and imperfect conditions that analysts encounter in the real world.

Bolstered by an expanded scope, updates to its case studies, and refinements to its central arguments, the second edition of *Policy Analysis as Problem Solving* remains an excellent go-to resource for students and aspiring analysts in policy analysis and public policy courses.

Rachel Meltzer is the Plimpton Associate Professor of Planning and Urban Economics at Harvard University's Graduate School of Design. Her research concentrates on urban economies, economic development, housing, land use, and local public finance. Dr. Meltzer's work has been supported by grants from the National Science Foundation, Social Science Research Council, the U.S. Department of Housing and Urban Development, and the Lincoln Institute of Land Policy, among others, and her research and writing appear in the top journals spanning policy, economics, and urban studies.

Alex Schwartz is Professor of Urban Policy at the New School. His research focuses on housing and community development, including public housing and other affordable housing programs, and community development corporations. Dr. Schwartz is the author of *Housing Policy in the United States*, now in its fourth edition (Routledge 2021), and his research and writing appear in journals such as the *Journal of Urban Affairs*, the *Journal of the American Planning Association*, *Housing Policy Debate*, and *Cityscape*, among others.

"The second edition of this innovative textbook leverages an interdisciplinary perspective and intuitive approach to policy analysis as 'evidence-based advice-giving'. I like the way it continues to integrate the latest insights from the behavioral sciences and design thinking and their application to public policy. And I appreciate how the book not only inspires deeper learning about policy analysis but also teaches practical skills that students can take with them as they confront the challenges of real-world policy design and implementation."

Gregg Van Ryzin, *Professor, School of Public Affairs and Administration, Rutgers University–Newark*

"Meltzer and Schwartz deliver an accessible, well-organized, and contemporary introduction to public policy analysis. I use their book to teach theory courses on public policy, and the text offers just the right mix of solid scholarship and practical application. Replete with excellent examples and two running policy cases, the narrative arc of the book fits well with my students' own development as policy professionals—they grow with Meltzer and Schwartz as the book progresses over nine chapters."

Justin Hollander, *Professor of Urban & Environmental Policy & Planning, Tufts University*

"*Policy Analysis as Problem Solving* is the ideal handbook for students seeking the skills to engage in social and public health policy analysis in real-world contexts. By integrating the conventional rational model of analysis with approaches that reflect the true complexity of politics and human behavior, Meltzer and Schwartz have crafted an accessible, flexible, and actionable framework for generating evidence-based policy recommendations that advance the social and economic determinants of health."

Linnea Laestadius, *Associate Professor of Public Health Policy, University of Wisconsin Milwaukee*

"Meltzer and Schwartz have quickly become an authority on how to help students get started. They explain the classic steps of policy analysis, show how it fits into the bigger picture of policymaking, and relate it to a push to democratise policy design. By combining these insights, Meltzer and Schwartz help students to compare policy analysis ideals and real-world dynamics."

Paul Cairney, *Professor of Politics and Public Policy, University of Stirling, UK*

"The first edition of *Policy Analysis as Problem Solving* proved to be an excellent counterpoint to standard textbooks that focused too narrowly on the economics of policy analysis and the role of market incentives in modeling policy alternatives. The Second Edition expands with new case studies and illustrations. It provides a superior alternative textbook for instructors and students concerned about fairness and equity in producing evidence-based policy recommendations. The critique of conventional policy analysis methods is balanced and lucid and should be required reading for every serious practicing policy analyst."

Samuel L. Myers, Jr., *Director and Professor, Roy Wilkins Center for Human Relations and Social Justice at the Hubert H. Humphrey School of Public Affairs, University of Minnesota*

Policy Analysis as Problem Solving

A Flexible and Evidence-Based Framework

Second Edition

Rachel Meltzer and Alex Schwartz

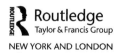

NEW YORK AND LONDON

Designed cover image: naqiewei/iStock

Second edition published 2025
by Routledge
605 Third Avenue, New York, NY 10158

and by Routledge
4 Park Square, Milton Park, Abingdon, Oxon, OX14 4RN

Routledge is an imprint of the Taylor & Francis Group, an informa business

© 2025 Rachel Meltzer and Alex Schwartz

The right of Rachel Meltzer and Alex Schwartz to be identified as authors of this work has been asserted in accordance with sections 77 and 78 of the Copyright, Designs and Patents Act 1988.

All rights reserved. No part of this book may be reprinted or reproduced or utilised in any form or by any electronic, mechanical, or other means, now known or hereafter invented, including photocopying and recording, or in any information storage or retrieval system, without permission in writing from the publishers.

Trademark notice: Product or corporate names may be trademarks or registered trademarks and are used only for identification and explanation without intent to infringe.

First edition published by Routledge 2018

Library of Congress Cataloging-in-Publication Data
Names: Meltzer, Rachel, author. | Schwartz, Alex F., 1957– author.
Title: Policy analysis as problem solving : a flexible and evidence-based framework / Rachel Meltzer and Alex Schwartz.
Description: Second edition. | New York, NY : Routledge, 2025. | Includes bibliographical references and index.
Identifiers: LCCN 2024042108 (print) | LCCN 2024042109 (ebook) | ISBN 9781032493893 (hardback) | ISBN 9781032493886 (paperback) | ISBN 9781003432753 (ebook)
Subjects: LCSH: Policy sciences. | Problem solving.
Classification: LCC H97 .M4464 2025 (print) | LCC H97 (ebook) | DDC 320.6—dc23/eng/20241024
LC record available at https://lccn.loc.gov/2024042108
LC ebook record available at https://lccn.loc.gov/2024042109

ISBN: 978-1-032-49389-3 (hbk)
ISBN: 978-1-032-49388-6 (pbk)
ISBN: 978-1-003-43275-3 (ebk)

DOI: 10.4324/9781003432753

Typeset in Times New Roman and Copperplate
by Apex CoVantage, LLC

CONTENTS

ACKNOWLEDGMENTS   IX

INTRODUCTION   1
Organization of the Book   5
Case Studies: Child Support Debt and Electoral
    Participation   7
References   13

CHAPTER 1   WHAT IS POLICY ANALYSIS?: MAINSTREAM AND
ALTERNATIVE PERSPECTIVES   15
What Is Policy Analysis?   15
Policy Analysis as Part of the Larger Policy Process   16
The "Rational Model" of Policy Analysis   20
Critiques of the Rational Model   23
Alternative Models of Policy Analysis   26
Summary: Using the Rational Model Flexibly   33
References   34

CHAPTER 2   DEFINING THE PROBLEM AND SETTING THE STAGE   37
The Rationalistic Approach   38
Alternative Perspectives   39
How to Establish a Problem Statement   40
Using Evidence to Frame the Nature of the Problem   53
Summary   56
Child Support Debt Case: Defining the Problem   57
References   63

CONTENTS

Chapter 3	Devising Alternative Policy Options	67
	Approaches for Generating Alternatives	69
	Modeling Alternatives on Existing or Previous Programs and Policies	70
	Alternative Strategies for Developing Alternatives	75
	Insights From Behavioral Economics and Related Fields	81
	Insights From the Field of Design	93
	Summary	96
	Child Support Debt Case: Alternative Policy Options	97
	References	106
Chapter 4	Objectives and Criteria	109
	What Are Criteria?	109
	Where Do Criteria Come From?	111
	Constructing Effective Criteria and Measures	117
	Two Common Pitfalls	137
	The Analytical Matrix	138
	Summary	139
	Child Support Debt Case: Criteria	140
	References	143
Chapter 5	Technical Aspects of Policy Analysis: Discounting, Cost-Benefit Analysis, and Cost-Effectiveness Analysis	145
	Discounting: Accounting for Time Value of Money	146
	CBA Introduced	155
	What Is CBA?	157
	Why CBA Is Hard to Do in Practice	177
	Using CBA Flexibly and Pragmatically	183
	An Alternative to CBA: Cost-Effectiveness Analysis	186
	Summary	189
	References	190
Chapter 6	Analysis and Making Recommendations	193
	Prediction and Estimation	194
	Additional Considerations When Projecting Outcomes	205
	Comparison of Outcomes	206
	Making Recommendations	215
	Summary	217

	Child Support Debt Case: Analysis of Policy Options and Recommendation	219
	References	232
Chapter 7	RESEARCH AND POLICY ANALYSIS	235
	The Role and Purpose of Research in Policy Analysis	235
	The Research Plan	236
	Documents	240
	Interviews and Focus Groups	247
	Public Events and Site Visits	256
	Data Sets	257
	Surveys	263
	Case Studies and "Best Practices"	266
	Summary	268
	Child Support Debt Case: Research Methods and Data Sources	269
	References	272
Chapter 8	POLICY ANALYSIS IN PRACTICE	275
	Where Do Policy Analysts Work?	275
	Policy Analysts Need Good Communication Skills	284
	An Ethical Code for Policy Analysts?	288
	Ethical Analyses Versus Ethical Practices	289
	Challenges to Incorporating Ethics Into Policy Analysis	291
	How to Conduct Ethical Policy Analysis	293
	Summary	296
	Child Support Debt Case: Ethical Dilemmas	297
	References	299
Chapter 9	EPILOGUE	303
	What's Next?	304
Appendix I	CASE FOR ANALYSIS: WATER SHORTAGES IN THE LOWER AND UPPER BASINS OF THE COLORADO RIVER	307
Appendix II	CASE FOR ANALYSIS: REGULATING SHORT-TERM RENTALS	321
Index		331

Acknowledgments

A big thank you to Vicki Turetsky for bringing us up to date on the child support debt situation since the publication of the first edition of this book and for answering our many questions as we revised the child support case study. As with the first edition, we are incredibly fortunate to draw on Vicki's extensive first-hand knowledge of the nation's child support system. We are also very grateful to Aaron Bierstein for his work on the new case studies on Arizona's water crisis and short-term home rentals. He conducted thorough research and drafted the cases with authority and flair. Thanks too to Michael Zajakowski Uhll and Tyler White for their research assistance. Finally, we thank the many students at the New School and Harvard who have taken Policy Analysis with us. This book could not have been written without them.

INTRODUCTION

Our goal in writing this book is to provide a straightforward yet flexible framework for conducting policy analysis. We provide tools for collecting and organizing disparate information on policy options and coming up with a cohesive course of action. We present the key elements in policy analysis and discuss the many ways by which they can be defined and implemented.

Two premises are at the heart of this book. First, the development and analysis of public policy should be logical and to the extent possible based on evidence. Second, policy analysis is open to, and benefits from, multiple scholarly fields and should not be limited to the perspectives and methods of a single discipline. It may seem obvious that public policy should be shaped by evidence and a logical course of argument, but unfortunately it is not difficult to find examples of policies promulgated repeatedly in the total absence of empirical support:

- Decrease income taxes to stimulate economic growth—or oppose any increase in taxes on the grounds that doing so will stifle economic growth.
- Rely exclusively on abstinence education (prohibiting provision of contraceptives) to reduce unwanted and/or teenage pregnancies.
- Promote carbon-based energy sources and deny the role of greenhouse gases as a key cause of climate change.

- Refuse to extend Medicaid eligibility because doing so would reduce one's incentive to work.

We believe that policies should be developed and debated with evidence and cogent arguments. Such evidence, however, can include many forms, from financial data to anecdotes. In this book we discuss how to marshal a diverse array of evidence so that analysts can make a compelling case for the policy options they recommend.

The second premise—that policy analysis benefits from multidisciplinary perspectives and methods—contrasts with the current dominance of economics. Most textbooks on policy analysis are couched in terms of economics; most articles published by the primary scholarly journal in the field examine policy issues from a market-based perspective; the federal government requires all major proposed regulations to be subject to cost-benefit analysis, a method rooted in microeconomics. As will be discussed in more detail in Chapter 1, while economics has much to offer policy analysis, its individualistic perspective can also be limiting.

In particular, we question economics' assumptions that individuals are primarily motivated by a desire to maximize their economic well-being and that policies should be judged by the degree to which the number of people who benefit exceeds the number who do not—or by comparing the total benefit and total monetary cost. We also question the efficacy of some of the techniques, such as cost-benefit analysis, that economists use to evaluate public policy. We believe that other disciplines—including design, psychology, political science, and sociology—also offer important insights for policy analysis.

Texts on policy analysis usually take the form of either instruction or critique. The former usually present a version of the "rational model" for conducting policy analysis and describe various techniques for carrying out each step of the process. The latter highlight key theoretical and practical limitations of the rational model.

The rational model typically takes on the following form, or a closely related variation:

1. Define the problem.
2. Identify potential policy options (alternatives) to address the problem.

3   Specify the objectives to be attained in addressing the problem and the criteria to evaluate the attainment of these objectives as well as the satisfaction of other key considerations (e.g., equity, cost, equity, feasibility).
4   Assess the outcomes of the policy options in light of the criteria and weigh trade-offs between the advantages and disadvantages of the options.
5   Arrive at a recommendation.

Critiques of policy analysis, on the other hand, question the assumptions inherent to the rational model, and highlight shortcomings of the dominant analytic methods.

However, these critiques offer little guidance on how to carry out policy analysis in light of the weaknesses of the dominant model. If the rational model is fatally flawed, as some suggest, how should policy ideas be developed and assessed?

In this book we aim to offer guidance on how to make evidence-based decisions about policies while also recognizing and responding to the many critiques of traditional policy analysis. Like other authors of policy analysis texts, we draw on a basic framework, the "rational model." By this we mean that policy analysis involves a series of steps, starting with problem definition and concluding with a recommendation. In between, one must decide on the objectives to be attained, the criteria to evaluate potential policies, and the policy options to be considered. One must then compare the strengths and weaknesses of these alternative policies in light of the criteria.

We depart from more traditional texts in that we emphasize the open-ended quality of each of these steps. We argue that there are numerous ways of framing a problem, that analysts have discretion in both deciding on the criteria used to evaluate policy options and, as importantly, in defining these criteria. We also argue that analysts have much latitude in deciding on the alternative policies that can be considered. The choices analysts make in carrying out policy analysis can reflect the sensibilities of different academic disciplines as well as different values and priorities.

While we show that the basic framework for policy analysis is flexible and open to multiple perspectives and values, we also argue that it demands logic and evidence. In order to be persuasive, and credible, analysts must situate the problem; defend their evaluative criteria; and be able to demonstrate that their policy recommendation is superior, on balance, to other alternative options in addressing the problem, as defined by the analyst. At a minimum, the analyst needs to present a clear and defensible ranking of options to guide the decisions of the policy makers.

Throughout the text, we will illustrate key concepts and the different ways by which they may be approached through a discussion of case studies. Two primary case studies are threaded throughout the book. The first one concerns policies enacted by numerous states and localities in the 1980s and 1990s to make noncustodial fathers more likely to meet their child support obligations. During this period, the news media carried numerous stories about "deadbeat dads" and the financial distress of single-parent families. States across the country took up the issue and passed legislation to sanction fathers who failed to meet their child support obligations. Many of these measures criminalized fathers living in poverty and had the unintended consequence of making it more difficult for fathers to find jobs or maintain relationships with their children (a summary of the case is presented at the end of this chapter).

The second case focuses on the politically charged issue of voter participation. Since 2013, when the US Supreme Court invalidated key components of the Voter Rights Act, states have diverged in their approach to voting policy. Some states and localities have sought to increase voter participation, prompted by declining or stagnant turnout. Other states, citing concerns over electoral fraud, have put in place measures such as voter ID laws that make it more difficult for some citizens to vote. We look at various strategies to strengthen voter registration and turnout in the United States and beyond.

We will use these cases to illustrate the different ways by which problems can be framed and the kinds of policies and criteria that may flow from these alternative framings. We will also use them to discuss alternative options for reducing child support debt and increasing voter turnout. We use the cases to examine the types of criteria that could be used to evaluate these options and the kinds of evidence and arguments that might be used in comparing the strengths and weaknesses of the options.

Organization of the Book

Chapter 1 provides an overview of the field of policy analysis, focusing both on mainstream and alternative perspectives. It describes the context in which policy analysis takes place and distinguishes policy analysis from related fields such as the legislative process and policy research. The chapter summarizes the key steps and assumptions of the traditional (rational) model of policy analysis and discusses alternative models.

The next five chapters examine specific elements in the rational model of policy analysis. Problem definition is the subject of Chapter 2. The chapter shows how different ways of describing a policy problem can lead to very different policy options and recommendations. It also provides practical guidance for framing a problem and identifies common pitfalls to avoid.

Chapter 3 turns to the policy options to be evaluated and compared. It discusses various ways to identify and refine alternative policies, including insights from the fields of design and behavioral economics. The chapter discusses how possible alternatives may be adapted from other policy domains and from other geographic locations. It reviews various generic policy responses to policy problems and how they can be refined. It examines how the elements of a given policy option can be reconfigured and combined into multiple discrete options. It discusses challenges of identifying and adapting "best practices" to inform alternative options.

Chapter 4 focuses on objectives and criteria. Objectives refer to the broad goals that the analyst wishes to achieve in addressing the problem, criteria to the specific measures used to assess the attainment of these objectives, as well other key considerations. Policy analysis almost always includes criteria such as effectiveness, equity, cost, and feasibility. How these criteria are defined and operationalized can vary widely. This chapter, making use of the child support case study and other examples, provides guidelines for developing criteria in light of several key challenges.

Chapter 5 builds on Chapter 4 by focusing on several analytic techniques frequently used to measure the efficiency and effectiveness of alternative policy options. These techniques include cost-benefit and cost-effectiveness analysis. In addition, Chapter 5 also introduces the concept of the time value of money, explaining how monetized costs and benefits that occur in the future must be discounted into their present value. This procedure is essential for both cost-effectiveness and cost-benefit analysis and for estimating the total cost of any option that involves expenditures over time. In addition to describing the procedures for carrying out these analytic techniques, the chapter also examines and critiques their key assumptions. Consideration is given both to the advantages of these techniques and their pitfalls.

In Chapter 6 the book examines the process of analysis—how to assess the most likely outcome of each policy option if it were adopted and how to compare these outcomes. The chapter will discuss the methods that policy analysts often use to estimate the outcomes of policy alternatives. It also shows how the results of the research and analysis can be summarized in a matrix to facilitate comparison of the outcomes and highlight key trade-offs.

Chapter 7 focuses on the types of research that can inform policy analysis. It reviews the key sources of secondary data and it provides guidance on conducting interviews, focus groups, and surveys. It also discusses the challenges of "best-practice" research—basing policy options on past or current initiatives in other jurisdictions and drawing lessons from their outcomes.

In Chapter 8, the book turns from guidance on how to carry out policy analysis to a discussion of policy analysis in practice. The chapter examines the types of jobs in the public, nonprofit, and private sectors that involve policy analysis. It discusses how the "policy environment"—including the nature of the relationship between the analyst and client, the analyst's employment security, and the client's predisposition towards the issue at stake—can constrain or promote certain types of analysis. Finally, the chapter considers several ethical issues in policy analysis.

Chapter 9 is a brief epilogue that summarizes the book's basic approach to policy analysis and discusses several ways of developing skills and experience through practice.

Throughout the book, we offer numerous examples to illustrate the elements of policy analysis and the key challenges they involve. These examples include the earlier mentioned child support and voting issues and others dealing with a variety of topics, including environmental protection, affordable housing, pedestrian safety, and health care.

To further help students develop policy-analytic skills, the book contains additional cases in the appendices that cover two contemporary policy issues. One case describes the history, context, and implications of a worsening water shortage in the western United States. The second case deals with the rise of short-term rental platforms and how they have affected local housing markets and accommodation businesses. Both cases include prompts at the end to guide analytical exercises and discussions using the material from the cases. The cases can easily be supplemented with additional data and sources to expand the assignment, but the limited and imperfect nature of the content is also instructive. The cases set up scenarios where students must grapple with realistic constraints when conducting their policy analysis.

Case Studies: Child Support Debt and Electoral Participation

Case Summary: Child Support Debt in the United States

On April 4, 2015, a police officer in North Charleston, South Carolina, fatally shot Walter Scott in the back. Unarmed, Mr. Scott had fled from the police officer after being pulled over in his car for a broken brake light. Mr. Scott was one of numerous African American men who have been shot by the police with little or no apparent justification. The killing has been cited as yet another instance of racial injustice in the criminal justice system. It soon became evident, however, that Mr. Scott's death also underscored profound inequities in another aspect of society: the way by which the government determines and enforces child support responsibilities. Mr. Scott had been jailed several times for failing to pay child support for his children, and he had run away from the police officer on April 4 because he dreaded being jailed again.

Low-income fathers such as Mr. Scott have often been incarcerated for failing to pay child support, although the frequency of incarceration for child support violations has diminished in recent years. It is especially common in the South, above all in South Carolina, where about one in eight inmates are jailed for child support violations (Brito 2012: 618; see also Robles & Dewan 2015). Incarceration is the most severe penalty for child support violations. Its incidence varies from state to state, and also within individual states, with some judges being more inclined than others to send noncustodial parents to jail for violating their child support orders (Haney 2022). A growing number of states rarely use civil contempt and the threat of jail to enforce child support, but incarceration remains a real possibility in others.

The child support program was created in 1975 with the twin goals of preventing families from needing to go on welfare (originally Aid for Families with Dependent Children; after 1996, Temporary Assistance for Needy Families [TANF]) and of recovering some of the cost of providing welfare and other types of public assistance. The program is voluntary for families that do not receive welfare; they pay a small fee for the government to collect child support payments from noncustodial parents. The program is mandatory for families who receive welfare. However, in this case, the government is entitled to retain the child support payments it collects to recover some of the costs of providing welfare, and in some cases Medicaid and foster care. In other words, child support payments collected on behalf of parents who receive TANF often do not go to them but to the government instead (Haney 2022; Turetsky and Waller 2020).

Through a series of laws starting in the 1970s, and particularly with the Personal Responsibility and Work Opportunity Reconciliation Act of 1996 ("welfare reform act"), federal and state governments instituted a series of increasingly stringent measures to force noncustodial parents to make financial contributions towards the welfare of their children. These measures included mandating genetic testing to verify the paternity of noncustodial parents; establishing national databases of recently hired employees to make it easier to identify parents who have not paid child support; facilitating ways of automatically withholding income and assets from parents who owe child support (e.g., payroll withholding); and imposing various penalties against parents who do not pay child support, including cancelation of driver's licenses and professional licenses, credit bureau reporting, and passport denial (Turetsky and Waller 2020; Haney 2022; Legler 2003).

These policies resulted in a significant increase in support paid to families but also resulted in unintended consequences for low-income noncustodial parents, including long-term debt, impoverishment, unemployment, incarceration, and estrangement from their children.

Governments justified their efforts to strengthen child support enforcement as a way of getting noncustodial parents—usually but not always fathers—to help address the material needs of their children and to face the responsibility of parenthood. These efforts also reflected a desire to provide additional income to keep families off of welfare and to recoup some of the cost of providing welfare benefits to low-income female-headed families.

In the heyday of welfare reform, noncustodial parents who did not provide financial support for their children were often called "deadbeats" (Mincy & Sorensen 1998)—people who can afford to help support their children but refuse to do so. While the use of the term "deadbeats" has faded in the past decade, inherent in the term is the idea that parents who fail to pay child support do so to evade their obligations. However, most parents who do not meet their support obligations lack the financial means to pay what is ordered. Approximately 25 percent of all noncustodial parents are poor, and the large majority of them struggle to pay child support if they pay at all (Office of Child Support Enforcement 2023: 2; Sorensen & Zibman 2001). Indeed, these parents may more aptly be called "deadbroke," not "deadbeats" (Brito 2012). A study of nine large states found that 70 percent of all child-support arrears is owed by parents earning less than $10,000 a year. It also found that only 3 percent of all parents with incomes over $10,000 did not pay child support in the past year (Sorensen et al. 2007).

The problem of unpaid child-support debt is large. More than 6 million parents were in arrears on their child-support obligations in 2022, owing $114 billion (Office of Child Support Enforcement 2023: 95). Much of these arrears are owed by relatively few parents who owe large amounts. For example, parents owing $100,000 or more in child support account for 22 percent of total child support debt but only 3 percent of all parents with child support debt (Putze 2017).

In the intervening decades since welfare reform, most states have moderated their child support policies and practices with respect to low-income parents, largely in response to research on child support debt (Sorensen 2016). States are more likely to consider the noncustodial parent's actual earnings and ability to pay in setting child support orders and are more likely to reduce orders during periods of unemployment and incarceration. These trends are reflected in the Flexibility, Efficiency, and Modernization in Child Support Programs Final Rule that the Obama administration adopted in 2016 to address many of the inequities and hardships experienced by low-income noncustodial parents. Among other provisions, the rule requires that child support orders be based on the noncustodial parent's ability to pay and essentially requires states to reduce or suspend child support payments in the event of incarceration (Office of Child Support Enforcement 2017a, 2017b).

As a result of these changes in child support policy, current support obligations, on the whole, are more realistic, and unpaid arrears are accumulating at a less rapid pace than in the past (Sorensen 2021). However, noncustodial parents who fell behind on support payments charged under the older policies still owe the money, regardless of whether they had the ability to satisfy the original orders. Neither the Final Rule nor previous reforms reduce child support arrears incurred by low-income parents.

We use the issue of **child support debt** as a case study to illustrate various aspects of policy analysis. Each chapter will conclude with a discussion of the case as it pertains to the aspects of policy analysis covered in the chapter. The client is a (hypothetical) state Department of Social Services. In Chapter 2, we examine the evolution of child support policy, the growth of child support debt, and the impact of that debt on noncustodial parents and their children. In Chapter 3, we present several potential alternative policies to reduce child support debt. The criteria for evaluating these alternatives are presented in Chapter 4. In Chapter 6, we assess the alternatives in light of the criteria and arrive at a recommendation. We also refer to the case in the other chapters as well.

Case Summary: Voter Participation

The right to vote and participate in the democratic process has been both sacred and contentious for centuries. Indeed, the preservation of democratic systems relies on fair and open elections. The battle between voter suppression and enfranchisement continues to this day, elevated by the expansion of social media and increasingly rapid and unfiltered platforms for disseminating information. The division in perspectives is very clear cut. And, as the federal government has retreated from regulatory oversight over voting rights, the divisions largely fall along state lines at this point.

There are those who are concerned about voter fraud. The states dominated by this view have largely turned to voter restrictions as the remedy. Then there are those who assert that access to voting is unduly, and unfairly, restrictive. These critics point out that there is vanishingly little evidence to support claims of voter fraud and argue that strict voter requirements are a thinly veiled attempt to reduce access to the polls for poor, young, and minority voters (Brennan Center 2018; Berman 2017). Even though voter turnout has increased in recent elections—nearly 67 percent of the voting age population participated in the 2020 presidential election compared to 55.7 percent in 2016—the U.S. still consistently boasts a lower turnout than half of modern democracies (Desilver 2022). Local elections historically have had even lower turnouts. The states keen on expanding voting access are exploring various ways of making sure recent gains don't reverse.

There is little agreement on why people actually vote or on what policies work best to increase electoral participation. Instrumental or rational approaches view the decision to vote as the result of a personal cost-benefit calculation (Downs 1957), but this approach has limited predictive ability when it comes to actual voting behavior. As a single vote is unlikely to sway election results, the costs will invariably outweigh the benefits, leading to the "paradox of voting." Resource theories build on the rational approach, hypothesizing that individuals with more resources—namely education, time, and money—are more likely to vote (Smets and van Ham 2013). This concurs with voting trends in the United States and globally: older, more educated, and wealthier citizens vote at consistently higher rates. What it doesn't explain is the downward trend in voting across advanced democracies even as income and education levels rise.

More contemporary theories recognize a sense of civic duty, a belief that voting is "the right thing to do." People with a strong sense of duty are 70 percent more likely to vote, and voting is higher in places where civic culture is strong. However, civic duty remains a hazy concept, difficult to define and measure, and even more difficult to influence (Smets and van Ham 2013; Bierschbach and Kaul 2016; Blais and Galais 2017).

In contrast, sociological approaches are concerned with the external forces that shape voting behavior. Voting is understood not as an individual decision but as one influenced by families, neighbors, and communities at large (Pacheco 2008; Aldritch 2011; Smets and van Ham 2013). Social networks can have negative effects on voting behavior; for example, people with low incomes living in segregated communities are less likely to vote than their peers in economically mixed areas (Bartle et al. 2017). But social networks, even those created in online spaces, can also be leveraged to lift turnout (Fowler and Goodman 2017). Pressure to comply with social norms is a powerful motivator and can be used to influence voting behavior (Gerber et al. 2008; Davenport 2010; Coppock and Green 2016). It has been argued that the overall decline in voting turnout across advanced democracies is attributed to changes in the way political campaigns are organized, with more use of mass marketing and less reliance on direct outreach by friends and neighbors (Goldstein and Ridout 2002).

The influence of how political information gets disseminated and verified should not be understated. Increasingly, social media has become a primary source of news among younger adults, and the technology has enabled the very rapid spread of information (Pew Research Center 2023), with relatively few mechanisms for verifying the truth of the content. And while it does not explain the root causes, the proliferation of social media may exacerbate the polarization of politics, and in turn what information users access related to voting access (Barrett et al. 2021).

There are also legal and institutional barriers to voting. The United States' unique system of registration laws, which puts the onus on individuals to register and to report any restricted access, has historically depressed turnout by an estimated 14 percent (Powell 1986; Avery and Peffley 2005; Smets and van Ham 2013).

Throughout this book we will examine the issue of voter participation in the United States. In Chapter 2, we explore the problem of low voter participation in more detail. In Chapter 3, we examine several options for increasing voter turnout. In Chapter 4, we develop criteria for evaluating these options, and in Chapter 6, we use these criteria to assess the policy options.

References

Aldritch, John H. 2011. *Why Parties?* Chicago: University of Chicago Press.
Avery, James M., and Mark Peffley. 2005. "Voter Registration Requirements, Voter Turnout, and Welfare Eligibility Policy: Class Bias Matters." *State Politics and Policy Quarterly 5*, *1*: 47–67.
Barrett, Paul, Justin Hendrix, and Grant Sims. 2021. "How Tech Platforms Fuel U.S. Political Polarization and What Government Can Do About It." *Brookings Institution*. www.brookings.edu/articles/how-tech-platforms-fuel-u-s-political-polarization-and-what-government-can-do-about-it/
Bartle, John, Sarah Birch, and Mariana Skirmuntt. 2017. "The Local Roots of the Participation Gap: Inequality and Voter Turnout." *Electoral Studies 48* (August): 30–44.
Berman, Ari. 2017. "A Big Win for Voting Rights in Texas and a Big Loss for Trump." *The Nation* (April 11). www.thenation.com/article/a-big-win-for-voting-rights-in-texas-and-a-big-loss-for-trump/
Bierschbach, Briana, and Greta Kaul. 2016. "The Five Reasons Why Voter Turnout in Minnesota is So High." *MinnPost* (September 29). www.minnpost.com/politics-policy/2016/09/five-reasons-why-voter-turnout-minnesota-so-high
Blais, Andre, and Carol Galais. 2017. "Measuring the Civic Duty to Vote: A Proposal." *Electoral Studies 41* (March): 60–69.
Brennan Center. 2018. *Disbanded: Trump's 'Voter Fraud' Commission*. www.brennancenter.org/issues/trump-fraud-commission
Brito, Tonya L. 2012. "Fathers Behind Bars: Rethinking Child Support Policy toward Low-Income Fathers and Their Families." *Iowa Journal of Gender, Race & Justice 417*: 617–673.
Coppock, Alexander, and Donald P. Green. 2016. "Is Voting Habit Forming? New Evidence from Experiments and Regression Discontinuities." *American Journal of Political Science 60*, *4*: 1044–1062.
Davenport, Tiffany C. 2010. "Public Accountability and Political Participation: Effects of a Face-to-Face Feedback Intervention on Voter Turnout of Public Housing Residents." *Political Behavior 32*, *3*: 337–368.
Desilver, Drew. 2022. "Turnout in U.S. has Soared in Recent Elections but by Some Measures still Trails that of Many Other Countries." *Pew Research Center* (November 1). www.pewresearch.org/short-reads/2022/11/01/turnout-in-u-s-has-soared-in-recent-elections-but-by-some-measures-still-trails-that-of-many-other-countries/
Downs, Anthony. 1957. *An Economic Theory of Democracy*. New York: Harper & Row.
Fowler, Yara R., and Charlotte Goodman. 2017. "How Tinder Could Take Back the White House." *New York Times* (June 22). www.nytimes.com/2017/06/22/opinion/how-tinder-could-take-back-the-white-house.html
Gerber, Alan S., Donald P. Green, and Christopher W. Larimer. 2008. "Social Pressure and Voter Turnout: Evidence from a Large-Scale Field Experiment." *American Political Science Review 102*, *1*: 33–48.
Goldstein, Kenneth M., and Travis N. Ridout. 2002. "The Politics of Participation: Mobilization and Turnout over Time." *Political Behavior 24*, *1*: 3–29.
Haney, Lynn. 2022. *Prisons of Debt: The Afterlives of Incarcerated Fathers*. Berkeley, CA: University of California Press.
Legler, Paul. 2003. *Low-Income Fathers and Child Support: Starting Off on the Right Foot*. Denver, CO: Policy Studies, Inc. www.issuelab.org/resources/10140/10140.pdf

Mincy, Ronald B., and Elaine J. Sorensen. 1998. "Deadbeats and Turnips in Child Support Reform." *Journal of Policy Analysis and Management* 17, *1*: 44–51.

Office of Child Support Enforcement. 2017a. *Final Rule Resources: Flexibility, Efficiency, and Modernization in Child Support Programs Final Rule*. www.acf.hhs.gov/css/resource/final-rule-resources

Office of Child Support Enforcement. 2017b. *Overview—Final Rule 2016 Flexibility, Efficiency, and Modernization in Child Support Programs Final Rule*. www.acf.hhs.gov/sites/default/files/programs/css/overview_child_support_final_rule.pdf

Office of Child Support Enforcement. 2023. *Preliminary Report FY2022*. Washington, DC: Author. www.acf.hhs.gov/sites/default/files/documents/ocse/fy_2022_preliminary_report.pdf

Pacheco, Julianna S. 2008. "Political Socialization in Context: The Effect of Political Competition on Youth Voter Turnout." *Political Behavior* 30, *4*: 415–436.

Pew Research Center. 2023. *New Platform Fact Sheet* (November 15). www.pewresearch.org/journalism/fact-sheet/news-platform-fact-sheet/

Powell, G. Bingham Jr. 1986. "American Voter Turnout in Comparative Perspective." *The American Political Science Review* 80, *1*: 17–43.

Putze, Dennis. 2017. "Who Owes the Child Support Debt?" *Analyze This (Blog of the Federal Office of Child Support Enforcement)* (September 15). www.acf.hhs.gov/css/ocsedatablog/2017/09/who-owes-the-child-support-debt

Robles, Frances, and Shaila Dewan. 2015. "Skip Child Support. Go to Jail. Lose Job. Repeat." *The New York Times* (April 19).

Smets, Kaat, and Carolien van Ham. 2013. "The Embarrassment of Riches? A Meta-Analysis of Individual-Level Research on Voter Turnout." *Electoral Studies* 32, *2*: 344–359.

Sorensen, Elaine. 2016. *Child Support is a Good Investment*. Washington, DC: Office of Child Support Enforcement.

Sorensen, Elaine. 2021. *Most Arrears Were Submitted to OCSE More Than Five Years Ago*. Washington, DC: Office of Child Support Enforcement. www.acf.hhs.gov/css/ocsedatablog/2021/09/most-arrears-were-submitted-ocse-more-five-years-ago

Sorensen, Elaine, Liliana Sousa, and Simon Schaner. 2007. *Assessing Child Support Arrears in Nine Large States and the Nation*. Washington, DC: The Urban Institute. www.urban.org/sites/default/files/publication/29736/1001242-Assessing-Child-Support-Arrears-in-Nine-Large-States-and-the-Nation.PDF

Sorensen, Elaine, and Chava Zibman. 2001. "Getting to Know Poor Fathers Who Do Not Pay Child Support." *Social Service Review* 75, *3*: 420–433.

Turetsky, Vicki, and Maureen R. Waller. 2020. "Piling on Debt: The Intersections Between Child Support Arrears and Legal Financial Obligations." *UCLA Criminal Justice Law Review* 4, *1*: 117–141.

1

WHAT IS POLICY ANALYSIS?
MAINSTREAM AND ALTERNATIVE PERSPECTIVES

What Is Policy Analysis?

We define policy analysis as evidence-based advice giving and as the process by which one arrives at a policy recommendation to address a problem of public concern. Policy analysis almost always involves advice for a client—whether an elected official, the head of a governmental agency or department, or the executive director of a nonprofit organization.

Policy analysts may work under the direct purview of the client or as a consultant.[1] In either case, the policy analyst advises the client on how to address a particular issue or problem. The policy analyst is seldom the decision maker but rather the purveyor of the information that bolsters certain choices over others. The client may be in a direct position to address the problem; he or she may have the authority to implement the recommendation with little or no approval from others. For example, a parks commissioner may be able to adopt the recommendation of a staff policy analyst to expand recreational programming in parks located in low-income neighborhoods without consulting with other government officials. On the other hand, other clients may have little or no authority to implement a policy recommendation. A city council member, a state representative, a member of Congress, or an advocacy organization may draw on policy analysis to decide on what legislation to support with regard to a particular issue. In some cases, the client for policy analysis is less obvious or tangible. Advocacy organizations and think tanks, for example, often employ policy analysts—and publish policy analysis—to draw attention to particular issues and to lend support to particular solutions. In this context, the client may be construed as the public at large or particular governmental bodies or officials. Policy analysis here is less about advising a government agency or nonprofit organization on a particular course of action to address a problem and more about influencing public debate over the issue.

In the first section of this chapter, we begin by positioning policy analysis within the overarching domain of policy studies and policy making. In the second section, we present the "rational model" of policy analysis. We introduce the traditional versions of this approach and explain their similarities and differences with the framework we adopt in this book. Like the traditional model, we believe that policy analysis requires the systematic comparison of alternative policy options in light of various evaluative criteria. However, our approach differs from the more orthodox versions in that it is open to multiple ideological and disciplinary perspectives. The third section briefly discusses major critiques of the rational model, and the fourth section summarizes alternative models for policy analysis based on the concepts of design and incrementalism. The final section summarizes our approach to policy analysis in this book.

Policy Analysis as Part of the Larger Policy Process

Policy analysis is part of a much broader field of policy studies. In addition to policy analysis, which concerns the determination of policies to recommend, policy studies encompass program or policy evaluation, studies of policy or program implementation, and more broadly, studies of the policy-making process (Howlett et al. 2009).

Policy analysis is different from program evaluation. The latter assesses how well a program or policy (which may have been recommended by a policy analyst) has met its objectives. Sometimes, program evaluations lead to changes in the design or implementation of the program, or to its elimination altogether[2]—and policy analysis often relies on program evaluations to help compare policy options. Evaluations can provide information on the effects of a program, how it operates in the field, and its underlying logic, all of which contribute to policy decision making (Greenberg et al. 2000).

Policy analysis is also distinct from the study of program implementation—which may be part of program evaluation. Implementation concerns the ability of an organization and its partners to carry out the steps proscribed by the policy. For example, Pressman and Wildavsky (1984), in their classic study of the implementation of an economic development and job training program in Oakland, California, emphasize the need to consider "clearance points"—the steps in the implementation process for which agreement is required by other entities, such as other government agencies or private businesses. The more clearance points there are, and the greater the number of participants whose approval is required, the more likely implementation will be delayed or fail altogether. Pressman and Wildavsky also stress the position of the participants in the clearance points with regard to the policy at hand: specifically, whether they are likely to support or oppose it, the intensity of their support or opposition, and the resources that they can bring to bear in support or opposition.

Implementation studies may be included in program evaluation, especially in formative evaluations that seek to find ways of improving the performance of a given program. They are not part of policy analysis, since they come after the policy has been decided (the outcome of policy analysis). However, policy analysts are wise to keep the lessons of implementation studies in mind when comparing alternative policy options. These studies can shed light on the administrative feasibility of these alternatives. We discuss implementation in more detail in Chapters 4 and 6.

Policy Analysis and Policy Making

Policy analysis concerns the process of making policy recommendations. It is part of a larger, more encompassing, process of policy making. By policy making, we refer to the ways by which policy proposals gain traction and are eventually embraced by elected officials and legislatures. It also refers to the legislative process, the deal making that often enables proposed laws to attract a sufficient number of supporters. Many policy ideas may linger for years if not decades before they are recognized as viable options, and many ideas remain forever on the fringes of political acceptability. Similarly, even if a policy idea has significant political support, it may take years to be passed into law—and it may never succeed in doing so. In other words, that a policy analyst recommends a particular course of action to address a problem does not mean that the recommendation will ever be approved or implemented. This is especially true when the recommendation requires legislation. John Kingdon, for example, in his classic text, *Agendas, Alternatives, and Public Policies*, tells the story of a senator who, on receiving a draft bill from a legislative aide, tells him that while he will introduce the legislation "tomorrow," he sees no reason to read it now since "it will take twenty to twenty five years for it be brought into being" (Kingdon 2003: 116).

There is an extensive literature in political science and related fields on this broader context of policy making. Several theories have been put forth to explain why policy ideas that once languished in the political wilderness can suddenly gain currency and become credible policy options. Others attempt to explain how legislators can forge alliances to win passage of laws authorizing new policies. We discuss a few of the most prominent frameworks here, touching only the surface of a wide-ranging field.

One of the most influential frameworks of how governments come to recognize certain issues as problems to be addressed and adopt particular policy solutions to address them is John Kingdon's "multiple streams." He discusses how openings to policy changes—"policy windows"—occur at particular moments and usually last for brief periods. Some policy windows open at regular intervals, such as the beginning of a new presidential administration. Others may appear during times of crisis. He describes the policy-making process as an "organized anarchy" where processes are somewhat structured but not linear or predictable. Kingdon discusses how "policy entrepreneurs" capitalize on these policy windows and elevate particular issues and/or policy solutions to the fore. He also discusses how problems, policies, and politics constitute separate but also interrelated "streams" that are shaped by their own rules and dynamics. Policy entrepreneurs, when appropriate policy windows open up, "couple" these streams—connecting particular problems and solutions, and increasing the likelihood that legislators and other policy makers will adopt the desired policy.

Frank Baumgartner and Bryan Jones's punctuated equilibrium theory (PET) is another theoretical conception of the policy-making process. Baumgartner and Jones attempt to explain why public policies occasionally shift from incremental adjustments to radical changes in approach. Whereas public policies are usually quite stable—seeing minor, mostly incremental, changes over time—they are sometimes altered in fundamental ways, or replaced altogether. Stasis, they argue, is maintained by "policy monopolies" that resist change, and change is induced by a breaking down of those monopolies. In other words, extended periods of stability or stasis are occasionally punctuated by moments of far-reaching change (Baumgartner et al. 2018).

Another conceptual approach to understanding policy adoption is the advocacy coalition framework (ACF) developed by Paul Sabatier and Hank Jenkins Smith. The ACF, as the name implies, examines advocacy coalitions within specific policy "subsystems" defined by particular topics (e.g., transportation, criminal justice), territorial jurisdictions, and the actors who influence the subsystem dynamics. Under this framework, emphasis is placed on the aggregation of individuals and organizations within a policy subsystem into discrete coalitions. These coalitions are "defined by actors sharing core beliefs who coordinate their actions in a nontrivial manner to influence a policy subsystem" (Jenkins-Smith et al. 2018: 195). Major policy changes, according to the framework, typically flow from changes in the composition and stability of the advocacy coalitions, external shocks, such as crisis or regime changes, and from negotiated agreements between "previously warring coalitions" (p. 203).

In addition to various theoretical conceptions of policy change, journalists and historians have offered important insights into the legislative process and the cultivation and use of political power. Robert Caro (2003, 2012), for example, in his multi-volume biography of Lyndon Johnson, examines in detail how he cobbled together legislative majorities to support landmark civil rights bills. Caro highlights how as majority leader of the US Senate and as president, Johnson managed to convince lawmakers to vote for the legislation despite their sometimes stark ideological and political differences. Journalist Jane Mayer (2016), in *Dark Money*, also describes how certain very wealthy individuals influence public discourse and electoral politics on a number of social and economic issues through their donations of large sums to right-wing think tanks and through their contributions to political action committees. We mention these examples to emphasize the point that policy analysis is by no means the only, or the most influential, shaper of public policy.

While the literature on the broader political and institutional context in which policy ideas are adopted and implemented is certainly germane to policy analysis, and in some cases needs to be considered in the analysis of certain policy options, in this book we focus more narrowly on the methodology of policy analysis itself. That is, we examine the steps involved in framing a policy issue, identifying possible solutions, and evaluating them. The recommendations produced through policy analysis may or may not be adopted, and, if they are adopted, it may take years for that to happen. The more fundamental point is that most policy proposals, whether or not they move onto the legislative agenda, or are given serious consideration for executive action, are subject to some form of policy analysis. Policy analysis provides the empirical and conceptual support for the recommendation, and explains why the recommendation is superior to other possible courses of action. In addition, policy debates draw heavily on policy analysis. Among other things, participants in the debates argue about the nature of the problem being addressed and about the positive and negative consequences of the proposed solutions—and policy analysis can be used as input into decision-making processes within government, large nonprofit organizations, and community-based groups.

The "Rational Model" of Policy Analysis

Policy analysis, as discussed earlier, involves the systematic comparison of the strengths and weaknesses of alternative ways of addressing a given problem. Although scholars have presented several different formats of the rational model of policy analysis, these are essentially distinctions without a difference.

In this book we adopt a five-step framework:

1 Define the problem.
2 Identify potential policy options (alternatives) to address the problem.

3   Specify the objectives to be attained in addressing the problem and the criteria to evaluate the attainment of these objectives as well as the satisfaction of other key considerations (e.g., equity, cost, equity, feasibility).
4   Assess the outcomes of the policy options in light of the criteria and weigh trade-offs between the advantages and disadvantages of the options.
5   Arrive at a recommendation.

Other policy analysis texts present similar frameworks. As shown in Table 1.1, they may differ in terms of the sequencing of some of the steps in the analytic process, and they may combine some steps into a single step or split one step into multiple components. For example, Bardach and Patashnik's model omits explicit consideration of objectives, melding them with criteria, and breaks analysis into two steps ("project outcomes" and "confront trade-offs"). It also distinguishes between the recommendation stage ("stop, etc.") and the exposition of the recommendation ("tell your story").

Notwithstanding minor differences in terminology, and in the number and composition of the steps in the analytic process, these models of policy analysis are quite similar. Each requires alternative policy options to be compared in terms of various criteria—criteria that gauge the effectiveness of the options in addressing a given problem while taking into account other key concerns. Their fundamental objective is to arrive at a well-reasoned solution to a well-defined problem. All expect the analyst to capture the essence of the problem to be addressed, to identify a number of possible ways of addressing this problem, to estimate as best as possible the likely outcomes of these alterative options, and to compare these outcomes in light of specific criteria. Ultimately, after assessing the strengths and weaknesses of each alternative, including any trade-offs, the analyst must recommend which policy option to pursue.

Most formulations of policy analysis share a similar emphasis on rationality and, regardless of their variations, are commonly known as the "rational model." That is, they prescribe a rational approach to policy analysis, and they define rationality in similar ways. They view rationality from a neoclassical economic perspective. The unit of analysis is the individual, and individuals seek to maximize their economic

Table 1.1 Alternative Versions of the "Rational Model" of Policy Analysis

Bardach and Patashnik (2015)	Patton et al. (2013)	Stokey and Zeckhauser (1978)	Hammond et al. (1999)	Wiemer and Vining (2005)
1. Problem definition 2. Assemble some evidence 3. Construct the alternatives 4. Select the criteria 5. Project the outcomes 6. Confront the trade-offs 7. Stop, narrow focus, deepen, decide! 8. Tell your story	1. Problem definition 2. Determination of evaluation criteria 3. Identification of alternatives 4. Evaluation of alternatives 5. Comparison of alternatives 6. Assessment of outcomes	1. Establish the context. What is the underlying problem? What specific objectives are to be pursued? 2. Laying out the alternatives 3. Predicting the consequences 4. Valuing the outcomes 5. Making a choice	1. Problem 2. Objectives 3. Alternatives 4. Consequences 5. Trade-offs	**Problem Analysis** 1. Understanding the problem 2. Choosing and explaining related goals and constraints (in addressing it) 3. Selecting the solution method **Solution Analysis** 1. Choosing impact categories for goals (criteria) 2. Specifying policy alternatives 3. Predicting impacts of alternatives 4. Evaluating impacts of the alternatives 5. Presenting recommendations

welfare. The impacts of alternative policy options are assessed by aggregating their estimated effects, and their costs and benefits, on individuals (Stokey and Zeckhauser 1978; Wiemer and Vining 2005). In addition to an economistic interpretation of rationality, some versions of the rational model presume that analysts have sufficient time and information to identify and assess a comprehensive set of potential policy options. They also prescribe a "stagist" methodology, in which analysts move through each step of the analytic process in sequence, not moving to the next one until the current one is completed.

As discussed later, our version of the rational model is amenable to alternative notions of rationality. Economic efficiency is but one of many perspectives that can be applied in evaluating alternative policy options. We argue that policy analysts, depending in part on their relationship to their client (Jenkins-Smith 1982), have considerable latitude in deciding on the values and principles to be emphasized in the analytic process. In other words, analysts must apply logic and evidence in comparing the strengths and weaknesses of alternative policy options, but logic and evidence need not be steeped in microeconomics or in any other specific discipline.

In addition, we do not presume that analysts must possess "perfect information" or that the alternatives they consider are necessarily comprehensive. We also emphasize that the analytic process is highly iterative, with analysts cycling back and forth between the various steps as they gain new information and insights.

Critiques of the Rational Model

Numerous scholars have criticized the rational model over the decades (Fisher 2003; Lindblom 1959; Stone 2012). These criticisms concern certain (presumed) assumptions, the positivistic quality of the approach, and its emphasis on economic models. As we discuss, we believe these criticisms pertain more to the way the rational model is sometimes presented and to how it has been employed than to its essential character. We believe that the model is far more flexible and open ended than its critics recognize.

Cognitive Limits

One of the oldest criticisms of the rational model is that it demands too much of the human intellect and fails to recognize the limited resources and time available to policy analysts. Herbert Simon and Charles Lindblom wrote in the 1940s and 1950s about the cognitive limitations that prevent people from imagining and considering the full range of possible options to solve a given problem. In addition, analysts seldom if ever have available to them the monetary or staff resources to fully investigate all of the possible policy options or the time that would be required if they did have these resources.

Simon (1997) famously coined the phrase "bounded rationality" to convey the idea that people can apply reason to assess different potential solutions but that these potential solutions are a subset of all that are possible and that the application of reason may be limited by incomplete information and by the inability of the analyst to consider the full range of possible consequences. Within these parameters, analysts can apply a well-reasoned, evidence-based rationale for a recommended course of action. Although the argument for the recommendation may have its limitations, it suffices.

As we discuss later in our discussion of Lindblom's model of incremental policy analysis, we do not believe that the rational model actually demands a comprehensive set of policy options or their exhaustive evaluation. Policy analysis always involves a limited set of options. Analysts have discretion to decide which options are worthy of consideration. As will be discussed in Chapter 3, the selection of alternative policies, what to include and what to exclude, reflects the values and priorities of the analyst and his or her client. If certain options are "off the table," they will not be subject to analysis and will not be recommended. The rational model requires comparison of two or more potential policies, but it does not specify the number to be considered or which potential solutions should be selected for consideration.

Positivist and Economistic Emphasis

The rational model has also been criticized for being overly narrow, mechanistic, and positivistic. Some scholars argue that the model tends to focus on narrowly defined problems and employs a narrow set of parameters, preventing a broader more open-ended discussion. The model is said to be mechanistic in that analysis is prescribed to proceed in a specific sequence of steps, and that the analysis of potential solutions gives undue emphasis to numeric ratings. There is little room for nuance, subtlety, and ambiguity. Critics also fault the rational model for its positivistic character, its emphasis, as Frank Fisher puts it, "on rigorous quantitative analysis, the objective separation of facts and values, and the search for generalizable findings" (2003: 3). This approach, critics contend, overlooks the vital role of narrative and argument in shaping the way an issue is understood and how possible options are perceived. Rather than try to insulate policy analysis from politics, analysts need to understand how the basic assumptions and processes of policy analysis are inherently political (Stone 2012; Fisher 2003).

The rational model of policy analysis is also, in a related vein, criticized for the dominance of the assumptions and methods of traditional neoclassical economics. Deborah Stone, for example, argues that conventional policy analysis favors an economic model of society, in which all social relationships are governed by a calculus of market-based transactions. Policies are to be chosen on the basis of economic efficiency, preferably through cost-benefit analysis. According to the economic mindset, the unit of analysis is always the individual. Policies should be evaluated by the number of individuals who benefit or by the total benefits accrued by individuals less the total costs accrued by other individuals. Stone argues that this individualistic, economistic mode of thinking ignores the fact that people live in political and cultural communities. People do not only think about how a given problem and its proposed solutions affect them economically as individuals but also in terms of the various communities to which they belong. Whereas the market-based model of society defines the public interest to be the sum of individual interests, it can also be seen as what people view as being good for their community.

Texts on policy analysis often emphasize economic perspectives. Some require a basic understanding of microeconomics. Even less technical books, such as Bardach and Patashnik's widely used *Practical Guide for Policy Analysis*, embrace the individualistic perspective of economics. Bardach and Patashnik equate the aggregate of individual welfare with the public interest. They argue that measures of efficiency based on estimates of "individual citizens' construction of their own welfare" is "thoroughly democratic:"

> Indeed, siding with efficiency . . . is a way to produce more humanistic policy results, too. . . . [P]olicy decisions failing to consider efficiency very often fail to take account of the little guy at all. The little guy may be little, but in a proper efficiency analysis, he at least shows up to be counted. Efficiency analysis imposes a moral check. . on political visionaries eager to relocate entire populations so as to make room for dams, and on special interests eager to impose seemingly small price increases on large numbers of consumers.
> (Bardach and Patashnik 2015: 29)

To be fair, Bardach and Patashnik also recognize that since measures of efficiency often rest on "willingness to pay," they can favor individuals with higher incomes and can underestimate the importance of values that "have few or no human defenders and therefore no human pocketbooks to back an estimate of willingness to pay" (pp. 29–30).

Alternative Models of Policy Analysis

Although the rational model of policy analysis has been criticized for decades, this criticism does not seem to have inspired scholars or practitioners to suggest many alternative approaches to policy analysis. Notwithstanding its conceptual and other shortcomings, the rational model is by far the predominant framework for conducting policy analysis. In this section we discuss two of the few alternative approaches. The first is inspired by basic methods in the field of design. The second, originally articulated by political scientist Charles Lindblom, replaces the rational model with an incremental approach.

Design-Based Approaches and Policy Analysis

From the field of design has come a somewhat different model of policy analysis, one that also proceeds in stages. Over the past two or so decades, a number of practitioners and scholars have sought to distill from the design process key principles that can be applied beyond the traditional domain of design. Often termed "design thinking," "service design," and "human-centered design" (Bason 2017; Trippe 2021), these principles have been adapted to improve business management, public services, and public policy. Advocates of design-based approaches argue that the ways by which designers tackle design problems—whether in architecture, product design, fashion, or other realms of design—can not only be applied outside the traditional field of design but can also lead to better outcomes. Although there is no standard definition of "design thinking" and related concepts, these approaches share several core elements. These principles include the importance of viewing problems from the perspective of people who face them directly, the benefit of devising potential solutions in collaboration with the people who would be most affected by them, and the importance of experimentation (Bason 2017; Gordon and Mugar 2020).

There are clear parallels between the rational model of policy analysis and design thinking. For example, Bernard Roth, Academic Director of the Hasso Plattner Institute of Design at Stanford University and one of the first proponents of design thinking, defines the concept as a five-step process (2015):

1 Empathize.
2 Define the problem.
3 Ideate.
4 Prototype.
5 Test and get feedback from others.

Like the "rational model" of policy analysis, this version includes a problem definition (in this case, it encompasses two elements: empathy and problem definition) and development of potential alternatives (again split into two stages: "ideation" and prototype). "Analysis" in Roth's version of design thinking involves the testing of prototypes and solicitation of feedback on them. Through the testing and refinement of prototypes, one arrives at the solution. The main difference between design thinking and the rational model of policy analysis is that the evaluative criteria may not be clearly stated or stated at all. The analysis of alternatives rests mostly on how well the alternatives (or prototypes) "work" or test out.

Roth's is by no means the only version of design thinking. Other scholars and designers offer models that can differ in certain respects. For instance, several of the contributors to *Design for Policy* (Bason 2014) argue that design should do more than address problems. Instead of being reactive to specific problems, it is a means to "envision a desirable future and developing a way for this future to become a reality" (Bason 2014: 299).

Although design-centered approaches to policy are not synonymous with the rational model of policy analysis, they do share similar concerns, especially the need to assess alternative ways of solving a problem. While design thinking and related approaches offer relatively little guidance with regard to how alternatives should be evaluated (what is the measure of success in testing prototypes?) and seems to limit analysis of potential policies to the comparison of prototypes, the framework provides important insights on how alternative options might be conceived. Perhaps most important, the concept emphasizes the need for analysts to be empathic—to try to understand as thoroughly as possible how the issue affects individuals, communities, and organizations—and to involve people affected by the issue in the process of devising possible solutions.

The Incrementalist Model of Policy Analysis

The most prominent alternative to the rational model, incrementalism, was formulated by Lindblom in 1959 in his seminal article, "The Science of Muddling Through." Lindblom claims that the traditional model of policy analysis, which he calls the "rational-comprehensive" approach, is inherently unrealistic. It demands too much of the human intellect, and it requires too much time and resources to be feasible. Lindblom says that the need to be comprehensive, to envision all manners of potential solutions to a problem, is not humanly possible. He also says that it is difficult, if not impossible, to specify the objectives or criteria on which alternative solutions should be evaluated. First, different people and groups may disagree on the values or objectives that should be emphasized in analyzing policy options. Second, there is no clear way of knowing how to rank these values and objectives when they are in conflict.

Lindblom argues that while the rational-comprehensive approach is widely prescribed, it is honored in the breach. Instead, he says, policy analysts follow a different, incrementalist method. Lindblom says that this method is not only more feasible than the rational-comprehensive approach, but also it is conceptually superior. Lindblom describes the elements of this incrementalist method and explains how it avoids the limitations of the rational-comprehensive approach.

Rather than attempt to establish a wide array of alternative policy options to address a problem and specify various objectives and criteria for their evaluation, Lindblom argues that in practice policy analysis involves the comparison of a small number of alternatives that vary slightly from the policies that are currently in place. This method greatly limits "the number of alternatives to be investigated and also drastically simplifies the character of the investigation of each" (p. 84). Under this incremental approach it is not necessary to estimate the full range of potential effects of the alternatives; all that matters is "how the proposed alternative and consequences differ from the status quo." In addition, rather than compare the alternatives against a set of values and objectives on which analysts and policy makers may not agree, the incrementalist approach requires only that the analysts and policy makers agree on a particular alternative; they do not have to agree about the goals to be achieved in deciding on the policy or on how these goals should be measured or weighted. In other words, in comparing alternative policy options, one is also comparing the values and goals; they are embedded in the alternatives themselves.

Conceptually, Lindblom argues that this incremental approach avoids key shortcomings of the traditional version of policy analysis. In particular, it eliminates the need to arrive at a comprehensive set of possible policies to address a problem. By limiting the analysis to options that differ only slightly from the status quo, it is far easier, less time consuming, and less costly to develop the alternatives and to assess their potential consequences. Even though individual policy analysts only examine alternatives that deviate slightly from current policies, Lindblom claims that a semblance of comprehensiveness is achieved in the aggregate. Numerous analysts work on any one issue, whether working for the same or different policy makers or serving as an advocate. With each analyst considering different options, the overall assortment of alternatives under consideration may be larger and wider ranging than what any individual analyst could conceive on his or her own. Moreover, the multiplicity of analysts and decision makers also means that a wide array of values and goals are at play.

Another advantage is that the incrementalist model does not require analysts or their clients to agree on the values, objectives to be achieved in addressing a problem, or how these values and objectives should be measured and weighted. Lindblom notes that people can agree on the same policy solution to a problem, but for different reasons. If they had to agree on the values and objectives first, they might not ever begin to consider the policy alternatives. According to Lindblom, "he chooses among values and among policies at one and the same time" (p. 82). Furthermore, in comparing marginally different alternatives, analysts "need not try to analyze any values except the values by with the alternative policies differ and not be concerned with them except as they differ marginally" (p. 83).

In our view, Lindblom's incrementalist approach may be preferable to the more traditional framework in certain circumstances. We also believe that in extolling the virtues of incrementalism, Lindblom exaggerates the defects of the rational model. Starting with the later point, Lindblom emphasizes two problems with the rational-comprehensive approach: the impossibility of compiling a truly comprehensive set of policy alternatives and of analyzing their probable consequences and the necessity of obtaining agreement on the values and objectives to be achieved in addressing the problem.

The need for comprehensiveness in policy analysis is much exaggerated. Lindblom is correct that it is psychologically and intellectually impossible for any individual to envision all possible solutions to a given problem. Indeed, ever since Simon wrote about "bounded rationality" in the 1940s it has been widely accepted that cognitive limitations prevent decision makers or analysts to consider all possible policy options. In addition, it is well known that nearly all analysts face constraints of time and resources. They must complete their analysis and arrive at a recommendation within a certain period of time, and their budget for research and analysis is also limited.

But is comprehensiveness necessary for the rational model? We agree that it is impossible to be truly comprehensive in identifying the universe of potential policy solutions, but that does not mean that all of the alternatives to be considered must be only marginally different from the policies currently in place. Why not consider a range of divergent options?

We also agree with Lindblom that it is often easier for people to agree on a policy to pursue than to agree on the objectives to be achieved in adopting the policy. People may agree on a policy for different reasons. We agree that it can be counterproductive to require agreement on values and objectives before deciding on alternative policies. Indeed, as Deborah Stone points out, political leaders often prefer ambiguity over precision in stating their goals for proposed legislation, policies, or programs. Ambiguous goals may broaden political support for the proposed policy while more explicitly stated goals may narrow the political constituency. "By labeling goals vaguely and ambiguously," argues Stone, "leaders can draw support from different groups who might disagree on specifics. Ambiguity can unite people who might benefit from the same policy but for different reasons" (2012: 252).

Yet, while precise statements of the values and objectives to be achieved in addressing a problem may be problematic from a political perspective, this does not mean that specificity is a liability for policy analysis. That is, it is one thing to promote a policy idea in a legislative body or in the public at large and another to evaluate the strengths and weaknesses of various policy options for an individual policy maker. Policy analysts advise policy makers on the optimum means of addressing a problem, taking into account various criteria that concern some measure of effectiveness as well as such other considerations as equity, feasibility, and cost. This analysis can help the policy maker determine which policies to support. The analysis may not always be used in full as a means of gathering political support for the proposed policy. The policy maker, in other words, may draw from the policy analysis in its complete form, in part, or not at all, in promoting the policy. He or she may find it advantageous to explain the benefits of the policy, or the weaknesses of alternative ones, in broader, more ambiguous terms than those found in the original policy analysis. For example, elected officials may prefer to justify legislation or executive decisions in general terms that can be interpreted in a variety of ways. A more specific justification might appeal to a narrower range of voters and could be opposed by voters who disagree with the more explicit objectives of the policy.[3] It is the analyst's job to convey relevant information, whether it supports or challenges the proposed alternative.

Finally, we believe that Lindblom exaggerates the incidence and virtue of incrementalism as the norm for policy analysis and policy making. We don't deny that many policy changes are incremental—for example, the duration of benefits for unemployment insurance or food stamps (the Supplemental Nutrition Assistance Program, or SNAP) may be shortened or lengthened, the amount of the Earned Income Tax Credit may be increased, or the maximum income of households eligible for the tax credit may be changed. However, it's not at all difficult to identify policy changes that are not incremental. The history of the federal government is rife with examples of fundamental policy changes. These include decisions to go to war, to create new safety-net programs, to protect the environment, and to recognize the civil rights of minority populations. Indeed, political scientists have long debated—and developed models to explain—why public policies periodically make sudden and large shifts in scale and focus. As discussed earlier in the chapter, Baumgartner and Jones' theory of punctuated equilibrium attempts to explain why large-scale policy changes occur, disrupting periods "marked by stability and incrementalism" (Baumgartner et al. 2018: 59).

We also disagree with Lindblom that incrementalism is wiser than more sudden fundamental policy changes. Lindblom rightly notes that incremental changes involve less risk. They are based on the knowledge of the effects of previous, closely related policy changes, and they can be quickly modified with subsequent incremental policy changes. However, there are times when incremental changes do not suffice. They can fall short during times of economic crisis, when the scale of unemployment, poverty, and related issues necessitates a major response—including increased subsidies but perhaps other changes too, such as regulatory reforms. Social movements, such as the civil rights movement of the 1960s, the environmental movement of the 1970s, and the more recent gay rights movement have led to decidedly nonincremental changes in legislation such as the Civil Rights Acts of 1964 and 1968, the creation of the Environmental Protection Agency, and more recent actions to recognize same-sex marriage.

Summary: Using the Rational Model Flexibly

In this chapter, we have positioned policy analysis within the broader field of public policy and presented our basic framework for policy analysis. We emphasize that policy analysis constitutes **evidence-based advice giving**. Policy analysts advise clients in government and in the private and nonprofit sectors on how to address issues of public concern. Of course, the client is not obligated to follow the analyst's recommendations and may decide on other courses of action.

Our framework for policy analysis closely resembles that of other texts. Policy analysis moves through various **stages**. The nature of the problem must first be articulated. The objectives to be achieved in addressing the problem must be defined, and the criteria for ascertaining the achievement of these objectives must be specified. Alternative options for addressing the problem must be identified and evaluated in light of the criteria. One or more of these alternatives will be recommended.

Our framework for policy analysis differs from other models, however, in that it does not prescribe a specific definition of rationality. The model provides a template for comparison and assessment of alternative ways of addressing an issue. It does not prescribe how that issue should be defined. It does not dictate the objectives or criteria to be employed or how they should be specified. It does not determine which alternatives should be considered or how they should be analyzed in light of the criteria. Just because analysts often apply the economic concept of efficiency as the key criterion, this does not mean that efficiency must always be a criterion. Nor does it mean that efficiency, or any other criterion, must be defined in a particular way. Our version of policy analysis does not insist on the primacy of neoclassical economics. We believe that policy analysis is not bound to any one academic discipline or ideological position.

The model does require that the analyst be consistent and systematic in comparing the alternatives and base that comparison on evidence and logical argumentation. As we discuss throughout the book, each step in the rational model, from problem definition through recommendation, is **flexible and open-ended**. No ideological or political perspective need be excluded. Analyses based on the rational model can easily arrive at diametrically opposite recommendations—the results are contingent on the assumptions and decisions made in each step.

We also argue that the model is less rigid and mechanistic than is often presumed. While the model implies a linear progression from problem definition to policy recommendation, this linearity is for expository purposes. In practice, policy analysis is **iterative**: analysts cycle back and forth across the steps, revising them in light of new knowledge and insights gained in other phases of the analysis. For example, an analyst may revise his or her conception of the problem after researching potential policy options. He or she may modify the criteria in the course of comparing the policy options. The first set of alternatives to be considered can bear little resemblance to the ones in the final analysis.

Finally, policy analysis must be **persuasive**. It must be sensitive to political, institutional, and cultural contexts. It must marshal many forms of evidence and logic to demonstrate why the recommended policy (or policies) is on balance superior to other options.

Notes

1 See Chapter 8 for a review of the various settings in which policy analysts work.
2 There is a voluminous literature on program evaluation. A classic introduction is Rossi and Lipsy 2003.
3 See Stone 2012 on the uses and value of ambiguity in public policy.

References

Bardach, Eugene, and Eric M. Patashnik. 2015. *A Practical Guide for Policy Analysis* (5th Edition). Los Angeles, CA: Sage Publications.
Bason, Christian (ed.). 2014. *Design for Policy*. New York: Routledge.
Bason, Christian. 2017. *Leading Public Design: Discovering Human-Centred Governance*. Bristol (UK): Policy Press.
Baumgartner, Frank R., Bryan D. Jones, and Peter B, Mortensen. 2018. " Chapter 3: Punctuated Equilibrium Theory: Explaining Stability and Change in Public Policymaking." In *Theories of the Policy Process* (4th Edition), Paul A. Sabatier, and Christopher M. Weible (eds.). New York: Routledge.

Caro, Robert A. 2003. *Master of the Senate: The Years of Lyndon Johnson*. New York: Vintage Books.

Caro, Robert A. 2012. *The Passage of Power: The Years of Lyndon Johnson*. New York: Viking.

Fisher, Frank. 2003. *Reframing Public Policy: Discursive Politics and Deliberative Practices*. New York: Oxford University Press.

Gordon, Eric, and Gabriel Mugar. 2020. *Meaningful Inefficiencies: Civic Design in an Age of Digital Expediency*. New York: Oxford University Press.

Greenberg, D., M. Mandell, and M. Onstott. 2000. "The Dissemination and Utilization of Welfare-to-Work Experiments in State Policymaking." *Journal of Policy Analysis & Management 19*: 367–382.

Hammond, John S., Ralph L. Keeney, and Howard Raiffa. 1999. *Smart Choices: A Practical Guide to Making Better Decisions*. Boston, MA: Harvard Business School Press.

Howlett, Michael, M. Ramesh, and Anthony Perl. 2009. *Studying Public Policy* (3rd Edition). New York: Oxford University Press.

Jenkins-Smith, Hank C. 1982. "Professional Roles for Policy Analysts: A Critical Assessment." *Journal of Policy Analysis and Management 2*: 88–100.

Jenkins-Smith, Hank C., Daniel Nohrstedt, Christopher Weible, and Karin Ingold. 2018. "Chapter 6: The Advocacy Coalition Framework: Foundations, Evolution, and Ongoing Research." In *Theories of the Policy Process* (4th Edition), Paul A. Sabatier, and Christopher M. Weible (eds.), New York: Routledge.

Kingdon, John. 2003. *Agendas, Alternatives, and Public Policies* (2nd Edition). New York: Longman.

Lindblom, Charles. 1959. "The Science of Muddling Through." *Public Administration Review 19*, *2*: 79–88.

Mayer, Jane. 2016. *Dark Money: The Hidden History of the Billionaires Behind the Rise of the Radical Right*. New York: Anchor Books.

Patton, Carl V., David S. Sawicki, and Jennifer J. Clark. 2013. *Basic Methods of Policy Analysis and Planning* (3rd Edition). Boston, MA: Pearson.

Pressman, Jeffrey, and Aaron Wildavsky. 1984. *Implementation* (3rd Edition). Berkeley, CA: University of California Press.

Rossi, Peter H., and Mark W. Lipsy. 2003. *Evaluation: A Systematic Approach* (7th Edition). Los Angeles, CA: Sage Publications.

Roth, Bernard. 2015. *The Achievement Habit*. New York: Harper Business.

Simon, Herbert A. 1997. *Administrative Behavior* (4th Edition). New York: Free Press.

Stokey, Edith, and Richard Zeckhauser. 1978. *A Primer for Policy Analysis*. New York: W. W. Norton.

Stone, Deborah. 2012. *Policy Paradox: The Art of Political Decision Making* (3rd Edition). New York: W. W. Norton.

Trippe, Helena Polata. 2021. "Policy Instrumentation: The Object of Service Design in Policy Making." *Design/Issues 37*, *3*: 89–100.

Wiemer David. L., and Aidan R. Vining. 2005. *Policy Analysis: Concepts and Practice* (4th Edition). Upper Saddle River, NJ: Prentice Hall.

2
DEFINING THE PROBLEM AND SETTING THE STAGE

Policy analysis cannot start in earnest without an understanding of the problem at hand. Although this task may seem simple and straightforward, it can often occupy a considerable amount of time and research. Indeed, one cannot narrow in on policy options or evaluative standards without having set the parameters of the central problem. Or worse, efforts could go towards solving the wrong problem entirely (Dunn 1988). In very tangible terms, this could mean lost time and resources and missed opportunities. While the goal is to establish a concise and accessible problem statement, it is complicated by the historical and political context of an issue, the particular audience for the overall policy analysis, and the experiences and biases of the analyst. In this chapter we discuss the goals and challenges of defining the problem and present a strategy for developing an effective problem statement.

As we do throughout the book, we draw from the case on child support enforcement and debt accumulation presented in the introduction. We imagine the client to be a state Department of Social Services, the arm of the government that typically administers and oversees child support debt collection. This case immediately raises questions about how to frame the central problem. At first, police brutality, against men of color in particular, stands out as the immediate problem. However, when we learn more, the circumstances behind Mr. Scott's arrest warrant, and the confrontation with the police officer that followed, raise other central problems. By better understanding and collecting evidence on the events leading up to Mr. Scott's death, a discrete problem emerges, one that traces back to how child support enforcement policies are designed and administered. This case provides an instructive example of how the framing of an issue matters and how problem definitions can bear consequences even decades later. We refer to this case throughout the chapter and do a more in-depth application at the end.

Disentangling a clear and pointed problem statement is no easy feat. How can the analyst distinguish one problem from another? Which one is actually relevant? Is there one that will more effectively mobilize attention around the issue at hand? We will address these tactical questions later on in the chapter. First, we briefly review some theoretical underpinnings to problem definition.

The Rationalistic Approach

As we discussed in Chapter 1, the "rational model" of policy analysis is the most prominent approach to policy-related decision making. While the rational model has been formulated in various ways, the first stage is universally "defining the problem"; the stages that follow proceed under the assumption that the problem has been set clearly and definitively. In order to achieve a well-defined problem, the rational model makes a set of rigid assumptions about the intent and capacities of the analyst and the information available to them. Although not often observed in practice, the spirit of the rational model relies on single decision makers with access to perfect information and infinite resources to collect and process that information. The model relies on an objective construction of the problem statement. A common critique of the rational model is that the reliance on comprehensive information and resources is unrealistic. Arguing that it imposes excessive cognitive burdens on the decision maker, Simon (1986) proposed a "bounded rational" approach. His model relaxes the assumptions related to perfect information and unlimited processing capacities. The product, however, is still a well-defined, and singular, problem statement.

Most appealing about the rationalistic approach to problem definition is the intent: establishing a clear, concise, and evocative problem statement to ground the analysis is a crucial first step. As we discuss in more detail, doing so facilitates not only a focused analysis but also effective communication about the project to clients, other policy makers, and the public more broadly. However, the rational model provides little guidance on how to get to a well-defined problem statement, especially in the context of decision makers and institutions that do not conform to rationalistic assumptions.

Alternative Perspectives

Contrary to what the rational model implies, problems are rarely, if ever, objectively construed. Problem formulations are laden with values and are a product of the analyst's creativity and the overarching contexts. Dery put it well when he described problems as "products of imposing certain frames of reference on reality" (1984: 4). Deborah Stone (2012) most notably made mainstream a similar critique of the rationalistic model of decision making in her book, *Policy Paradox*. In the polis (her political counterpart to the rationalistic market), problems are strategically defined, and their interpretations are ambiguous. Interests are competing, and therefore goals and expectations are fluid and contradictory. Problems still identify "too much" or "too little" of something, but standards of acceptability are subjective and socially constructed. This is consistent with Giandomenico Majone's assertion that "norm-setting" is actually the first step in defining the problem (1988). Therefore, the process of establishing a clear problem definition necessitates persuasion and argumentation. In addition, the problem statement is not fabricated by the policy maker or analyst in an isolated setting but rather shaped out of the political and social institutions that perpetuate either positive or negative social constructions of people and issues (Schneider et al. 2014). Inherent to "the problem" is that some standard or expectation is not being met; however, these standards always presuppose some set of norms, which are typically a product of the social and institutional context within which they operate.

Stone's work is also important in understanding that problems are defined and promulgated through narratives and stories that have plots, characters, and morals (Stone 2012; Jones and McBeth 2010). These narratives use symbols, imagery, and numbers to "pit forces of evil against forces of good" (Stone 2012: 138) and to guide discourse around the communication of a particular problem. Design processes also prioritize "collecting stories" to build empathy with the potential user (or recipient) of the public policy or service (Bason 2017). Indeed, future design (policy) solutions are a direct translation of user or citizen experiences. This framework suggests that the definitions of problems are malleable depending on the narratives or contexts at play. John Kingdon (2003) goes further to assert that problems are created to bolster (and offer targets for) existing solutions. Kingdon presents a model of policy making that is nonlinear and chaotic, akin to the Garbage Can Model where a decision opportunity is a "garbage can into which various kinds of problems and solutions are dumped by participants as they are generated" (Cohen et al. 1972: 2). Identifying the problem is not systematic but rather random and circumstantial.

Therefore, while the rationalistic approach is limited in the messy and subjective world of policies and politics, it does bring home the importance of starting with a clear problem definition. This does not mean that it will be objective and free of ideological influence. This makes the process of problem definition more complex. The analyst needs to assess and navigate the various frames and, notwithstanding, come up with a singular and clear problem statement. We now present a strategy for doing this.

How to Establish a Problem Statement

What we propose here is an approach to problem definition that maintains the importance of a focused and succinct statement, while incorporating the messy, subjective realities of policy decision making. Policy analysis is done in many different contexts and for a wide range of audiences. *Who is defining the problem? And for whom?* These are important questions to answer when articulating the problem statement. Is the problem definition driven by a client with very specific objectives, or is it taken from a broader public debate and crisis? Is the audience attuned to the technical nature of the problem, or do they have a more generic awareness of the issue? Is the client equipped to handle a broadly defined problem, or are they better suited to address a more narrowly defined one?

The child support case presents a good example of how the context of the policy's framing can shift how the problem itself is defined. The federal enforcement of child support through the Child Support Recovery Act of 1992 was initially a response to payment evasion by noncustodial parents with the means to pay. The media reinforced this narrative, running stories about affluent executives intentionally neglecting their obligations. But policy makers also picked up on similar themes. President Bill Clinton highlighted the tendency of "deadbeat" parents to "skip from state-to-state" to avoid child support obligations in his speech introducing the Deadbeat Parents Punishment Act of 1998. The policy was initially presented as economic restitution for children and mothers, an issue that crossed class lines and garnered broad-based support. Changes in laws, both federal and state, were concerned with calibrating a level of punishment that would deter the behavior. The child support system also became increasingly automated (Brito 2012). Over time, however, child support enforcement (CSE) policies had both ideological and tangible effects on families. It reinforced a notion of the nuclear family that prioritized the (financial) stability of married two-parent households over single-parent homes. At the same time, enforcement policies discouraged noncustodial parents from staying connected with their children and families (Brito 2012; Garfinkel et al. 2001; Haney 2022). In reality, these different family structures were also portrayed by stark income and race disparities. And the tangible effects fell along these lines as well: CSE policies have disproportionately affected low-income men of color, who are less likely to be able to pay child support and unable to afford lawyers to defend them in court and are therefore more likely to end up incarcerated (Brito 2012; Garfinkel et al. 2001; Turetsky and Waller 2020; Haney 2022).

Over time, the narrative around CSE policies has changed, paying more attention to the implications for overall child and family well-being rather than solely economic restitution. Noncustodial parents were being incarcerated for nonpayment, which weakened any parent–child ties that did exist, exacerbated the parents' unemployment troubles, and often embroiled the parents in the criminal justice system. Some policy makers eventually realized that it was important to differentiate between those parents who *could not* and those who *would not* pay their child support obligations and to recognize the barriers to fulfilling child support obligations. Policies increasingly differentiate between "can't pay" and "won't pay" noncustodial parents and have adjusted the severity and rigidity of the legal response for the former. For example, a 2016 final rule at the federal level safeguarded due process in proceedings related to civil contempt by incorporating criteria related to the noncustodial parent's ability to pay.[1] The commissioner of the federal Office of Child Support Enforcement summarized this shifting perspective in a *New York Times* article on the topic:

> While every parent has a responsibility to support their kids to the best of their ability, the tools developed in the 1990s are designed for people who have money. . . . Jail is appropriate for someone who is actively hiding assets, not appropriate for someone who couldn't pay the order in the first place.
>
> (Robles and Dewan 2015: 3)

While some CSE policies still rely on incarceration as a threat for nonpayment, the stated problem has become more nuanced (and there is anecdotal evidence to suggest that the implementation of the policies reflects this new framing as well). Today, after years of reforming the policies to address unfair child support burdens, remaining problems focus on the management of child support debt held by poor, and typically black and Hispanic, noncustodial parents. While policy reforms have increasingly used ability to pay to determine child support obligations (thereby mitigating unreasonable child support burdens moving forward), noncustodial parents are still saddled with past child support debt. Furthermore, enforcement policies around child support have seriously impeded individuals' abilities to manage the debt (this is discussed in more detail in the case summary at the end of this chapter).

In the case of child support, the problem has transformed over time. It started with a punitive lens: *too many fathers are evading their child support responsibilities*. The assumption was that fathers could pay and were intentionally neglecting their children, custodial parents, and the state. As the nature of the issue changed, the problem became more restorative: *too many noncustodial parents cannot pay child support and the children and families suffer*. Currently, the problem is even more focused on *the unbearable burden of accrued debt for noncustodial parents from unpaid child support obligations*. These differences are important because of the policy responses that follow. These have also changed over time and will be discussed in Chapter 3.

Researching the Nature of the Problem

In order to situate the problem, the analyst needs to do a good deal of research. As Stone (2012) asserts, the goal is not to find a definitive problem framing, but, rather, to understand the problem from multiple perspectives and become fluent in these varied "languages" (p. 135). The analyst should arrive at the problem statement fully aware of the biases and assumptions that inform it. To acquire this awareness, the issue at hand first needs to be understood within its historical, political, institutional, and social contexts.

Here, the economic lens of "market failure" can be an informative way to approach the problem. Market failures can often justify public attention and government intervention. The rationale for government intervention is either when the market is not performing well or isn't performing at all or when there are goals other than efficiency (Stokey and Zeckhauser 1978).[2] There are six main reasons for market failure, which offer various frameworks for problem definition.

1. Externalities: these emerge when individual decisions do not take into account the costs and benefits experienced by others. Therefore, the prices reflected in the private market will not capture the costs or benefits to society generated by individuals consuming or producing a particular good or service. For example, the firm's costs of producing certain goods may not incorporate the costs to the environment in the form of pollution emitted during the production process.
2. Public goods: these are goods or services that "benefit the common interests of citizens" (Stokey and Zeckhauser 1978). A single person will get such a small share of the benefits from a public good that he or she will be unlikely to purchase it on his or her own. In addition, they are characterized as (i) nonrival (one person's consumption of the good does not diminish the enjoyment of the good by another person) and (ii) non-excludable (it is impossible or impractical to exclude someone from the consumption of the good). Some

examples of public goods are national defense, certain wilderness areas, and scientific knowledge (Stokey and Zeckhauser 1978).

3 Imperfect information: in a well-functioning market, information exchange is costless. Market failure occurs when information asymmetries take place to a large degree—that is, when one party is privy to more or different information than the other party in any transaction. For example, the dealer of a used car better knows the quality of the car than the buyer. Without some mechanism for making the quality information equally accessible to the consumer, the purchase will either not take place or take place at a price that does not reflect the actual quality of the good.

4 High transaction costs: in a well-functioning market, transaction costs (i.e., the costs of making trades happen) are small to nonexistent. If these costs are non-negligible, then transactions will not take place. For example, the cost of writing up a contract for a purchase (such as a piece of property) incurs a transaction cost; if this cost is too high then the purchase will not take place. Trades that are potentially beneficial will be forgone.

5 Nonexistent or unpredictable markets: some markets do not exist or involve so much uncertainty that transactions are prevented from taking place. For example, private markets for insurance often do not function efficiently. One of the main reasons is because of *adverse selection*, where those with worse-than-average performance (for example, in terms of health) are more likely to subscribe to the insurance, making it more costly to sustain. A second reason is *moral hazard*, where the insurance encourages behavior that prevents individual loss but at a cost lower than what they would have incurred without the insurance (like visiting the doctor more often than necessary because the copay for each visit is less costly to that individual person but incurs costs for the policy overall). Both of these threats make insurance markets, for example, more costly and less likely to induce beneficial transactions.

6 Monopolies (and oligopolies): a well-functioning market assumes many producers that don't have any individual influence over prices. A monopoly is a single producer in a market where the only constraint is the demand for the good or service (and not the production capabilities of a large number of competing producers). An

oligopoly is where the market is shared by a small set of producers. These types of producers can control the price in the market, often at a level that is higher than what would have been achieved through a well-functioning, competitive market.

Bardach and Patashnik (2015) note, however, that, in the absence of systemic market failures, "private troubles" are not always best addressed by government (p. 3). Indeed, government intervention can sometimes introduce more problems: "government failure," or government's inability to "advance the social good" (p. 4) may be a problem in and of itself (Weimer and Vining 2011).

Box 2.1 Insights From Service Design Research

Design research methods emphasize the importance of exploration in the problem definition phase (Bason 2017). Some go as far to say that "policymaking as designing begins with an inquiry, not a problem" (Junginger 2016: 62). One of the important implications of this approach is that the analyst's (or designer's) initial perspective and comprehension of the issue can evolve. There are several useful insights to keep in mind from this perspective:

- "Exploratory inquiry" (Halse et al. 2010) means letting go of pre-established hypotheses and possibly learning about unexpected circumstances and futures.
- There is just as much value of drawing on "hunches" (Rowe 1991) as there is in "structured information gathering" (Bason 2017). This makes sure the design (of the problem) is open and flexible.
- User-centric research helps to unearth root causes of the central issue, also known as the "architecture of problems" (Bason 2017).

Determining the nature of the problem is a process akin to what Dunn called "problem sensing" (1981), in which analysts become aware of diffuse or emergent signs of distress before they concretize them into clear problem statements. Let's consider an issue that has worsened in recent years: homelessness. According to the Bipartisan Policy Center (Torres 2023), approximately 582,500 people were unhoused on a single night in January 2022, of which about a quarter were chronically homeless. Homelessness, a complex and sprawling problem, has been framed in different ways depending on the perspective of the concerned party and on the perceived root cause.

Box 2.2 Different Problem Frames for Homelessness in the U.S.

1 How Can the Government Decrease the Number of Unhoused Individuals?

The problem can be framed as the injustice of homelessness itself—the fact that there are people without shelter is something in and of itself that needs to be remedied. Therefore, any solution needs to lower the number of unsheltered people. This framing, however, does not identify the causes of homelessness or differentiate among the various degrees of homelessness based, for example, on duration or frequency.

2 How Can the Government Increase the Production of Affordable Housing?

Others assert that homelessness is a housing problem (Colburn and Aldern 2022). This framing suggests that any solution needs to tackle the production and preservation of affordable housing. In particular, this framing requires spatial considerations, since the availability of affordable housing depends very much on local conditions. Therefore, any solution for homelessness needs to also take into account local and regional variation in housing supply and availability.

3 How Can the Government Improve Social, Mental Health, and Employment Services for Indigent Individuals?

An alternative explanation for homelessness is that it is a product of the social economic or health-related instability of those individuals who end up unhoused. This view prioritizes individual characteristics and circumstances over institutional factors like housing infrastructure. More conservative views on homelessness often consider its prevalence a public nuisance and point towards solutions that criminalize it (for example, making it illegal to sleep in public places). Although, it can be the case that those individuals confronting social, economic, or health-related challenges may also be more vulnerable to systemic drivers into homelessness, like discrimination or domestic violence. Altogether, this framing suggests that any intervention needs to be at the individual or household level and by addressing the root causes of the instability like employment and mental health services.

The decision to assume a particular lens is often political or strategic rather than analytic; a robust analysis, however, involves a multi-perspective approach to the issue. Box 2.2 displays some questions to guide this part of the analysis.

Box 2.3 Probing the Nature of the Problem

How Did the Problem Arise and Evolve Over Time?

1. Can you trace out a timeline of milestones in the history of the problem? What were the landmark events in it?
2. Who are the stakeholders? What exactly do they have at stake with respect to the problem?
3. What are the "boundaries" of the problem? That is, is the problem situated in a specific moment in time? In a particular geography or organization? In a particular political circle?

Why Does the Problem Warrant Attention?

1. What will happen if the problem is not addressed now?
2. Why should your particular audience care about the problem?
3. Why should another, related, audience care about the problem?
4. Why might an audience not care about the problem?

Identifying the Central Problem

Researching the core policy issue will likely unearth a series of associated problems; it is the analyst's job to identify the *central* problem and distinguish it from *related* and *underlying* problems. The *central* problem is the focus of the analysis—this is the issue that proposed options will directly address. A *related* problem is one that either runs parallel to the central problem or emerges as a side effect from it. An *underlying* problem, on the other hand, is a sweeping problem that may have important implications for the central problem and how it is addressed, but is also too large and endemic to be solved by the current analysis.

Let's consider the central problem that child support enforcement officials face today, the excessive debt incurred by noncustodial parents. We can articulate the *central* problem as follows: *how to reduce the debt burden for noncustodial parents?* A *related* problem would be the obstacles to payment—an issue critically connected to the central

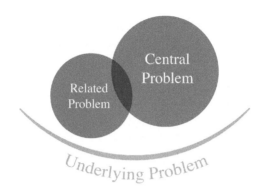

Figure 2.1 Different kinds of problems

problem but specifically as a precursor to it. This information will end up being central to the design and analysis of potential policy solutions. Another related problem is the excessive police violence against men of color, like Mr. Scott. This problem, while important, is more peripheral to the central problem articulated earlier. While the likelihood of fatal police incidences for noncustodial parents could be mitigated by addressing child support nonpayment and accumulation of debt, an intervention in the former would not solve the latter (and vice versa).

Finally, an *underlying* problem in this case would be broader determinants of divorce, poverty, and participation in the criminal justice system. The issue of child support enforcement is clearly situated in these broader systems, but the central problem, as stated, does not ask the analyst or policy maker to effect change on these systems in a comprehensive way. Differentiating the types of problems is an important and instructive exercise: it "bounds the problem" (Wagner 2014) or identifies which issues are within the scope of the analysis and, at the same time, reminds the analyst that problems should not be considered in isolation.

At this point in the analysis it is common to formulate ideas about the cause(s) of the central problem. This is natural, but we recommend that analysts *avoid a single causal story* at this stage. It is useful to log alternative causal pathways to help inform possible policy solutions. Acknowledging and articulating multi-causal problems can also help to engender broad-based support for an issue (Light 1985). However, if the analyst commits to a single causal story, the result could be "misdiagnosis" and a lack of scrutiny of the assumed causal path (Bardach and Patashnik 2015: 7). This approach could narrow the analysis to its detriment and, worst case, take it in a counterproductive direction. We discussed how the initial conception of child support nonpayment was couched in evasion (rather than inability to pay). The presumption of this cause led to a particular framing of the problem, which proved to be a misdiagnosis of the range of circumstances under which noncustodial parents do not fulfill their child support obligations.

Box 2.4 Mapping Out Problem Causation

When tackling problem definition, one of the first tendencies is to determine its origins. How did we get here? What led to current conditions? Rochefort and Cobb (1993) offer up a useful "anatomy" of problem definition for answering these questions, and we draw from their rubric here.

Questions to Determine Problem Causation
1. Is the problem a result of "personal" (i.e., individual) or "impersonal" (i.e., structural, institutional) decisions and behavior?
2. Is the problem an intended or unintended result of decisions or behavior on the part of individuals or institutions?
3. Can blame be placed on a particular individual or institution?
4. Is the causal path simple and straightforward or multi-pronged?

Understand the Audience

Another equally important purpose of conducting research at this stage is to understand the client (or whoever the target audience may be). Specifically, what is their stake in and capacity to directly address the issue? What is the span and nature of the client's authority to effect change? What are the time and resource constraints to solving the problem? For example, if the analysis were being conducted for a state legislator, the problem could be framed in a way to elicit legislative responses. However, if the client were a nonprofit advocacy group or a community-based service provider, the problem would have to be framed to reflect the more prescribed capacities of these organizations.

Let's consider a different issue: access to food subsidies, which in the United States are primarily provided through the Supplemental Nutrition Assistance Program (SNAP, formerly known as food stamps). A range of clients could face a similar central problem: *how to increase access to SNAP subsidies*. However, their abilities (and comparative advantages) to address it vary substantially. It is sometimes useful to frame the problem statement to reflect those differences. For example, *How should the organization advocate for changes to the SNAP program to broaden its application?* or *How can the organization increase access to SNAP benefits in their local community?* These distinctions are important for both methodological and political reasons. The problem statement will serve as the anchor of the analysis, and therefore it should set the parameters for the policy options. If the client engages in advocacy, then a solution that expects them to execute a particular policy change is not consistent with what they can do. Rather, solutions should involve strategies to organize around and promote an issue. For example, an advocacy organization would be unequipped to provide direct services around food access, but it could coordinate and lead efforts to lobby for increased public funding or changes in the design of policies related to those services. Having a tailored problem statement keeps the analysis grounded, and it also provides a clear signal to the client of the project's goals.

Finally, the analyst needs to do some self-reflection, to understand his or her own biases around an issue. Specifically, what are the analyst's assumptions about the nature of the problem and the stakeholders involved? For example, in the context of the food subsidy issue, the analyst should engage in some self-study of his or her own assumptions about food justice and what role the government should play in directing personal eating choices. Are the analyst's personal perspectives obscuring alternative lenses? If the analyst leans towards more interventionist approaches towards food policy, it would benefit the project to research and talk with individuals who advocate for more laissez-faire approaches.

Extensive research on the policy problem not only is a key part of focusing the analysis for the analyst, but it also contributes to how the issue will be framed in the final presentation of the analysis and recommendation(s). The final presentation of the analytical product can take on various forms: a memo, an extensive report, or an oral presentation. Whatever the medium, the problem needs to be motivated and situated for the audience. This framing is even more important for audiences who are not well informed on the topic or are predisposed to the opinion that the problem is not one that requires policy attention. For example, the analyst would need a coherent and compelling framing of the problem for those who view current food subsidies as satisfactory or even too generous.

Articulating the Problem Statement

In reality, the construction of an effective problem statement is more of an art than a science. Effective statements can take on various forms. However, in order to both ground the analysis and convey a focused policy intent, the statement should achieve five things. First, it should be **concise and digestible**. Wordy and dense statements are hard to follow and parse; the problem statement should be absorbed without much effort. Formatting also matters: problem statements are often most compelling when framed as questions. When presented as a question, it sets up the expectation for an answer, which will ultimately come out of the analyst's recommendation. Let's consider the child support case again. For example, it is the difference between stating *Excessive debt needs to be reduced* and asking *How can the government reduce the debt burden for noncustodial parents?* This distinction is also important methodologically. As we will discuss in Chapter 4, the status quo is always an option under consideration. By framing the problem as a question that needs to be answered, it leaves open the possibility that the status quo is the best way to proceed.

Second, the problem statement (or question) should, at the same time, be **meticulously worded**; indeed, every syllable matters when space and attention spans are at a premium. The degree to which jargon or technical language is included will depend on the audience.

Third, the statement should be "analytically manageable" (Veselý 2007), that is, **neither too broad** as to dilute the rigor of the analysis **nor too narrow** as to crowd out a reasonable range of options. For example, an alternative way to formulate the problem question is *How* *can the government forgive the debt for noncustodial parents?* The word *forgive* conveys something much more specific than *reduce* and doesn't leave options open for solutions that may not involve debt forgiveness. Conversely, the question could be framed too abstractly: *How can the government address the debt of noncustodial parents?* This formulation does not provide quite enough precision for guiding a focused analysis. While it leaves more options open for the proposed alternatives, it also avoids the real goal of reducing (or eliminating) the burdensome debt.

Fourth, the problem statement itself should **avoid any prescription** of a cause or solution. This point relates to the previous one, in that it can blind the analyst to a wider range of policy options. Consider if the problem were framed as *How can the government reduce debt by refinancing it?* Then the analysis is set up to ignore any solutions that do not involve refinancing.

Finally, the problem statement should be **open-ended**. These last two points are related in that they both ensure consideration of the widest range possible of options. An effective problem statement should not be framed as a yes-or-no question. For example, in the child support case, the question is most effectively framed as *How can the government reduce debt for noncustodial parents?* rather than *Is it possible to reduce debt for noncustodial parents?*. The former elicits the presentation of multiple options, which will be weighed against each other. The latter sets up a yes–no response, which is not only limiting but also often impossible to achieve. Box 2.4 summarizes common pitfalls when articulating an effective problem statement.

Box 2.5 Common Pitfalls in Articulating an Effective Problem Statement

1 The language is too jargony or technical for the audience.
2 The problem statement or question is too wordy or dense.
3 The problem is defined too broadly.
4 The problem is defined too narrowly.
5 The problem statement or question is prescriptive (assigning a solution to the stated problem).
6 The problem statement is not open-ended.

Using Evidence to Frame the Nature of the Problem

Defining the problem is more than simply stating it. The problem needs to be framed, or situated. Framing the issue "is a way of selecting, organizing, interpreting, and making sense of a complex reality" (Rein and Schön 1996: 11). It is often the analyst's job to make the case for focusing on one particular problem at a specific moment in time: *why this problem, and why now?*

This is the first instance in the process of policy analysis where the analyst will marshal evidence to make their case. The analyst needs to boil down often complex and messy issues into accessible and convincing statements and scenarios. In researching the nature of the problem, the analyst will come across many kinds of evidence. Quantitative data can be used to convey historical trends and patterns across various groups or places. Document and literature reviews can provide important qualitative context for the current state of the problem. First-hand stories and anecdotes can provide texture and familiarity to an issue that might otherwise seem unrelatable (Fischer and Forester 1993; Stone 2012). Regardless of the mode of information, visualizing the trends, relationships, and systems can be a powerful form of communication, especially when processes or inter-connections are complex. For example, design researchers create "service journeys" to convey the experiences of how citizens interface with public services and institutions over time (Bason 2017).

Rochefort and Cobb (1993) propose five dimensions that influence the degree to which a problem gains public attention. For our purposes, these can be used as guidelines for presenting data and information on the nature of the problem.

1. The degree of severity of the problem: the analyst should address the seriousness of the problem and what the implications might be should it not be addressed immediately. For example, groups opposing the Affordable Care Act used rising premiums and health care costs to motivate reform. The term "death spiral" was chosen carefully to convey a serious and uncontrollable situation in need of immediate policy attention.

2. The trend and location of incidence of the problem: the analyst needs to document the nature of the problem over time and whether or not there are places or people who disproportionately bear the burden of the problem. For example, gun control policies have repeatedly gained (often fleeting) prominence in the wake of school shootings. Gun control advocates have used the increasing number of mass school shootings, usually committed by teenagers or young adults, to bring attention to gun violence and put pressure on gun rights lobbies. Most recently, legal advocates have reinvigorated the strategy of holding parents criminally accountable for the crimes committed by their children.
3. The novelty of the problem: the analyst can highlight the unprecedented nature of the problem to promote its urgency. This can also help to motivate innovative solutions, since standard policies may not suit such a new problem. For example, policies around sustainability have gained more traction over the past decade due to what is presented as a "new normal." Policy makers and scientists use data to convey that threats from climate change and extreme weather events are unprecedented in their scale and frequency.
4. The proximity of the problem: the degree to which the problem affects someone's interests depends on the person or organization. Once the audience is identified, it can be very effective to convey how the problem "hits home." For example, homelessness (see Box 2.2) can be presented as a housing supply or a mental health problem, depending on the frame. Evidence supporting one particular frame over another will impact how closely the issue resonates with a particular audience.
5. The connection to crisis or emergency: crises call for immediate action and can help move an issue up the agenda. Does the problem itself constitute an emergency? Does it relate to or emerge out of some other nationally recognized emergency? For example, efforts to bring attention (and funding) to opioid addiction have framed it as a national crisis that needs immediate attention.

Box 2.6 Voting Case: Defining the Problem

We develop here a problem statement for the issue of voter turnout, which is motivated and summarized in the introduction of this book. Like the child support case, we will apply the analytical model to the problem framed here. The client for this analysis is an advocacy organization that is looking to develop and lobby state and local governments for interventions to increase voter turnout.

Framing

In a democratic nation, public policy decisions are shepherded and executed by elected officials. They often affect large swaths of people and institutions, and in most cases without their direct input (either in the election of the public official or the decision-making process itself). There tend to be two perspectives on how to approach electoral participation. One is to make sure that the right to vote is not abused and restrict participation in order to prevent voter fraud and maintain control over the composition of the electorate. The opposite perspective is that voting participation is too low and needs to be increased; maximum participation is ideal.

What Is the Problem?

There is scant evidence of rampant voter fraud. This argument has more often been a talking point or the product of isolated cases that have never been proven pervasive enough to change the outcomes of elections. There is more convincing (albeit varied) evidence on the merits of enabling an engaged electorate. For example, reducing barriers to voting, such as shortening distances to a polling station or extending polling site hours, can significantly improve voter turnout. And when voting participation increases among certain identity groups or constituencies, there are policy and economic changes that directly benefit them (Aneja and Avenancio-León 2020; Ang 2019; Cantoni 2020). The numbers around voter participation also speak for themselves: although voter turnout for the 2020 election was the highest in a century, it still only reached about two thirds of the U.S. voting population (Desilver 2022). Therefore, *How can the government increase voter turnout?*

Summary

In this chapter we discussed the challenges with and strategies for identifying a clear **central problem** to guide the analysis. Problem definition is a crucial first step. However, the first formulation of the problem is seldom the final one. Rather, defining the problem is an **iterative** and reflective process. It is not unusual for the analyst to circle back to revise the problem statement after considering alternatives and evaluative criteria. Information gathering occurs throughout the analytical process, and this feedback can help to refine the problem statement and strengthen the link between its intent and the proposed policy options. We recounted an example of this with the child support enforcement issue, where reasons for nonpayment were understood differently as time went by; the analyst may go through similar calibrations of an issue in even shorter periods of time.

We emphasized that problem statements need to be crafted in a way that acknowledges the client's objectives and interests. Evidence, both quantitative and qualitative, can be used to **frame the problem** and make a compelling case for why it warrants attention. Policy makers have limited resources and must make choices about which issues to espouse; an effective problem definition can help to garner support and attention around a problem. Problem statements should be **concise**, **digestible**, and **focused**, but **not overly narrow or prescriptive**. The goal is to set the stage for considering a range of options and for approaching the problem from various perspectives and strategies.

We also discussed the importance of identifying **related** and **underlying** problems, which can inform criteria and alternatives down the line. While the analyst will spend most of his or her time on a singular central problem, it rarely exists in isolation. Problems can beget other problems, and solutions to one problem can exacerbate another separate problem—the analyst needs to be aware of all of these complications (even if they cannot all be solved).

A well-defined problem is a crucial anchor for the analysis. It needs to be well articulated, backed up by evidence, and situated in the appropriate political and institutional contexts. Indeed, the coherence of the rest of the analysis hinges on a clear understanding of the central issue being addressed. It is harder to make the case for effective policy options when the problem under scrutiny is vague or unconvincing.

> **Box 2.7 Case Applications**
>
> We now take the concepts discussed earlier and apply them to actual cases, one related to child support debt and another related to voting in US elections. (See the text box on p. 55 for the voting case summary.) Each of the cases illustrates how to do the following:
>
> - Frame and situate the issue.
> - Use evidence to motivate the relevance and urgency of the issue.
> - Articulate a clear and concise problem statement.

Child Support Debt Case: Defining the Problem

Child support enforcement has a long and complicated history. The context for this policy issue is provided at the end of the introduction of this book. We draw from that case in order to frame and present a central policy problem. In the chapters that follow, we will apply the analytical model to address the problem developed here. The client for our analysis is a state Department of Social Services, where most child support agencies are housed.

Framing

How Prevalent Is Child Support?

The federal government, in partnership with states and local governments, collects nearly $27 billion annually from noncustodial parents to help support their children and also to reimburse the government for the cost of providing certain welfare benefits. In 2022, the child support program assisted 12.8 million children, about 18 percent of all children in the United States (Office of Child Support Enforcement 2023). The program is a large and growing source of financial support for low-income families. In 2007, it accounted for 40 percent of total household income for families that received child support, up from 29 percent in 1997 (Sorensen 2010). The child support program provides more financial assistance to children than these five major federal programs combined: Women with Infant Children (WIC), Social Security, Temporary Assistance for Needy Children, Child Care Development

Fund, and Supplemental Security Income (SSI). Only Medicaid and SNAP (food stamps) serve more children than the child support program (Office of Child Support Enforcement 2022).

How Does Child Support Work?

The child support system steers child support payments both to custodial parents and to state and local governments. Custodial parents receive the funds to help support their children, and governments receive the funds to reimburse themselves for some of the costs of providing "welfare" benefits to the children and custodial parents. Specifically, federal and state governments may be reimbursed for their expenditures to the family under the Temporary Assistance for Needy Families program, foster care maintenance payments funded by the federal government under Title IV-E of the Social Security Act, and Medicaid.

When Congress enacted the welfare reform act that replaced Aid for Families with Dependent Children with the time-limited TANF program, as much as 20 percent of child support payments went to the government and not to custodial parents. However, as welfare rolls have fallen precipitously since the early 2000s, custodial parents have received a growing share of child support payments. In addition, "family first" policy changes to child support reimbursement rules in 1996 and 2006 resulted in a significant drop in child support assigned to government to reimburse TANF assistance. In 2022, families received 96 percent and the government kept 4 percent of child support collections.

Similarly, most child support debt is now owed to custodial parents as opposed to the government (Sorensen 2014). As of 2022, about 17 percent of all child support debt is owed to the government for reimbursement of TANF expenditures (Office of Child Support Enforcement 2023), down from 51 percent in 2002 (Sorensen et al. 2007).

What Happens When Child Support Is Not Paid?

Most noncustodial parents with child support orders meet their obligations. However, a large minority does not, at least some of the time. As of 2022, the federal Office of Child Support Enforcement, a unit of the US Department of Health and Human Services now called the Office of

Child Support Services, reported about 9.3 million cases of child support arrears, totaling more than $14 billion (Office of Child Support Enforcement 2023). These cases include parents who are in arrears on their current child support obligations and parents who still have outstanding child support debt for children who have reached adulthood. The unpaid arrears total represents a cumulative amount back to the beginning of the program in 1975 and not an annual amount. Most of it is uncollectible but remains on the books and subject to government enforcement efforts. In 2021, 88 percent of total child support arrears involved debt that had been incurred more than five years before, including 29 percent that had been on the books for 20 or more years (Sorensen 2021). The older the arrears, the less likely they will ever be paid (Sorensen et al. 2007).

Until 2016, when the federal government issued new rules for the child support system, the ways by which some state governments determined child support obligations and enforced payment of child support made it especially hard for low-income parents to satisfy their requirements. Indeed, the methods for determining child support payments virtually guaranteed that many parents could never afford to pay, and the enforcement methods greatly exacerbated the problem (Brito 2019). These include basing obligations on imputed income (usually based on a full-time, minimum wage job, which is often higher than the negligible income that many of these fathers earned); including retroactive child support debt obligations; and charging interest on unpaid obligations, penalties that impede the fathers' chances to gaining employment or staying on top of payments (such as license suspensions or incarceration), and lack of effective legal defense (Brito 2012; Haney 2022). See Box 4.5 for a detailed description of the common debt drivers.

Box 2.8 Common Causes of Child Support Debt

Imputed Income

When a noncustodial parent is unemployed or works sporadically, as is often the case among indigent fathers, and/or fails to appear in court, judges often applied an "imputed" income to determine child support payments. Most often, imputed income was based on a full-time, year-round, minimum wage job. This imputed income often bore no connection to the parent's actual income or to his or her ability to earn such an income. One national study, for example, found that only 30 percent of poor noncustodial parents who did not pay child support worked, and those who worked did so for an average of 20 weeks a year (Sorensen and Zibman 2001: 423–434). Another 29 percent were institutionalized (overwhelmingly incarcerated) and thus unable to earn any income.

Retroactively Determined Obligations

When the initial child support amount is determined retroactively, the parent is required to reimburse the government for months or years of welfare payments, and in some cases for the costs of childbirth covered by Medicaid. As a result, the initial child support obligation can total thousands of dollars, far beyond the means of noncustodial parents with low incomes (Bartfield 2003; Haney 2022; Turetsky and Waller 2020).

High Interest Rates

When noncustodial parents fall behind their child support payments, the unpaid balance is often charged interest—and some states impose very high interest rates—causing child support debt to increase rapidly. In many cases, half or more of the total child support debt owed by noncustodial parents derives from accumulated interest charges (Bartfield 2003). As of 2022, 35 states charged interest on child support debt, at a rate ranging from 1 to 12 percent (Haney 2022: 66–70).

Enforcement Methods

Penalties for parents who fail to satisfy their child support requirement further exacerbate their ability to pay. Suspension of driver's licenses can impede one's ability to seek, obtain, or retain employment. Revocation of professional licenses prevents one from working in his or her trade. Incarceration is most damaging of all. Parents often lose their jobs when they are jailed and of course earn essentially no income while incarcerated. Employers are often reluctant to hire people who have been incarcerated, whether or not they have felony convictions (Brito 2012; Haney 2022).

Limited Legal Recourse

Noncustodial parents have limited legal recourse to challenge their child support obligations or appeal their incarceration or other penalties. In many cases, courts determine child support obligations without the noncustodial parent being present; in some cases, the parent is unaware of the child support order (Brito 2012; Haney 2022). Moreover, noncustodial parents are seldom provided with free legal counsel since their cases are usually treated as a civil and not a criminal matter (Turetsky and Waller 2020). Without an attorney, it is extremely difficult for parents to appeal jailing or persuade courts to decrease child support payments in response to reduced economic circumstances. Indeed, courts frequently considered incarceration or employment "voluntary" and therefore insufficient grounds for child support adjustment (Brito 2012; Haney 2022).

The distribution of child support debt is highly skewed. More than half of all noncustodial parents in arrears owe less than $10,000, but they account for less than 10 percent of the total debt. In contrast, 15 percent of all parents with more than $40,000 in child support debt are responsible for 55 percent of total arrearage. Three percent of noncustodial parents owe $100,000, but they account for 22 percent of all child support debt (Putze 2017). Overall, parents with incomes of less than $10,000 owe most of the outstanding child support debt (Turetsky and Waller 2020: 120).

Noncustodial parents with large amounts of child support debt are disproportionately likely to have little or no incomes. In a study of child support arrears in nine large states, Sorensen et al. (2007) found that three-quarters of all "high debtors (with arrears in excess of $30,000) had no reported income or reported incomes of $10,000 or less. These noncustodial parents accounted for 70 percent of total child support arrears in the nine states" (Sorensen et al. 2007: 3).

What Is at Stake?

Child support debt is harmful in several important respects. For the noncustodial parent, it puts him or her at risk of incarceration, reduces the opportunity to secure gainful employment, and can drive him or her into the underground economy. For the children, it can weaken or eviscerate their relationship with their noncustodial parents, and reduce the amount of financial support they receive from them. For the custodial parent, it can aggravate tensions and conflicts with the noncustodial parent. For the government, it leads to unnecessary expenditures for criminal justice, and other social services (Turetsky and Waller 2020; Haney 2022).

Noncustodial Parents
Child support debt makes it very difficult for low-income parents to obtain and keep jobs. Incarceration for failing to pay child support often causes parents to lose their jobs (as happened to Walter Scott), and employers are often reluctant to hire people with criminal records. The loss of driver's, professional, and occupational licenses can further diminish a parent's employment prospects. The suspension of driver's licenses is among the most common and onerous enforcement measures taken against noncustodial parents with child support debt. About 80 percent of all workers in the US commute to their jobs in their cars. Without a car, workers are usually dependent on public transportation, which is unevenly available and often unreliable. Being dependent on public transit can greatly increase the time it takes to get to work, and it increases the risk of arriving late—and of getting fired. Suspended driver's licenses also make people ineligible for many jobs that require driving. Not having a car can also make it more difficult for noncustodial parents to see their children. If noncustodial parents are caught driving with a suspended driver's license, they may be incarcerated—especially if they are on parole (Haney 2022).

Noncustodial parents with large child support-debt burdens (defined as more than 50 percent of income) are less likely to work than otherwise similar men, and when they are employed, they work fewer hours (Miller and Mincy 2012; Cancian et al. 2009). Child support debt "discourages fathers from taking and keeping jobs in the mainstream economy and increases the likelihood that they will generate illegal income to make child support payments or to support themselves" (Turetsky 2017).

Custodial Parents and Children
Child support debt is not merely a problem for noncustodial parents. It can exacerbate already fraught relations with the custodial parent and can lead noncustodial parents to become disengaged if not estranged

entirely from their children (Haney 2022; Legler 2003). Children not only lose financial support from their fathers but also their emotional and social support as well (Um 2019).

What Is the Problem for the Government to Consider?

Unpaid child support has financial implications for the government and can threaten the economic and social viability of noncustodial and custodial parents and their children. While collections of child support have improved over time, many low-income noncustodial parents remain saddled with debt that will never be collected. Many of the negative by-products of child support nonpayment and debt can be addressed by targeting debt reduction. Therefore, *how can the government reduce the debt burden for noncustodial parents?*

Notes

1 See www.acf.hhs.gov/css/resource/final-rule-flexibility-efficiency-and-modernization-in-child-support-enforcement-programs.
2 We present an admittedly brief discussion of market failures. For a more detailed discussion of market failures, see Weimer and Vining (2011).

References

Aneja, Abhay, and Carlos Fernando Avenancio-León. 2020. "The Effect of Political Power on Labor Market Inequality: Evidence from the 1965 Voting Rights Act." *Washington Center for Equitable Growth, Working Paper*. https://equitablegrowth.org/working-papers/the-effect-of-political-power-on-labor-market-inequality-evidence-from-the-1965-voting-rights-act/

Ang, Desmond. 2019. "Do 40-Year-Old Facts Still Matter? Long-Run Effects of Federal Oversight under the Voting Rights Act." *American Economic Journal: Applied Economics 11*, *3*: 1–53. https://doi.org/10.1257/app.20170572

Bardach, Eugene, and Eric M. Patashnik. 2015. *A Practical Guide for Policy Analysis: The Eightfold Path to More Effective Problem Solving* (5th Edition). Washington, DC: CQ Press.

Bartfield, Judi. 2003. *Forgiveness of State-Owed Child Support Arrears*. Madison, WI: Report Submitted to Wisconsin Department of Workforce Development by the Institute for Research on Poverty, University of Wisconsin. https://www.irp.wisc.edu/wp/wp-content/uploads/2020/06/sr84.pdf

Bason, Christian. 2017. *Leading Public Design: Discovering Human-Centred Governance*. Policy Press.

Brito, Tonya L. 2012. "Fathers Behind Bars: Rethinking Child Support Policy Toward Low-Income Noncustodial Fathers and Their Families." *Iowa Journal of Gender, Race & Justice 15*: 617.

Brito, Tonya L. 2019. "The Child Support Bubble." *UC Irvine Law Review 9*: 953–988.
Cancian, Maria, Carolyn J. Heinrich, and Yiyoon Chung. 2009. *Does Debt Discourage Employment and Payment of Child Support?: Evidence from a Natural Experiment*. Madison, WI: Institute for Research on Poverty.
Cantoni, Enrico. 2020. "A Precinct Too Far: Turnout and Voting Costs." *American Economic Journal: Applied Economics 12, 1*: 61–85. https://doi.org/10.1257/app.20180306,
Cohen, Michael D., James G. March, and Johan P. Olsen. 1972. "A Garbage Can Model of Organizational Choice." *Administrative Science Quarterly 17, 1*: 1–25.
Colburn, G., and C.P. Aldern. 2022. *Homelessness is a Housing Problem: How Structural Factors Explain US Patterns*. University of California Press.
Dery, David. 1984. *Problem Definition in Policy Analysis*. Lawrence: University Press of Kansas.
Desilver, Drew. 2022. "Turnout in U.S. has Soared in Recent Elections but by Some Measures still Trails that of Many Other Countries." *Pew Research Center* (November 1). www.pewresearch.org/short-reads/2022/11/01/turnout-in-u-s-has-soared-in-recent-elections-but-by-some-measures-still-trails-that-of-many-other-countries/
Dunn, William N. 1981. *An Introduction to Public Policy Analysis*. Englewood Cliffs, NJ: Prentice Hall.
Dunn, William N. 1988. "Methods of the Second Type: Coping with the Wilderness of Conventional Policy Analysis." *Review of Policy Research 7, 4*: 720–737.
Fischer, Frank, and John Forester. 1993. *The Argumentative Turn in Policy Analysis and Planning*. Durham, NC: Duke University Press.
Garfinkel, Irwin, Daniel R. Meyer, and Sara S. McLanahan. 2001. "A Brief History of Child Support Policies in the United States." In *Father Under Fire*, Irwin Garfinkel, Sara S. McLanahan, Daniel R. Meyer, and Judith A. Seltzer (eds.). New York: Russell Sage Foundation.
Halse, Joachim, Eva Brandt, Brendon Clark, and Thomas Binder. 2010. *Rehearsing the Future*. The Danish Design School Press.
Haney, Lynn. 2022. *Prisons of Debt: The Afterlives of Incarcerated Fathers*. Berkeley, CA: University of California Press.
Jones, Michael D., and Mark K. McBeth. 2010. "A Narrative Policy Framework: Clear Enough to be Wrong?" *Policy Studies Journal 38, 2*: 329–353.
Junginger, Sabine. 2016. "Towards Policymaking as Designing: Policymaking Beyond Problem-Solving and Decision-Making." In *Design for Policy*. Routledge.
Kingdon, John W. 2003. *Agendas, Alternatives, and Public Policies*. New York: Longman.
Legler, Paul. 2003. *Low-Income Fathers and Child Support: Starting Off on the Right Track. Final Report*. Denver, CO: Policy Studies, Inc.
Light, Paul Charles. 1985. *Artful Work: The Politics of Social Security Reform*. New York: Random House.
Majone, Giandomenico. 1988. "Policy Analysis and Public Deliberation." In *The Power of Public Ideas*, Robert Reich (ed.). Cambridge, MA: Harvard University Press.
Miller, Daniel P., and Ronald B. Mincy. 2012. "Falling Further Behind? Child Support Arrears and Fathers' Labor Force Participation." *Social Service Review 86, 4*: 604–635.

Office of Child Support Enforcement. 2022. "2022 Child Support: More Money For Families." *(Infographic)*. www.acf.hhs.gov/sites/default/files/documents/ocse/2022_infographic_national.pdf

Office of Child Support Enforcement. 2023. *Preliminary Report FY2022*. Washington, DC: Author.

Putze, Dennis. 2017. "Who Owes the Child Support Debt?" *Analyze This (Blog of the Federal Office of Child Support Enforcement)* (September 15). www.acf.hhs.gov/css/ocsedatablog/2017/09/who-owes-the-child-support-debt

Rein, Martin, and Donald Schön. 1996. "Frame-Critical Policy Analysis and Frame-Reflective Policy Practice." *Knowledge and Policy 9, 1*: 85–104.

Robles, Frances, and Shaila Dewan. 2015. "Skip Child Support. Go to Jail. Lose Job. Repeat." *New York Times* (April 19).

Rochefort, D.A., and R.W. Cobb. 1993. "Problem Definition, Agenda Access, and Policy Choice." *Policy Studies Journal 21, 1*: 56–71.

Rowe, Peter G. 1991. *Design Thinking*. MIT press.

Schneider, Anne L., Helen Ingram, and Peter DeLeon. 2014. "Chapter 4: Democratic Policy Design: Social Construction of Target Populations." In *Theories of the Policy Process*, Paul A. Sabatier, and Christopher M. Weible (eds.). New York: Routledge.

Simon, Herbert A. 1986. "Rationality in Psychology and Economics." *Journal of Business 59, 4* (Part 2): S209–S224.

Sorensen, Elaine. 2010. *Child Support Plays an Increasingly Important Role for Poor Custodial Families*. Washington, DC: Urban Institute.

Sorensen, Elaine. 2014. "Major Change in Who is Owed Child Support Arrears." *US Office of Child Support Enforcement, Child Support Fact Sheet Series, Number 4*. www.acf.hhs.gov/sites/default/files/programs/css/changes_in_who_is_owed_arrears.pdf

Sorensen, Elaine. 2021. *Most Arrears Were Submitted to OCSE More Than Five Years Ago* Washington, DC: Office of Child Support Enforcement. www.acf.hhs.gov/css/ocsedatablog/2021/09/most-arrears-were-submitted-ocse-more-fi ve-years-ago 1/4

Sorensen, Elaine, Liliana Sousa, and Simon Schaner. 2007. *Assessing Child Support Arrears in Nine Large States and the Nation*. Washington, DC: The Urban Institute. www.urban.org/sites/default/files/publication/29736/1001242-Assessing-Child-Support-Arrears-in-Nine-Large-States-and-the-Nation.PDF

Sorensen, Elaine, and Chava Zibman. 2001. "Getting to Know Poor Fathers Who Do Not Pay Child Support." *Social Science Review* (September): 420–434.

Stokey, Edith, and Richard Zeckhauser. 1978. *A Primer for Policy Analysis*. New York: W. W. Norton.

Stone, Deborah. 2012. *Policy Paradox: The Art of Political Decision Making* (3rd Edition). New York: W. W. Norton.

Torres, Francis. 2023. "Housing Supply and the Drivers of Homelessness." *Bipartisan Policy Center*.

Turetsky, Vicki. 2017. "The High Price of Unmanageable Child Support Debt." *Presentation at Conference Sponsored by New York City Office of Child Support Enforcement*, September 26.

Turetsky, Vicki, and Maureen R. Waller. 2020. "Piling on Debt: The Intersections Between Child Support Arrears and Legal Financial Obligations." *UCLA Criminal Justice Law Review 4, 1*: 117–141.

Um, Hyunjoon. 2019. *The Role of Child Support Debt on the Development of Mental Health Problems among Nonresident Fathers, Working Papers wp19–05-ff*. Center for Research on Child Wellbeing, Princeton University. https://ffcws.princeton.edu/sites/g/files/toruqf4356/files/documents/wp19-05-ff.pdf

Veselý, Arnošt. 2007. "Problem Delimitation in Public Policy Analysis." *Central European Journal of Public Policy 1*, *1*: 80–101.

Wagner, Travis P. 2014. "Using Root Cause Analysis in Public Policy Pedagogy." *Journal of Public Affairs Education 20*, *30*: 429–440.

Weimer, David L., and Aidan R. Vining. 2011. *Policy Analysis*. Boston, MA: Longman.

3
DEVISING ALTERNATIVE POLICY OPTIONS

A policy recommendation can be no better than the policy options under consideration. If an option is not "on the table," it cannot be recommended. Policy analysis involves the identification and comparison of different ways of addressing a particular problem. While the analysis should arrive at the best of these policy alternatives, there can always be an alternative that is better still but was never considered. It is therefore crucial to identify a wide range of possible options and select the most promising of these options for further analysis.

The number of possible solutions to a problem is limited by one's imagination—as well as by the time available to conceive of them. Ultimately, the goal of the analyst should be to develop a portfolio of options that would address the problem in distinctive ways. In identifying possible options, it is always important to ask *how* they would address the problem or how they would meet the objectives you've established for addressing it (Hammond et al. 1999: 50). In asking *how*, you can home in on the mechanisms inherent to the alternative that would enable it to achieve your objectives. Otherwise, you run the risk of proposing alternatives that are tangential to the issue at hand. They may be interesting, and perhaps address some aspect of the issue, but do not get at the heart of the matter.

In Chapter 2 we discussed how problems can be framed in many ways and that the way in which problems are depicted reflects the values and goals of policy analysts and their clients. The same is true for the presentation of policy alternatives. While there will be times when the policy analyst and/or the client has no preconceived notion of how a particular issue should be addressed, and is open to a wide range of possible options, there may be others when the analyst or client seeks to promote particular approaches and/or keep others out of consideration.

The names given to alternatives and the contrasts between the alternatives under consideration can influence how they are perceived in ways that supersede their actual analysis. Deborah Stone, for example, discusses how the names given to possible policies can trigger positive or negative emotional responses (2012). For example, calling the inheritance tax a "death tax" implies that such taxes are fundamentally unfair, as if the government is taxing, or exploiting, everyone at the moment of their death—even though the federal inheritance tax is currently (as of 2024) subject only to estates worth more than $13.6 million—less than 0.2 percent of all estates.[1]

Also, the juxtaposition of alternatives can help persuade others of the analyst's desired outcome. We started this chapter with the observation that if alternatives are left "off the table" they will not be subject to analysis or considered as potential solutions. Therefore, one strategy is for the analyst to omit policies that might otherwise be viewed as credible alternatives to his or her preferred approach. In addition, the analyst can couple his or her preferred policy option with ones that are blatantly undesirable so that the client or other audiences will be drawn to the former. In other words, the analyst may pose the alternatives as a "Hobson's choice" between one realistic option and others that are seriously flawed and unacceptable (Stone 2012).

In this book we assume that policy analysts recommend policies based on a good-faith assessment of their strengths and weaknesses. That said, we also recognize that the choice of alternatives to be considered is always subject to the values and priorities of the analyst and his or her client. The range of alternatives to be considered is never comprehensive, and is always circumscribed in some way. In the following sections we assume that the analyst and client wish to examine multiple options for addressing a problem, and we introduce several ways of identifying and developing them.

Approaches for Generating Alternatives

Policy analysis usually involves comparison of three to five or so alternatives, including the status quo. Consideration of a larger number of options can quickly become unwieldy. However, that three to five options are subject to a full analysis does not mean that these were the only options to be identified or considered. It is almost always wise to start by identifying a large and wide-ranging set of possible options. The analyst can then choose among these options for further analysis. In some cases, two or more potential alternatives can be combined to form a new alternative; conversely, other options might be split apart to form multiple, more narrowly defined options. Sometimes, alternatives can be adopted in whole cloth from other contexts (places, organizations, times). More often, they must be adopted to fit local circumstances. In some cases, analysts must design policy options from scratch or combine elements of two or more approaches.

How does one identify possible policy options? There are numerous possibilities. In this chapter we discuss several ways to identify and develop policy alternatives. Some of these methods involve incremental adjustments to the status quo or the identification of programs or policies adopted in other places or at other times to address similar or analogous issues. Other approaches are more inductive in nature, involving adaptation of basic modes of government intervention, various kinds of "thought experiments," or the application of principles from such fields as behavioral science and design (see Box 3.1 for summary of approaches). We conclude the chapter by considering possible alternative policies to reduce child support debt.

Box 3.1 Common Sources for Ideas About Alternatives

- Status quo
- Incremental changes to the status quo
- Client suggestions
- Policies in other places that address similar issues
- Past policies addressing similar issues
- Analogous policies

- Dimensions: turning one alternative into several
- Standard modes of government intervention
- Brainstorming
- Building off an ideal
- Behavioral economics
- Design solutions

Modeling Alternatives on Existing or Previous Programs and Policies

Status Quo

One option that should almost always be considered is the status quo of sticking with the current policy and letting current trends continue. Policy changes could cause conditions to worsen. Some problems may prove to be temporary or random. For example, a town might be better off choosing not to build new schools to reduce overcrowding if the school-age population is projected to shrink in the near future. At minimum, the status quo should be considered as a baseline for comparison with the projected outcomes of alternative policy options.

Incremental Changes to the Status Quo

Besides the status quo, analysts may also consider small incremental changes to current policies. Indeed, Charles Lindblom, in his classic essay "The Science of Muddling Through" (1959), argues that, in practice, policy analysis focuses mostly on incremental adjustments to the status quo (see Chapter 1). For example, one might modify the eligibility criteria for a particular program, change the amount of a subsidy, or stiffen a penalty for violating a regulation. Patton et al. (2013), building on the work of Alex Osborn, offer the following ways by which existing programs or policies might be modified:

Magnify: make larger, apply more often, duplicate
Minify: make smaller, narrower, omit, split apart
Substitute: change location, change sponsor, change components, change financing

Combine: combine approaches, combine sponsors
Rearrange: change sequence, change timing (speed up/slow down), change locations (centralize, decentralize; mobile vs. permanent)
(Patton et al. 2013: 233)

Client Suggestions

Often the client will have ideas or suggestions of possible policy options. In some instances the client may want analytic support for a particular policy or program. When this occurs, the client is less interested in advice on how to solve a problem than in receiving evidence and argumentation in support of a particular course of action and perhaps critiques of other potential solutions that other actors (e.g., government officials, lobbyists) might favor. These circumstances can, of course, put analysts in a difficult ethical position, especially if they do not view themselves as an advocate (Jenkins-Smith 1982). (See Chapter 8 for a discussion of the ethics of policy analysis.)

Policies in Other Places That Address Similar Issues

Another common method is to explore how the issue is addressed elsewhere. Analysts can look at the programs, policies, and other initiatives of other governments and organizations to address similar problems. For example, in researching how a city might stem growth in opioid use and abuse, analysts could look at how other cities and states are approaching the problem, and how their approaches might be adapted for the client. In addition to canvassing efforts undertaken by other cities and states in the United States, policy analysts could also learn from the activity of nongovernmental organizations as well as international jurisdictions. In Chapter 7 we will discuss various research methods and information sources for identifying and developing policy alternatives.

Past Policies Addressing Similar Issues

Besides investigating how other places and organizations are currently contending with the issue, it is also important to look at how the issue, or issues similar to it, has been addressed in the past. For example, previous efforts to reduce substance abuse (crack, heroin) might offer lessons for today's opioid crisis.

Analogous Policies

In addition to exploring how the same or similar issues are or have been addressed elsewhere, it is also helpful to consider how policies or programs that address quite different, even unrelated, issues could be adopted to the issue at hand. For example, one might think about how methods used by the armed forces to recruit volunteers could be adopted for the purpose of recruiting young adults for a youth mentoring program. Similarly, in considering ways of reducing child support debt, analysts might look to policies and programs aimed at educational, medical, and credit card debt as potential models.

A Cautionary Note on "Best Practices"

Oftentimes, analysts refer to the efforts taken by other governmental and/or nongovernmental organizations to address a particular issue as a "best practice," implying that it could be a model for the client. Unfortunately, it is usually impossible to know if such efforts are indeed "best" or even "good." Few programs are subject to rigorous or any evaluations, so it is simply impossible to know with any certainty that programs that have not been evaluated are actually effective. While analysts may be excited to discover other programs that are designed to tackle the same or similar problems, the existence of such programs does not denote success. Even if administrative data suggest positive outcomes, such as reductions in opioid-related hospitalizations, these results may not be indicative of success or effectiveness.

Even if a program has been thoroughly and rigorously evaluated, it still may not be a "best practice" for the current situation. If it was implemented in a much smaller (or larger) jurisdiction with a very different political culture, with different population characteristics, or with different technical and financial capabilities, the program or policy may not be appropriate or suitable—although certain modifications to reflect differences in the overarching context might make it so.

Bardach and Patashnik (2015), in their discussion of "smart practices," emphasize the need to isolate the key factors and causal links that make a given program or policy successful. By focusing on these factors and the elements that support them, analysts may be able to see whether the policy or program can be adapted to fit the demographic, political, and institutional context of the client's jurisdiction.

Bardach and Patashnik stress the need to identify the basic mechanism through which a program or policy achieves its success. Analysts must then distinguish between the basic *functions* "involved in getting the mechanism to work and the particular features of the programs that embody those functions" (Bardach and Patashnik 2015: 132). Whereas the functions are usually indispensable, the features are not. For example, Bardach and Patashnik point to Riverside County, California's Greater Avenues for Independence (GAIN) welfare-to-work program of the early 1990s. The program distinguished itself from other welfare-to-work programs of the period by setting high expectations about work for its participants. It emphasized societal norms and expectations about work and economic self-sufficiency, and it signaled in various ways to participants that program staff were confident that they would succeed in obtaining a job and leaving welfare. These two features (expectations, confidence) constitute the basic mechanisms of the GAIN program. However, the specific program design features that impart these mechanisms may be adapted in various ways.

Dimensions: Turning One Alternative Into Several

Any policy alternative can be modified into multiple variations. It is sometimes useful to think about how a given policy option might be altered or to create two or more separate alternatives based on the same basic option. In modifying an alternative or creating multiple variants, one varies one or more key components. For example, one can change the eligibility criteria for a program, the fees that would be charged, the scale of its operation, the timing of its implementation, its geographic scope, and many other elements.

Inclusionary zoning provides a useful example of how choices about key design elements can lead to quite different programs.

Inclusionary zoning (sometimes termed "inclusionary housing") refers to programs established by state and local governments to leverage private real estate development to produce affordable housing (housing affordable to low- and/or moderate-income households). Inclusionary zoning requires or offers incentives to designate a portion of the housing units in new developments for low- or moderate-income households.

Here are some of the key program elements:

- *Mandatory versus voluntary:* Should the program apply to all eligible private housing development without exception, or should it be a voluntary incentive?
- *Minimum development size:* What is the minimum size of the development subject to inclusionary zoning? Five units? Fifty?
- *Tenure:* Should both rental and condominium units be subject to inclusionary zoning? To what extent should the affordable housing produced be rental or for homeownership?
- *Affordable set-aside:* What percentage of the units in the development should be reserved for (made affordable to) low- and/or moderate-income households?
- *On- or off-site provision of affordable units:* Should the affordable units always be included within the market-rate development, or should developers have the option of providing the units elsewhere? If so, under what conditions?
- *Income targeting:* What income groups should the affordable housing be targeted to? If the units should be designated for a mix of incomes, what incomes, and in what proportion?
- *Longevity of affordability:* For how many years should affordability requirements remain in effect? Should affordability be permanent? Should longevity of affordability differ for rental and owner-occupied housing?
- *Program oversight and management:* Who should oversee compliance with the program and ensure that affordable units are created and allocated to qualified households and remain in compliance over time?

Reflecting the number of design elements, inclusionary zoning programs vary widely in the United States. Some are voluntary, providing incentives to developers if they provide affordable housing; others are mandatory for all development over a designated size. Some apply only to very large developments; others apply to smaller properties as well. Some apply only to rental housing developments, while others involve all multifamily residential development—rental and condominium—above a specific size. Some require all affordable units to be provided on-site, while other programs allow developers to build affordable units at other sites or to contribute to a housing trust fund that can enable other developers to build the affordable housing. Some target moderate or even middle-income households, while others give priority to lower-income households. Affordability restrictions can vary from a few as five years to perpetual affordability. Some governments oversee inclusionary zoning programs directly; others contract with nonprofit organizations for this purpose. The flexibility makes it easier to tailor the program to the needs of the municipality.[2]

Alternative Strategies for Developing Alternatives

Researching how other governments and organizations are currently addressing the issue and have done so in the past can yield various potential models and precedents for the case at hand. However, some of the most creative and perhaps most effective ideas may emerge from less empirical means.

In this section we examine several additional ways to devise potential alternatives. These methods are more inductive in nature than the approaches outlined in the previous section. Rather than adapt existing or previous programs or policies that aim to address issues similar to the one at hand, the approaches outlined next require the analyst to construct potential alternatives by adapting principles and ideas from various fields or by exercising one's imagination. We begin by discussing how the analyst can base alternatives on various generic governmental functions. We then review strategies to imagine potential alternatives. Next, we discuss how principles from behavioral sciences and design can be used to inform potential alternatives.

Standard Modes of Government Intervention

One way to identify potential solutions to a problem is to draw from the standard toolkit of government: the various ways by which it can influence behavior, provide services, and raise revenue. As illustrated in Box 3.2, governments write laws and regulations to restrict certain types of behavior on the part of individuals and businesses and impose penalties for violating these laws and regulations; governments may provide direct subsidies to support or encourage certain kinds of activities and services; they can incentivize or sanction certain activities through the tax code; they can provide services directly or decide to contract with nonprofit or for-profit organizations to deliver these services.[3]

Box 3.2 Standard Modes of Government Intervention

Taxation (e.g., Income Tax, Property Tax, Sales Tax, Gas Tax, Excise Taxes, Liquor Tax, Commuter Tax)

Purpose: encourage or discourage certain activities; raise revenue.

Examples: introduce new tax; eliminate tax; change terms of existing taxes (change tax rates, change income levels subject to particular tax rates; exempt certain goods from sales taxes; increase taxes on specified goods such as liquor ("sin taxes"); offer tax incentives (credits, deductions) for investing in specified activities or locations.

Grants and Subsidies

Purpose: provide funds to encourage certain behavior.

Examples: grants for medical and scientific research; subsidies for low-income housing; below-market rate loans; loan guarantees.

Criminalization/Decriminalization

Purpose: make certain activities illegal; increase penalty for violating laws and regulations; reduce or eliminate legal sanctions against certain behavior.

Examples: legalization of recreational and medicinal marijuana use; minimum prison sentences; increase in statute of limitations for prosecution of certain crimes.

Regulation

Purpose: require people and businesses to adhere to specific standards to ensure health and safety or meet other social, economic, or environmental goals.

Examples: zoning, building codes; product safety regulations; privacy protections; calorie-content disclosure requirements for restaurant menus; automobile mileage standards; privacy protections for social media users.

Service Provision

Purpose: provide public services directly or pay other organizations to provide them.

Examples: public schools; public hospitals; after-school programs; recycling; change eligibility standards for services.

Health care illustrates the many ways by which government can bring this toolkit to bear. The Affordable Care Act of 2010 (The Commonwealth Fund 2018; Henry Kaiser Foundation 2018; Starr 2018) embodies several distinctive forms of intervention, and debates before and after the passage of the legislation highlight other potential means of governmental action. (See Box 3.3 for an example of another policy arena open to several kinds of intervention.)

Box 3.3 Policy Application: Greenhouse Gas Emissions

A wide range of generic policy interventions is also evident in efforts to address climate change by reducing greenhouse gas emissions. Federal and state governments have long debated how to reduce carbon generated by motor vehicles and by electric utilities. By increasing mile-per-gallon **requirements** for cars and trucks, the government required automakers to reengineer their products so that motor vehicles burn less greenhouse-gas-generating fuel while traveling the same distance as before. Similarly, most states require annual **inspections** of all motor vehicles to, among other things, ensure that exhaust emissions comply with environmental standards. Another way by which government has sought to reduce greenhouse gas emissions is to encourage the use of hybrid and battery-powered vehicles. They do so, for example, by offering income **tax credits** for the purchase of battery-powered vehicles, thereby offsetting some or all of the higher purchase price of these vehicles. The government can also help **subsidize** research and development of battery technology and other means of making motor vehicles more fuel efficient.

Another option, proposed by the first Bush Administration and implemented by several states, is "cap and trade"—whereby the total amount of allowable greenhouse gas emissions are capped at a set amount. Utilities and other businesses receive credits for reducing their greenhouse gas emissions and can sell these credits to other businesses that exceed the allowable standards, essentially setting up a **market** for emissions.

Yet another option that advocates propose but that has not been implemented is to significantly increase **gasoline taxes**. If gas taxes in the United States approached that of most European countries, consumers might seek out more fuel-efficient vehicles, including battery-powered ones. In addition, some advocates argue that if higher gas prices were an established reality, and use patterns might change over time so that there is more integration of residential and commercial uses, and higher density of construction so as to reduce the amount of daily vehicle miles driven.

Coal-powered electric plants are among the single largest sources of greenhouse gas emissions. Controversy rages at present about how and whether coal-powered electricity should be curtailed. The federal and state governments could simply issue **regulations or laws** banning the use of coal as a fuel for electricity generation, going into effect after a specific period of time, as have such countries as Canada and the United Kingdom (Plumer and Popovich 2017). Governments could impose a **tax on carbon** generated by electric utilities and other users of carbon-based fuels. The tax would add to the cost of relying on carbon-intensive fuels such as coal, and encourage utilities to change over to natural gas, solar, wind power, and perhaps nuclear power.

The Affordable Care Act combines different types of **subsidies** and **regulations** to expand health insurance coverage and to lower the growth of health care costs. Until Congress repealed this aspect of the Act in 2018,[4] it **mandated** that all people acquire health insurance. It **expanded** the Medicaid program to cover all people with incomes of up to 138 percent of the poverty line (although the Supreme Court ruled that the expansion of the Medicaid could be decided only by the states), and it provided **subsidies** to help cover the premiums for individuals and families with incomes up to a certain level. The Act also involves numerous **regulations** including, among many other things the following: requiring all individuals to obtain health insurance, setting minimum standards of coverage for all insurance policies, requiring insurance companies to cover dependent children up to the age of 26, prohibiting insurance companies from denying coverage to people with preexisting medical conditions, and eliminating lifetime caps on insurance benefits.

The legislative debates prior to the passage of Affordable Care Act and the critiques that have been leveled against it afterwards highlight other alternatives that might have been considered to attain the same objective of universal health care but were not put on the proverbial legislative table. For example, the government could **insure health coverage directly**—as is done in many other countries such as Australia, Canada, and most of Western Europe, and as the United States does in its Medicare and Medicaid programs. At minimum, if a "Medicare for All" policy isn't possible, states could be allowed to offer a "public option" of state-administered insurance to compete with private, for-profit insurance.

The child support case also illustrates the application of several standard modes of government intervention. As discussed in Chapter 2, the government defined the problem in terms of the refusal of parents to provide financial support for their children, deeming such parents "deadbeats." Federal and state government agencies responded to the problem in the 1980s and 1990s by imposing stiffer **penalties** against parents who fail to pay child support, and to make it easier for governments to track down these parents and secure child support payments from them. The sanctions governments imposed against parents who owe child support included suspension of driver's licenses, professional licenses, passports, and in some cases incarceration. State and federal governments agreed to **share information** on the identities of parents in arrears and to **require** employers to share with child support agencies the identities of all new employees so that their wages can be **withheld** for child support. Financial institutions were similarly required to share information on their accounts so that the government can tap into the accounts of delinquent parents. Finally, the government **increased funding** for genetic testing to verify the paternity of noncustodial parents (Brito 2012).

Brainstorming

Brainstorming is the spontaneous, unfiltered generation of ideas. In thinking about how to address a problem (any kind of problem, not just policy issues), it's often helpful to imagine and free-associate all sorts of potential solutions. Brainstorming is usually most productive when done in collaboration with others, so that each can build on the other's suggestions. The point of brainstorming is to generate lots of ideas, not to evaluate them or specify them in detail. Just keep a running list of them. Afterwards, you can decide which ones are worthy of further development.

IDEO, an influential design firm, offers the following "rules" for successful brainstorming:

1. Defer judgment. You never know where a good idea is going to come from. The key is to make everyone feel like they can say the idea on their mind and allow others to build on it.
2. Encourage wild ideas. Wild ideas can often give rise to creative leaps. When devising ideas that are wacky or out there, we tend to imagine what we want without the constraints of technology or materials.
3. Build on the ideas of others. Being positive and building on the ideas of others take some skill. In conversation, we try to use "yes, and . . ." instead of "but."
4. Stay focused on the topic. Try to keep the discussion on target, otherwise you may diverge beyond the scope of what you're trying to design for.
5. One conversation at a time. Your team is far more likely to build on an idea and make a creative leap if everyone is paying full attention.
6. Be visual. In brainstorms we put our ideas on sticky notes and then put them on a wall. Nothing gets an idea across faster than a sketch.

7   Go for quantity. Aim for as many new ideas as possible. In a good session, up to 100 ideas are generated in 60 minutes. Crank the ideas out quickly and build on the best ones (Ideo.org 2015: 95).

Building off an Ideal—Or Imagining Policies Without Constraints

Another useful way of envisioning potential options is to think about the ideal solution to the problem, suspending consideration of costs, political feasibility, and other constraints. One can then consider ways of modifying this solution so that these constraints could be addressed. It also may be possible to envision ways of eliminating some of these constraints so that the ideal solution becomes viable. As Patton, Sawicki, and Clark put it, the value of developing an ideal solution "is not so much in stating a goal to be attained, but rather in causing us to think about alternative means to move toward the ideal" (2013: 230). The field of "futures thinking" also offers techniques for imagining potential solutions to various kinds of problems in the form of scenarios and visioning exercises (Waverly Consultants 2017).

One potential downside of alternatives that derive from brainstorming or similar creative exercises is that their unique or idiosyncratic qualities can make them difficult to assess and compare with other potential policy options. The lack of prior research on novel policy ideas can render it difficult to compare them with more established options. In a related vein, if alternatives are sketched out in broad strokes and leave many details undefined, it can be difficult to assess them credibly. In addition, the interpersonal dynamics in a brainstorming session may impede the generation of creative ideas. For example, more extroverted individuals may dominate the discussion, and participants may feel obliged to adhere to the salient ideas or patterns of thinking (Ballis 2014).

Insights From Behavioral Economics and Related Fields

Behavioral sciences offer a fertile source of ideas for policy alternatives. The closely related fields of behavioral economics and psychology have revealed patterns of perception, cognition, and behavior that can inform innovative policy options. The pioneering research of Danny Kahneman and Amos Tversky, followed by many others, shows that people often act and think in ways that depart markedly from the expectations of traditional economics. Moreover, they discovered that they depart in ways that are systemic and predictable. These insights can help identify and develop potential alternatives—the subject of this chapter—and analyze their potential impact, which is the subject of Chapter 6.[5]

A key insight of behavioral economics and related fields is that humans think in two basic ways. As Kahneman (2011) famously put it, people "think fast and slow." Thinking fast refers to the mental shortcuts people take in understanding problems and making decisions—snap decisions, quick assumptions, cognitive biases, intuition, and emotion. Thinking slow, on the other hand, refers to the more considered, deliberate, and analytic approach people may also take in solving problems and making decisions. Kahneman called the former mode of thought "System 1" and the latter "System 2." Richard Thaler, a pioneering behavioral economist (and a colleague of Kahneman) and co-author Cass Sunstein refer to them as "Automatic" and "Reflective" systems. The former is akin to a "gut feeling" and the latter to "conscious thought" (Thaler and Sunstein 2008: 21).

Regardless of the nomenclature, the point is that many decisions and actions result from thinking fast instead of slow. Researchers in the field have identified several specific characteristics of System 1, characteristics that often lead to errors, or decisions that would run counter to what System 2 would suggest. Policy analysts have marshaled these insights to devise a wide array of public policies. Before we discuss how behavioral economics and related fields can generate policy alternatives, we review several of the key findings of behavioral economics with relevance to public policy.

Status Quo Bias

People are reluctant to depart from their current situation. More often than not, they stick with their current position and do not change even if such changes would lead to an improvement.

Loss Aversion

The same item is worth more to people when they already own it than when they do not. If asked to sell a possession, they will ask a higher price than what they would be willing to pay to acquire it in the first place. Loss aversion reinforces status quo bias in that it fosters inertia—a desire to stick with current holdings, even if letting go of them, or trading them for other things, would lead to an improved situation.

Framing

Choices are often contingent on the way in which they are presented. People often prefer one option when the choices are framed one way, and a different option when they are framed in another way. For example, Sunstein notes that people are more likely to choose to have an operation if they are told that 90 of 100 people who had the operation previously are still alive after five years than if they are told that ten people are dead after five years—even though the two outcomes are identical.

Anchoring

People's assessment of things—whether quantitative or qualitative—is often influenced by the context in which they are presented. The starting point of the assessment can influence the conclusion. Initial prompts, even arbitrary ones, can suggest the direction and magnitude of the answer. Thaler and Sunstein give the example of someone being asked to estimate the population of Milwaukee. If that person is from Chicago and knows that Milwaukee is the largest city in Wisconsin, he or she may assume that Milwaukee's population is about one-third of that of Chicago's population of about 3 million, amounting to 1 million. However, if someone from Green Bay, Wisconsin, is asked the same question, she may assume that Milwaukee's population is about three times that of Green Bay, or 300,000. Depending on the anchor (Chicago or Green Bay), one can arrive at very different estimates.

Availability

When asked to estimate the likelihood of risks, people often think about examples of such risks and how recent they were. Perceptions of the risk of a plane crash, for example, tend to rise in the aftermath of a recent crash and decline afterwards. Perceptions of risk, in other words, can be based much less on probability than on one's memory of recent events. As a result, risks may be exaggerated or unduly minimized.

Confirmation Bias

People tend to search for information that confirms their beliefs and are less likely to seek out or consider information that runs counter to them.

Representativeness

People often reach conclusions about patterns and things based on their apparent similarity to something else. They often ignore basic probabilities in favor of stereotypes and other preconceptions. For example, people see patterns when the outcomes are random, since they do not appreciate the variety of forms that random sequences can take. Kahneman and Tversky once gave a group of people descriptions of "Steve," a retiring, shy and withdrawn man with a "need for order and structure and passion for detail." They were asked if he was more likely to be an engineer or a librarian. They found that people were far more likely to answer "librarian." His characteristics matched their stereotype of that profession, even though men are far more likely to be engineers than librarians (Oliver 2017: 26).

Optimism and Overconfidence

People tend to be unrealistically optimistic about their prospects and future behavior. They tend to believe, for example, that they are less likely than others to experience ill health or financial misfortune. Similarly, people tend to be overconfident about their abilities.

Behavioral Sciences and Public Policy: "Nudges"

Although behavioral economics emerged as a field in the 1970s, it was not until the 2000s that it began to influence public policy in earnest. Drawing on the insights of the behavioral sciences, policy analysts have devised policies to address a wide array of issues in many countries.

Many of these policies take the form of a "nudge," a way of steering people into decisions and actions that would benefit them if they had given the matter considered attention instead of automatic reasoning.

"Nudge" was coined by Thaler and Sunstein in their highly influential book of that name, published in 2008. They consider nudges to be a form of "libertarian paternalism." Nudges are paternalistic in that they encourage people to act in ways that the government considers to be in their best interest—and that people would presumably judge so themselves if they had "paid full attention and possessed complete information, unlimited cognitive abilities, and complete self-control" (Thaler and Sunstein 2008: 5). Nudges are libertarian in that they do not coerce people to act in the desired way but always give them the option of acting otherwise. Nudges typically involve policies that leverage the insights of behavioral economics—the mental shortcuts that underlie many decisions and actions. They usually do not involve subsidies (except perhaps nominal ones), regulations, or penalties.

Many nudges rearrange what Thaler and Sunstein call "choice architecture"—the way in which options are sequenced, labeled, and designed. The sequence by which people encounter various options and the way in which these options are presented can greatly influence which options are chosen.

The most basic element of choice architecture, the most fundamental nudge, concerns the "default" option. If people are given choices—whether or not to enroll in a retirement plan, and what kind of plan to choose; what type of health insurance policy to join—most will choose the default option, the one that requires the least effort to activate, and in many cases no effort at all. Therefore, a key question for public policy is what that default option should be. Should people be automatically enrolled in a retirement plan—or a retirement plan of a particular type—or should the default option be not to enroll? In other words, the default option can be to "opt in" and allow people to opt out if they choose, or it can be to "opt out" and give them the chance to opt in later if they prefer. Numerous studies have shown that people are more likely to choose to participate in a program or policy if that program or policy is the default option than if they must take the effort to sign up.

The strategic use of the default option takes advantage of status quo bias, one of the most persistent and fundamental features of thinking fast.

Governments around the world have recently incorporated behavioral economics into their policy making. In the United States, the Obama Administration appointed Sunstein, co-author of *Nudge*, to serve as the administrator of the White House Office of Information and Regulatory Affairs. In this capacity, he required federal agencies to apply the principles of behavioral sciences in the design of their policies (Halpern 2015; Sunstein 2014).

In the United Kingdom, the Conservative–Liberal Democratic Coalition Government of 2010–2015 established a Behavioral Insights Team to develop and assess government interventions premised on the behavioral sciences. Soon known as the "Nudge Unit," the team's remit was to "transform at least two areas of policy; spread understanding of behavioral approaches across Whitehall [the central government], and achieve at least a tenfold return on the cost of the unit" (Halpern 2015: 54). The Nudge Unit gave itself two years to achieve its objectives. By the end of this period the unit had launched and evaluated numerous policy changes and programs, which were shown to generate revenue and savings well in excess of ten times the cost of the unit. The unit's staffing grew steadily, and in 2014 it was spun off from the government into an independent organization that advises governments around the world.

David Halpern, the founding director of the Behavioral Insights Team, chronicles its approach and accomplishments in his book, *Inside the Nudge Unit* (Halpern 2015). In it, he presents a simple framework for applying behavioral principles into public policy:

- **E**asy
- **A**ttract
- **S**ocial
- **T**imely

Easy

"If you want to encourage something," writes Halpern, "make it easy." Eliminate as much "friction" as possible. Often, this means modifying the default option so that people need do nothing at all to achieve the desired result, or it means reducing the number of steps people must take. This can mean reducing the number and complexity of forms one must complete to apply for a program or pay a tax. For example, the Nudge Unit found that making a small change in a letter sent to taxpayers—including a direct link to a partially pre-filled tax form—increased the proportion of people completing their tax form by 22 percent (Halpern 2015: 74). In another example, Halpern discusses how the Nudge Unit encouraged homeowners to insulate their attics so as to conserve energy. They compared three approaches: a home insulation service at a low but standard cost; a home insulation service offered at a substantial discount if any neighbors also hired the service; and a home insulation service combined with an attic clearance service, at a significantly higher cost than insulation alone. The unit found that while the third option cost more to the homeowners than the other two, it generated three times more business than the basic offer. Moreover, homeowners were essentially no more likely to respond to the discount option than to the basic offer. Halpern concludes from this experiment that it was not the price of the insulation that was the barrier but rather the hassle of having to clear out one's attic in order to install it. At least in this context, subsidy was less effective as an incentive than a behavioral nudge.

Conversely, Halpern notes that sometimes policy objectives can be achieved by making actions or decisions less easy—that is, by increasing rather than reducing friction. For example, requiring customers to wait a day before using a credit card or other financial products can make them less likely to borrow beyond their means. Limiting the number of pills that pharmacists can dispense at once can reduce the incidence of overdoses. New York City's former mayor, Michael Bloomberg, in an initiative that was ultimately struck down by the courts, tried to address obesity by prohibiting the sale of soft drinks in cups of more than 16 ounces in restaurants, movie theaters, and other establishments. The law did not prevent people from consuming large quantities of soda, but it made it less easy to do so (Sunstein 2014).

Voting Case: "Easy" and Voting Rights

"Easy," the first element of the Nudge Unit's basic framework for incorporating behavioral principles into public policy, is vividly illustrated in current controversies around voting rights in the United States. On the one side, governments and advocacy organizations that wish to increase voter participation have promoted numerous ways to make it easier and more convenient to register to vote and to vote. On the other side, certain state and local governments (all Republican) and allied advocacy groups have sought to make voting more difficult. Put differently, one side has tried to reduce the "frictions" of the voting process, while the other side has sought to increase it (Rosenberg 2017). Some of the numerous ways that states can make voting easier (reduce the frictions) include the following:

- "Motor Voter" programs whereby citizens are automatically registered to vote when they obtain or renew driver's licenses or register their cars or who otherwise interact with government agencies. Eligible voters are automatically registered to vote unless they decline (i.e., the default option is to register).
- Same-day registration. People can register to vote on election day.
- Voter registration at birth (proposed but not enacted). All people born in the United States are registered automatically at birth, with the registration timed to go into effect at age 18.
- Automatically mail ballots to registered voters.
- Early voting. Registered voters are allowed to vote prior to election day at a time that is more convenient.
- Universal vote-by-mail, a strategy that was popularized and expanded, albeit temporarily in many places, during COVID-19 when voting in person posed health risks.
- Change election day to Saturday or Sunday (proposed) or make election days a holiday. If elections were held over a weekend or on a holiday instead of on a Tuesday or other workday, it would be easier for voters who work to find time to vote.

Governments and advocacy groups who wish to make voting more difficult—ostensibly to reduce voter fraud, but given the exceedingly low incidence of voter fraud, the actual reason is most likely to suppress voting among low-income and minority groups who are less likely to support Republican candidates (Astor 2018; Levitt 2007; Wines 2016)—do so in the following ways:

- Eliminating Motor Voter and other modes of automatic voter registration as well as same day registration.
- Requiring voters to provide specific types of government identification, such as driver's licenses and passports.
- Limiting excuses for absentee voting, reducing the number of drop-off boxes for absentee ballots, or requiring (multiple) notarized signatures on mail-in ballots.
- Reducing or eliminating early voting.
- Reducing the number of polling places so that long lines may form or that distance itself precludes access, discouraging people from voting.
- Banning drive-through voting and vote-by-mail.

Attract

Nudges can take advantage of the fact that "people are drawn to that which catches their attention and that which is attractive to them" (Halpern 2015: 149). This aspect of behavioral science is commonplace in the private sector (advertising) but much less prevalent in government. Halpern emphasizes two aspects of attraction: the need to make something stand out and to make it attractive or persuasive. For example, a personalized letter that includes the recipient's name will stand out more than a form letter addressed to "To Whom It May Concern." If the language is clear and direct and keeps boilerplate to a minimum, it may also stand out. In addition to the visual clarity, personalization, and other ways of "catching attention," interventions must also be attractive as well. People must assess them positively. Halpern provides various examples of how governments, or nonprofit organizations, can impart positive impressions. Appealing to emotions can be more effective than appealing to reason. The choice of "messenger" can also matter. Halpern writes:

> seeing a politician on the news suggesting your kids should be vaccinated may have little impact, but seeing the Chief Medical Officer, or a senior doctor, white coat and stethoscope around their neck, suggesting the same thing is much more likely to be acted on.
> (2015: 103)

If the intervention seems novel or fun, that too can make it more likely to succeed. Halpern found that initiatives that take the form of games (e.g., lotteries) can be especially appealing.[6]

Social

Tapping into social norms and networks can greatly influence behavior. Halpern provides several examples of how policy can incorporate various norms and other social dynamics. For instance, if people are informed that most of the population pays their taxes on time, they will be more likely to pay their taxes on time. In another example, Halpern discusses the Nudge Unit's efforts to increase charitable giving. The unit found that a personal email from a colleague, combined with his or her photograph, asking recipients to join them in deducting a portion of their monthly salary to charity produced significant increases in the number of people signing up to have funds deducted automatically from their paycheck to start payroll giving (Halpern 2015). These and similar approaches "triggered a sense of personal connection and reciprocity."

Timely

The final element of the Nudge Unit's framework takes into account several well-documented aspects of behavioral science that concern the inconsistent ways by which people value and perceive time. People tend to focus on the status quo and value the present over the future. As a result, it can be difficult for people to modify their behavior even if they know they would be better off in the future if they did so (e.g., exercising more, eating healthier foods, abstaining from smoking, saving money). Halpern discusses how nudges can take into account three distinct aspects of timing. The first aspect is that early interventions are usually more effective than actions taken later on when habits and behaviors are more entrenched. Second, even when habits are well established, there are certain moments—such as marriage, the birth of a child, the start of a new career, or the purchase of a new home in a new city—when people are particularly responsive to policy interventions. For example, Halpern points out that people who have recently moved to a new home are significantly more responsive than other people to campaigns to encourage people to reduce automobile usage:

> If you've just moved house, your journey to work habits have yet to fully form, and you will be much more open to the suggestion of an alternative option than if you have already been driving to work for the last five years.
>
> (2015: 134)

In another example, Halpern recounts how the Nudge Unit added a single line in the email instructions for people intended to take an online qualifying test to join the police. The Nudge Unit was asked to find ways to increase recruitment of ethnic and racial minorities into the police. One obstacle was that the pass rate for ethnic minorities on the exam was one-third lower than for white applicants. The team felt that one reason for the lower pass rate had to do with differences in expectations and motivations among the applicants. To test this possibility, they added a line to the email instructions for the test "asking applicants to reflect for a moment about why they want to join the police and why it mattered to the community." This sentence was placed just before the link to the online exam. The unit found that while the additional sentence had no effect on white applicants, it increased the pass rate for minority applicants from around 40 to 60 percent, "entirely eliminating the difference with whites" (Halpern 2015: 138). The timing of the prompt seemed to make a big difference. Halpern doubts that it would have produced results anywhere as large if it had been included in an email letter sent a week before the exam.

The third aspect of timing concerns what Halpern calls "time inconsistent preferences," or the tendency to prioritize the present. Halpern discusses how policy can help people resist temptations to indulge in the present by enabling them to "shape choices for their future selves" (2015: 141). For example, the Nudge Unit found that asking people to donate money to charity before they received the money was more effective than asking them to donate when they had the money in hand.

Limitations of Nudges

Not all problems are amenable to nudges. For the most part, they deal with issues of behavioral change at the individual level. The emphasis is on "changing behavior to benefit those who are nudged, not to reduce the harms that these behaviors may have on others" (Oliver 2017: 117). In keeping with the principles of "libertarian paternalism" expressed by Thaler and Sunstein, the basic idea is to steer people in the direction they would choose to go if they were to give the matter more thought and consideration, if they would think slow instead of fast. In some instances low-cost changes in the "choice architecture" can be more effective than major regulatory changes or large subsidies.

Nudges and other policies informed by behavioral science are probably less effective in dealing with large-scale, structural issues. Even Halpern, a leading proponent of nudges, recognizes that this approach is unlikely to "make more than a dent on carbon emissions" and climate change. Similarly, it's highly unlikely that nudges alone can be effective in addressing economic inequality or racial discrimination.[7]

The application of behavioral economics and "nudges" in public policy is not without controversy. Some scholars and policy analysts are concerned that behavioral approaches can enable governments to engage in manipulative and unethical practices. Robin Hambleton (2014), for example, objects to the idea that "it is acceptable, even essential, to try to change our behavior without us realizing that our behavior is being changed." Hambleton argues that "psychological tricks" by public servants or their policy advisers to manipulate behavior is inherently offensive. In addition, he believes that nudges and other applications of behavioral psychology "taint the honesty and integrity of government" and violate "basic notions of transparency" in public decision making.

Thaler, Sunstein, Halpern, and other behaviorally inclined policy analysts argue in turn that while their approach may be paternalistic (Thaler and Sunstein indeed call it "Libertarian Paternalism"), it is not coercive. Policies built on behavioral sciences may steer people to certain directions, but they do not force them to make such decisions. For example, "choice architects" may establish "default options" to encourage certain choices, but they also give people the option of making other choices. Moreover, it can be argued many programs and policies always involve some kind of default option, in which case the government is already encouraging some kind of decision or behavior—the question then becomes what kinds of decision or behavior should be encouraged.

Nudges can vary in their effectiveness in different national and cultural contexts. Different groups may be more responsive to nudges than others. For example, when British taxpayers received notices stating that the great majority of fellow taxpayers paid their taxes on time, a large proportion of the letter recipients paid their taxes, but when a similar letter was sent to US taxpayers, there was no subsequent increase in tax payments. Evidently, US taxpayers were swayed to a much smaller extent than their British counterparts by the prospect of violating social norms (Sunstein 2017). In general, Sunstein notes, automatic notifications and other reminders are effective in most countries, as are default rules. However, when "people begin with strong preferences, and don't like the direction in which they are being nudged, nudges are going to have a weaker effect" (Sunstein 2017).

Perhaps most fundamentally, some findings of behavioral economics have not been replicated outside of highly controlled settings. Critics have pointed out that some of the ideas of behavioral economics are based on experiments conducted among university students in which they were asked to assume certain roles. When the experiments were repeated in other, less controlled settings, the original findings were not consistently observed (Weatherby 2023). In applying behavioral economics in policy analysis, it is important to consider the extent to which the particular concepts have been validated.

Insights From the Field of Design

Designers offer several innovative ways of envisioning and developing policy alternatives. Some of the methods designers use to solve design challenges can be applied towards a wide variety of social, economic, and environmental issues. As discussed in Chapter 1, the notion of "design thinking" emerged in the 1990s and early 2000s to connote the broad applicability of design methodologies to subjects outside the conventional sphere of design. There is no single definition of design thinking, but most versions refer to similar means of "ideation"—the creation of design solutions, which can include policy alternatives. Design thinking is not the only term used to express these concepts and activities. Others include civic design, human-centered design, service design, and strategic design (Bason 2017: 5; Gordon and Mugar 2020; Trippe 2021).

Several elements stand out in the incipient literature on design and policy with respect to the creation and development of policy options. These include a need for "empathy," the "co-creation" of policy ideas with people directly affected by the policy or who would be involved in its implementation, and rapid prototyping and experimentation.

Empathy

Empathy refers to the ability to understand things from the perspective of others; to be able to put yourself in other people's shoes, to "enter into another person's feelings" (*Design Thinking for Public Service Excellence*, p. 8). In the context of policy analysis, empathy requires analysts to understand how the issue at stake impacts the people who are most closely affected. This kind of understanding usually involves sustained dialog with a variety of people who would be the focus of the policy. Other skills such as ethnography can also be vital in developing an empathetic understanding of the issue to be addressed (Bason 2014, 2017; IDEO.org 2015). Empathy is also essential for co-creation, the second key aspect of design-centered policy analysis.

Co-Creation

Co-creation refers to the collaboration of designers (or policy analysts) with a cross-section of individuals who are directly or indirectly affected by the policy issue and/or its potential solutions. The term refers to a broad array of ways by which designers may work with members of the public to discuss the nature of a particular issue and to explore alternative ways of addressing it. It can involve workshops and focus groups with various stakeholders or on-site visits to communities and organizations affected by the issue. Some designers have found that games, visualization tools, and simulations can be useful ways of generating new and innovative ideas for solving problems in collaboration with representatives of various groups (Bason 2017; Halse 2014).

Gordon and Mugar (2020), offer an alternative framework for the co-creation process, focusing on four key elements: "network building, holding space for discussion, distributing ownership, and persistent input."

- Network building refers to virtual or in-person convenings of various stakeholders "to explore critical issues and possible solutions. These discussions build "networks that further enable opportunities for sharing experiences and knowledge" (22).
- By holding space for discussion, Gordon and Mugger stress the need to provide ample time and opportunity for discussion, allowing for multiple perspectives, including dissent.
- Distributing ownership refers to the process by which stakeholders are given "clear pathways to participation" and given support and encouragement to devise policy solutions.
- Persistent input occurs when practitioners "not only ask people what they think, but they do so from a position of stability, continuity, and trust: asking once, and then being in the same place to ask again. This persistence is reflected in long term relationships between practitioners and the communities they work in" (22).

Prototyping

Prototyping and experimentation are integral to design, and to its applications for policy analysis. Prototyping refers to the development, testing, and refinement of possible solutions. A prototype is a preliminary model developed to test designs—or policies. After a prototype has been tried out for a period of time, designers can improve upon it in light of the knowledge and understanding gained from its implementation or discard it entirely and introduce new prototypes. The concept of prototype underscores the incremental character of policy analysis—and policy making. It is often better to experiment with a variety of approaches and tinker with them in response to experience rather than to think that one can produce the ultimate solution and presume that once created it will not require any modification.

The concept of prototype resembles that of a pilot project or program. At times, governments and nonprofit organizations launch small-scale and/or temporary initiatives to test and refine policies and programs. Such pilots may be followed by larger-scale and permanent interventions. However, if the pilot proves unsuccessful, its sponsor may decide against its continuation and pursue other options instead. The main distinction between prototypes and pilot programs is that whereas designers are inclined to prototype virtually all ideas before making a final decision and bringing them to scale, pilot programs are considered less often. While pilots can be indispensable for testing the value and effectiveness of new ideas—and the United Kingdom's Nudge Unit piloted nearly all of its interventions—sometimes policy analysts and their clients face immediate problems and do not have the time to devise and implement pilot programs and wait for the results. Furthermore, policy recommendations that do not involve pilots can almost always be improved upon during the course of implementation.

Summary

In this chapter we have considered a wide range of ways to identify and develop potential **policy options**. Some of these methods draw directly on precedents, on **current or past programs** or policies that address **similar** or **analogous issues**. Moreover, any one program or policy can be modified or reconfigured in almost limitless ways to address the problem at hand.

Policy analysis need not be bound to precedent in devising potential solutions. We have explored several methods by which analysts can formulate innovative options that may not have been tried before. These methods include the process of **brainstorming** and thinking about potential solutions in the absence of various constraints. Another approach is to consider how **generic powers of government** (e.g., regulation, taxation, subsidy) might be adapted. We have also discussed how principles from the **behavioral sciences** and from the field of **design** can be used to devise potential alternatives.

Ultimately, the analyst will want to consider a variety of options, options that would attack the problem through different means. Only a few alternatives will be put forth for detailed analysis, but in deciding which alternatives to consider, analysts will want to choose from a strong assortment of options. In reality, the client should be able to consider any option put forward; the analyst provides a strategy for comparing and ranking them. As noted at the start of the chapter, the final recommendation will be no better than the best of the alternatives that are put forth for analysis. If superior alternatives are "off the table," they cannot be recommended.

> **Child Support Debt Case: A Recap**
>
> In Chapter 2 we devised the *central problem statement*: *how can the government reduce the debt burden for noncustodial parents?*
> We also presented some background to the issue and data to *frame* its relevance and urgency:
>
> - Child support enforcement policy in the United States has often been extremely punitive towards noncustodial parents with low incomes, even as it has resulted in significant collections from better off noncustodial parents.
> - In 2016, the Obama Administration adopted the Flexibility, Efficiency, and Modernization in Child Support Programs Final Rule to address many of the inequities and hardships experienced by low-income noncustodial parents, including conditioning child support obligations on ability to pay (Office of Child Support Enforcement 2016, 2017a, 2017b). However, the rule does not address outstanding child support debt incurred by low-income parents.
> - States have the authority under federal law to adopt child support debt reduction ("compromise") policies. As of 2022, more than 9 million parents owe about $114 billion in accumulated child support arrears since the program's beginning. Of this amount, $19 billion is owed to states and other governmental jurisdictions, and $95 billion is owed to the custodial parents (Office of Child Support Enforcement 2023).

Child Support Debt Case: Alternative Policy Options

Federal law allows states to reduce the debt owed by noncustodial parents to the states for child support. States are not permitted to reduce the amount of child support owed to custodial parents without the custodial parent's consent. At least 36 states currently operate debt reduction ("compromise") programs on at least a pilot basis or settle arrearage on a case-by-case basis (Office of Child Support Enforcement 2022). A large proportion of these programs focus on cases in which the noncustodial parent has no current child support obligations (the children are grown) or when the debt is considered uncollectible.

States may have several objectives for their debt reduction programs. The two most basic goals are debt settlement and incentives to increase payment of current child support payments and reduce uncollectible debt. Settlement programs largely focus on reduction of uncollectible debt and decreasing the number of active cases with uncollectible debt (Ascend at the Aspen Institute & Good+Foundation 2020a; Bartfield 2003; Office of the Inspector General 2007).

Several states and other jurisdictions, however, have established programs that include parents with current child support obligations as well as those with no active cases. We based our alternative policy options for reducing child support debt on these existing programs, several of which are currently small in scale and/or pilots. In particular, we **adopted key aspects of their basic design**, including eligibility criteria, the timing and amount of debt reduction, requirements to receive debt reduction, and penalties for failing to satisfy them. In some cases, **we increased the scale** at which the programs operate.

Three alternatives involve "debt leveraging": in order to have their child support debt reduced, noncustodial parents must meet certain conditions and abide by a quid pro quo. For example, debt reduction may be conditional on regular payments of child support. A fourth alternative takes a different approach by writing off debt automatically and unconditionally when that debt was incurred when the noncustodial parent was incarcerated and was therefore unable to pay child support.

Participation Incentive Program

The Participation Incentive Program (PIP) is modeled closely after the state of Maryland's program of the same name. Created in 2008, PIP is open to noncustodial parents in arrears with current child support obligations as well as to those with no current obligations. The program forgives 50 percent of the arrears owed to the state after participants make 12 consecutive monthly payments of their child support and/or a portion of their child support arrearages. One hundred percent of the child support debt is forgiven after 24 months of consecutive payments. Participants are dropped from the program, and receive no debt reduction, if they fail to make three monthly child support payments during the two-year duration of the program.

Data are not available on the current size of the program. However, the Center for Policy Research found that 993 noncustodial parents had enrolled in the program by 2010 from the city of Baltimore, which accounts for most of the program's participants. More than 25 percent complied with their payment obligations and had $1.8 million of their debt forgiven. The program currently has two full-time staff dedicated to the program in Baltimore (Pearson et al. 2012). In the proposed alternative, total staffing would be increased to ten full-time positions.

Match Plus Outreach

Whereas the first alternative would forgive a set portion (50 percent or 100 percent) of a noncustodial parent's arrears after he or she satisfies their child support obligations over a specified period of time (12 to 24 months), Match Plus Outreach takes a different approach. For each dollar a participating noncustodial parent provides for child support, the state would reduce his or her child support debt by 50 cents. Unlike PIP, there is no penalty if the noncustodial parent misses any child support payments; in other words, debt reduction is not contingent on a series of regular child support payments. Instead, child support debt is reduced with each child support payment. If the parent fails to pay child support, his or her debt is not reduced, but he or she does not forfeit previous reductions.

Match Plus Outreach is modeled after Families Forward, a pilot demonstration program in Racine, Wisconsin, that started in 2005 and ran through 2008. The program was open to low-income noncustodial parents who were behind in their child support payments and owed at least $20,000 in child support debt. The program applied both to debt owed to the state and debt owed to custodial parents if the custodial parent provided consent. Participants who failed to make any payments during two consecutive quarters (six consecutive months) were removed from the program, and interest charges on their debt were reinstated (Heinrich et al. 2011: 4).

In total, 120 noncustodial parents participated in the program, about one-third of all eligible parents. About 75 percent of the participants had their state-owed debt reduced and 21 percent received debt forgiveness of debt owed to the custodial parent. Two participants received forgiveness of both state- and custodial-parent debt (Heinrich et al. 2011: 8). Two-thirds of the noncustodial parents in the program participated for 21 or more months (Heinrich et al. 2011: 13). An evaluation of the program found that compared to noncustodial parents with similar demographic and economic characteristics, participants made larger child support payments, were more likely to pay child support, and paid more frequently. They were also more likely to reduce their outstanding child support debt (Heinrich et al. 2011: 24).

While Match Plus Outreach emulates the basic approach taken by Families Forward in reducing child support debt in proportion to the noncustodial parent's child support payments, it does not replicate all aspects of this program. Whereas Families Forward required noncustodial parents to contact the custodial parent to ask if he or she was interested in participating in the program, Match Plus Outreach would employ staff to inform custodial parents about the program—this is the "outreach" component of the program. This feature follows suggestions made by Heinrich et al. in their evaluation of Families Forward. Focus groups with noncustodial and custodial parents revealed that it would be helpful to have a third party contact custodial parents and explain the program to them. Many noncustodial and custodial parents lack accurate contact information for the other parent, and many noncustodial parents had difficulty explaining the details of the program or were wary of asking the custodial parent to participate out of fear of escalating tensions between them (Heinrich et al. 2011: 26). Another key difference is that the scale of Match Plus Outreach would be larger. Whereas Families Forward was a pilot program that operated in a single county of Wisconsin, Match Plus Outreach would operate throughout the state.

Workforce Development

The previous two alternatives are premised on the assumption that an incentive to reduce child support debt will motivate noncustodial parents to meet their current child support obligations. PIP would forgive a portion of the parent's debt after he pays child support regularly over a specified period of time. MPO would reduce the debt in response to each child support payment. In other words, debt would be reduced after the noncustodial parent pays child support. Therefore, they assume that the parents can make the payments if given an appropriate incentive. The Workforce Development option does not make this assumption. This alternative would connect child support debt reduction to participation in a program designed to help participants find jobs that would enable them to pay for child support. This program would combine work preparedness, job training, and job placement and retention support with the aim of helping noncustodial parents obtain and keep jobs that would enable them to afford their child support obligations.

The Workforce Development alternative is modeled after two programs, Westchester County, New York's Responsible Employed Active Loving (R.E.A.L) Parenting Pilot for Stronger Families and the Center for Urban Families' (a nonprofit community-based organization) Baltimore Responsible Fatherhood Project.

R.E.A.L. is a small-scale pilot program started in 2016 by the Westchester County Department of Social Services. Limited to unemployed noncustodial fathers on public assistance with child support debt, the program requires participants to take 40 hours of classes over ten weeks on a range of topics, including work preparedness, career counseling, financial management, and parenting. On completion of the program, the county forgives 10 percent of the participants' debt. If they then find a job and retain it for 90 days, the county reduces the debt by an additional 25 percent. Finally, if participants pay child support in full and on time for 12 months, the county reduces the remaining debt to $500 (Wogan 2017).

Baltimore's Responsible Fatherhood Project, founded and administered by the Center for Urban Families, enables noncustodial parents to reduce their child support debt after completing a three-month program consisting of case management, support-service referrals, and educational workshops. The program engages cohorts of low-income fathers in workshops on employment readiness, parenting, co-parenting relationships, and related topics. The state of Maryland reduces the child support debt of participants who complete the program and obtain employment by up to 25 percent (Ludden 2015).

The Workforce Development alternative builds on R.E.A.L., the Responsible Fatherhood Program, and similar initiatives by combining employment readiness, job training, and case management to help low-income noncustodial parents secure living-wage jobs. The program would entail a ten-week workforce development course along with case management and job placement assistance. The state would forgive 25 percent of the participants' child support debt owed to the state on completion of the course. The state would forgive the remaining 75 percent of the debt if participants obtain and retain employment for six consecutive months.

Automatic Forgiveness of Arrears Due to Incarceration

Many noncustodial parents accrued child support debt while incarcerated. Nationally, 48 percent of men in federal and state prison have children under 18, and about 20 percent of them have child support orders (Haney 2022: 76). More broadly, counting people currently confined to prison, local jails, and those on probation or parole, roughly 50 percent of all fathers with child support orders "have some criminal justice background and roughly 20 percent of nonpaying, indebted parents were recently incarcerated" (Haney 2022: 76).

Although they had no way of earning income to pay child support, many did not have their child support orders modified to reflect the loss of income because of incarceration. As a result, parents who have been incarcerated accrue almost three times as much in arrears as those who were never in prison by the time their children are age 15 (Turetsky and Waller 2020: 125).

Until 2016, many states either regarded incarceration as "voluntary unemployment" and therefore ineligible for suspension or reduction of child support payments or deemed it a possible justification for modification, which required individual parents to request relief (Haney 2022;

Turetsky and Waller 2020). Even when parents had the right to have their child support orders reduced or suspended because of incarceration, many, as Turetsky and Waller (2020: 126) explain,

> do not understand the child support process or their rights to request review and adjustment of their child support orders and cannot easily contact the child support office. Because incarcerated parents are involuntarily confined, their access to the Internet or cell phones is often restricted due to security concerns. They may not have access to legal counsel or other community-based resources that could provide timely information. Consequently, their opportunity to seek information and request a review in time to prevent the accumulation of debts often is limited or nonexistent.

The Obama Administration's Final Rule of 2016 requires states to modify child support orders in the event of incarceration, which should reduce the accumulation of arrears. But, as noted, the rule does not affect arrears that had been incurred previously.

The Automatic Forgiveness of Arrears Due to Incarceration Alternative (AFAI) would eliminate all state-owed child support debt incurred by state residents while incarcerated in the state's prisons. The Departments of Social Services and Corrections would match their records to identify residents with child support debt who are currently or were formerly incarcerated in state prison. All child support obligations incurred while incarcerated would be forgiven. This would be an automatic procedure, requiring no action on the part of noncustodial parents. Several years ago, the state implemented a policy of automatically suspending child support orders for parents incarcerated for more than 60 days, but it did not modify the amount of debt that incarcerated parents had incurred previously. AFAI fills this gap. It is roughly analogous to student debt forgiveness programs that automatically write off college debt for people who meet certain criteria.

AFAI is modeled after several state programs that automatically suspend child support orders when non-custodial parents are incarcerated. For example, Oregon automatically suspends child support orders for people incarcerated for 180 days or more and for 120 days after release. The State's Child Support Program identifies parents with child support orders who are incarcerated through a "data match" with the Oregon Department of Corrections (Ascend at the Aspen Institute & Good+Foundation 2020b: 22). In addition to automatically suspending an incarcerated parent's child support obligations, the program also authorizes administrators or judges to "allow a credit and satisfaction against child support arrearages for each month that the obligor was incarcerated or that is within 120 days following the obligor's release from incarceration" (Ascend at the Aspen Institute & Good+Foundation 2020b: 22). Although we have not identified any jurisdictions that automatically reduce child support arrears incurred during incarceration, we are extrapolating from the current practice of some states to automatically suspend current child support orders during periods of incarceration (Ascend at the Aspen Institute & Good+Foundation 2020b; Turetsky & Waller 2020).

Box 3.4 Key Elements of Alternative Debt Reduction Options

Participation Incentive Program

Eligibility: all low-income noncustodial parents with child support debt.

Amount, timing, and type of debt reduction: 50 percent of outstanding debt is forgiven after 12 months of participation; 100 percent after 24 months; only state debt is reduced.

Participation requirements: consecutive monthly payments of child support.

Penalty for noncompliance: no debt reduction and removal from program if participants miss three monthly child support payments over the two-year duration of the program.

Match Plus Outreach

Eligibility: all low-income noncustodial parents with child support debt.

Amount, timing, and type of debt reduction: outstanding child support debt is reduced by 50 cents for every dollar paid in current child support; applies both to debt owed to the state and to custodial parent (with his or her consent).

Participant requirements: payment of child support.

> Penalty for noncompliance: no debt reduction if noncustodial parent misses monthly child support payments, but he or she can remain in the program, and previous debt reduction is not forfeited.
>
> **Workforce Development**
> Eligibility: all low-income noncustodial parents.
> Amount, timing, and type of debt reduction: 25 percent of outstanding debt is forgiven on satisfactory completion of ten-week workforce development course; remaining 75 percent is forgiven after retaining a full-time job for six consecutive months; only state debt is reduced.
> Participant requirements: successful completion of workforce development program, followed by full-time employment for a minimum of six consecutive months.
> Penalty for noncompliance: no debt reduction if requirements are not satisfied.
>
> **Automatic Forgiveness of Arrears Due to Incarceration**
> Eligibility: all low-income noncustodial parents who had incurred child-support debt while incarcerated in the state's prison system
> Amount, timing, and type of debt reduction: 100 percent of debt owed to the state incurred while incarcerated would be forgiven.
> Participant requirements: None
> Penalty for noncompliance: None (no compliance requirements)

Notes

1 Internal Revenue Service, "Estate Tax". 2024. www.irs.gov/businesses/small-businesses-self-employed/estate-tax and Joint Committee on Taxation. *History, Present Law, and Analysis of the Federal Wealth Transfer System*. Report Prepared for a Public Hearing of the Subcommittee on Select Revenue Measures of the House Committee of Ways and Means. March 8, 2015. www.jct.gov/publications.html?func=startdown&id=4744
2 See Schuetz et al. 2009; Wang and Balachandran 2023 for overviews of inclusionary zoning.
3 See Bardach and Patashnik (2015) Appendix B for a useful listing of "things governments do."
4 In its tax cut legislation of 2017, Congress repealed the ACA's mandate that all individuals and families have health insurance. Starting in 2019, people will be able to forego health insurance without penalty (Radnofsky 2018).
5 The literature on behavioral economics and its applications for public policy is large and growing fast. For more background on the subject, and examples of behavioral

approaches to public policy, see Kahneman 2011; Thaler and Sunstein 2008; Sunstein 2014; Halpern 2015; Oliver 2017; Thaler 2015; Lewis 2016, who provide accessible accounts of the development of the field. *Behavioral Science and Policy*, a peer-reviewed international journal, frequently includes articles on behavioral approaches to public policy.

6   See Rosenberg (2016) for examples of lotteries as tools for achieving public policy objectives.

7   Halpern discusses several innovative ways by which behavioral sciences have been effectively applied towards poverty reduction.

References

Ascend at the Aspen Institute & Good+Foundation. 2020a. "Implementing Sensible Debt Reduction Strategies." *Child Support Policy Fact Sheet*. https://ascend-resources.aspeninstitute.org/wp-content/uploads/2020/08/2_ChildSupport_Reducing_Arrears.pdf

Ascend at the Aspen Institute & Good+Foundation. 2020b. "Setting Realistic and Accurate Child Support Orders." *Child Support Fact Sheet*. https://ascend.aspeninstitute.org/wp-content/uploads/2023/11/3_ChildSupport_Right_Sizing_Orders.pdf

Astor, Maggie. 2018. "Seven Ways Alabama has Made It More Difficult to Vote." *New York Times* (June 23).

Ballis, Rochelle. 2014. "Brainstorming Doesn't Work—Do This Instead." *Forbes* (October 8). www.forbes.com/sites/rochellebailis/2014/10/08/brainstorming-doesnt-work-do-this-instead/#44deea7f6522

Bardach, Eugene, and Eric M. Patashnik. 2015. *A Practical Guide for Policy Analysis* (5th Edition). Los Angeles, CA: Sage Publications.

Bartfield, Judi. 2003. *Forgiveness of State-Owed Child Support Arrears*. Madison, WI: Report Submitted to Wisconsin Department of Workforce Development by the Institute for Research on Poverty, University of Wisconsin. www.irp.wisc.edu/publications/sr/pdfs/sr84.pdf

Bason, Christian (ed.). 2014. *Design for Policy*. New York: Routledge.

Bason, Christian. 2017. *Leading Public Design: Discovering Human-Centred Governance*. Bristol (UK): Policy Press.

Brito, Tonya L. 2012. "Fathers Behind Bars: Rethinking Child Support Policy toward Low-Income Fathers and Their Families." *The Journal of Gender, Race, and Justice* (Spring): 617–672.

The Commonwealth Fund. 2018. *The US Health Care System*. http://international.commonwealthfund.org/countries/united_states/

Gordon, Eric, and Gabriel Mugar. 2020. *Meaningful Inefficiencies: Civic Design in an Age of Digital Expediency*. New York: Oxford University Press.

Halpern, David. 2015. *Inside the Nudge Unit*. London: WH Allen.

Halse, Joachim. 2014. *Tools for Ideation: Evocative Visualizaiton and Playful Modeling as Drivers of the Policy Process*. C. Bason (ed.). New York: Routledge.

Hambleton, Robin. 2014. *Leading the Inclusive City*. Bristol, UK: Policy Press.

Hammond, John. S., Ralph L. Keeney, and Howard Raiffa. 1999. *Smart Choices: A Practical Guide to Making Better Decisions*. Boston, MA: Harvard Business School Press.

Haney, Lynn. 2022. *Prisons of Debt: The Afterlives of Incarcerated Fathers*. Berkeley, CA: University of California Press.

Heinrich, Carolyn, Brett Burkhardt, Hilary Shager, and Lara Rosen. 2011. *The Families Forward Program: Final Evaluation Report*. Madison, WI: Institute for Research on Poverty, University of Wisconsin-Madison. Report Prepared for Wisconsin Department of Workforce Development (January).

Henry, J. Kaiser Foundation. 2018. *Summary of the Affordable Care Act*. www.kff.org/health-reform/fact-sheet/summary-of-the-affordable-care-act/

Ideo.org. 2015. *The Field Guide to Human Centered Design*. San Francisco: Author.

Jenkins-Smith, H.C. 1982. "Professional Roles for Policy Analysts: A Critical Assessment." *Journal of Policy Analysis and Management 2, 1*: 88–100.

Kahneman, Daniel. 2011. *Thinking Fast and Slow*. New York: Farrar Straus and Giroux.

Levitt, Justin. 2007. *The Truth About Voter Fraud*. New York: Brennan Center for Justice. www.brennancenter.org/sites/default/files/legacy/The%20Truth%20About%20Voter%20Fraud.pdf

Lewis, Michael. 2016. *The Undoing Project*. New York: W. W. Norton.

Lindblom, Charles. 1959. "The Science of Muddling Through." *Public Administration Review 19, 2*: 79–88.

Ludden, Jennifer. 2015. "Some States are Cutting Poor Dads a Deal on Unpaid Child Support." *Morning Edition, NPR* (November 20). www.npr.org/2015/11/20/456353691/some-states-are-cutting-poor-dads-a-deal-on-unpaid-child-support

Office of Child Support Enforcement. 2016. "Flexibility, Efficiency, and Modernization in Child Support Enforcement Programs." *Final Rule. Federal Register 81, 244*: 93492–93569.

Office of Child Support Enforcement. 2017a. *Final Rule Resources: Flexibility, Efficiency, and Modernization in Child Support Programs Final Rule*. www.acf.hhs.gov/css/resource/final-rule-resources

Office of Child Support Enforcement. 2017b. *Overview—Final Rule 2016 Flexibility, Efficiency, and Modernization in Child Support Programs Final Rule*. www.acf.hhs.gov/sites/default/files/programs/css/overview_child_support_final_rule.pdf

Office of Child Support Enforcement. 2022. "Family and State Benefits of Debt Compromise Program." *Information Memorandum. IM-22-03* (August). www.acf.hhs.gov/css/policy-guidance/family-and-state-benefits-debt-compromise

Office of Child Support Enforcement. 2023. *Preliminary Report FY2022*. Washington, DC: Author. www.acf.hhs.gov/sites/default/files/documents/ocse/fy_2022_preliminary_report.pdf

Office of the Inspector General. 2007. *State Use of Debt Compromise to Reduce Child Support Arrearages*. Washington, DC: US Department of Health and Human Services. OEI-06–06–00070 (October). https://oig.hhs.gov/oei/reports/oei-06-06-00070.pdf

Oliver, Adam. 2017. *The Origins of Behavioural Public Policy*. Cambridge: Cambridge University Press.

Patton, Carl V., David S. Sawicki, and Jennifer J. Clark. 2013. *Basic Methods of Policy Analysis and Planning* (3rd Edition). Boston, MA: Pearson.

Pearson, Jessica, Nancy Thoennes, and Rasa Kaunelis. 2012. *Debt Compromise Programs: Program Design and Child Support Outcomes in Five Locations*. Report Submitted by Center for Policy Research to US Department of Health and Human Services, Administration for Children and Families, Office of Child Support

Enforcement (September). www.ywcss.com/sites/default/files/pdf-resource/debt_compromise_improving_child_support_outcomes_final_report_nov_14_2012.pdf

Plumer, Brad, and Nadja Popovich. 2017. "19 Countries Vowed to Phase Out Coal. But They Don't Use Much Coal." *New York Times* (November 16). www.nytimes.com/interactive/2017/11/16/climate/alliance-phase-out-coal.html

Radnofsky, Louise. 2018. "The New Tax Law: The Individual Health-Insurance Mandate." *Wall Street Journal* (February 13). www.wsj.com/articles/the-new-tax-law-the-individual-health-insurance-mandate-1518541795

Rosenberg, Tina. 2016. "For Better Scratch and Win." *New York Times* (October 11).

Rosenberg, Tina. 2017. "Increasing Voter Turnout for 2018 and Beyond." *New York Times* (June 13).

Schuetz, J., R. Meltzer, and V. Been. 2009. "31 Flavors of Inclusionary Zoning: Comparing Policies From San Francisco, Washington, DC, and Suburban Boston." *Journal of the American Planning Association* 75, 4: 441–456.

Starr, Paul 2018. "A New Strategy for Health Care." *The American Prospect* (January 4). http://prospect.org/article/new-strategy-health-care

Stone, Deborah. 2012. *Policy Paradox: The Art of Political Decision Making* (3rd Edition). New York: W. W. Norton.

Sunstein, Cass R. 2014. *Why Nudge? The Politics of Libertarian Paternalism*. New Haven: Yale University Press.

Sunstein, Cass R. 2017. "Some Countries Like 'Nudges' More than Others." *Bloomberg View* (July 19). www.bloomberg.com/view/articles/2017-07-19/some-countries-like-nudges-more-than-others

Thaler, Richard H. 2015. *Misbehaving: The Making of Behavioral Economics*. New York: W. W. Norton.

Thaler, Richard H., and Cass R. Sunstein. 2008. *Nudge: Improving Decisions About Health, Wealth, and Happiness*. New Haven: Yale University Press.

Trippe, Helena Polata. 2021. "Policy Instrumentation: The Object of Service Design in Policy Making." *Design/Issues 37*, 3: 89–100.

Turetsky, Vicki, and Maureen R. Waller. 2020. "Piling on Debt: The Intersections Between Child Support Arrears and Legal Financial Obligations." *UCLA Criminal Justice Law Review 4*, 1: 117–141.

Wang, R., and S. Balachandran. 2023. "Inclusionary Housing in the United States: Dynamics of Local Policy and Outcomes in Diverse Markets." *Housing Studies 38*, 6: 1068–1087.

WaverlyConsultants. 2017. *The Futures Toolkit: Tools for Futures Thinking and Foresight Across UK Government*. Report Prepared for the UK Government Office of Science. https://assets.publishing.service.gov.uk/government/uploads/system/uploads/attachment_data/file/674209/futures-toolkit-edition-1.pdf

Weatherby, Leif. 2023. "A Few of the Ideas About How to Fix Human Behavior Rest on Some Pretty Shaky Science." *New York Times* (November 30). www.nytimes.com/2023/11/30/opinion/human-behavior-nudge.html

Wines, Michael. 2016. "Some Republicans Acknowledge Leveraging Voter ID Laws for Political Gain." *New York Times* (September 16). www.nytimes.com/2016/09/17/us/some-republicans-acknowledge-leveraging-voter-id-laws-for-political-gain.html

Wogan, J.B. 2017. "A New Strategy for Collecting Child Support: Debt Forgiveness." *Governing* (June 27). www.governing.com/topics/health-human-services/gov-child-support-westchester-new-york-debt-foregiveness.html

4
Objectives and Criteria

Ultimately, the goal of any policy analysis is to present viable solutions for the stated problem. Sometimes the analyst can identify a single alternative to recommend, but it is also common for the analyst to present a narrowed list of several options. In either scenario, the options need to be ranked in some way; indeed, anyone can pull together a list of policies, but it is the analyst's job to do so in an informative and organized way. Most of the time, the potential strategies for addressing a problem are myriad and the analyst is faced with the task of narrowing them down to a manageable few or a preferred one. In this chapter we discuss how to do this in a logical and transparent manner by employing evaluative *criteria*.

What Are Criteria?

Before getting into the details of criteria, we need to discuss *objectives* and goals more broadly. Policy analysis is conducted to solve or mitigate an identified problem, but it is also done in pursuit of other broad goals, or *objectives*. Again, the child support case is a good example of how policy goals are wide ranging and shifting over time. Enforcement policies have been framed as critical in preventing child and family poverty and as important for maintaining the traditional nuclear family structure. They have also been framed as punitive and a means of securing economic reimbursement to the government for welfare money distributed to single-parent families in need. More recently, objectives have centered around minimizing the racial and economic inequities in how enforcement policies are designed and implemented. It is no surprise that these distinct framings led to very different policy approaches. Objectives represent the broader goals to be achieved in addressing the problem; they are the moral, ideological, and political touchstones for the project writ large. Methodologically, objectives provide a useful point of reference for the analyst as the possible solutions multiply. Politically, the stated objectives signal to the audience the moral framing of the analysis and the final policy recommendation(s).

Criteria are derivatives of the objectives and take on more concrete and measurable forms. A single objective can encompass one or several criteria. There is an important hierarchy to objectives and criteria: broader objectives and goals should first be identified before drilling down to more specific evaluative criteria. Criteria are also known as "impact categories" (Weimer and Vining 2011), as they capture the degree to which projected outcomes, or impacts, are likely to be achieved in each of the proposed alternatives. Criteria are the evaluative core of policy analysis; the analyst uses them to differentiate among the alternatives in terms of how well they will achieve the policy goals and objectives established at the onset of the project. Criteria will be used to determine which options are ranked higher and which one, if any, is dominant or more desirable. The number of criteria is not infinite, and they need to be carefully chosen to cover the right substance and range of priorities. If the criteria are poorly constructed and inconsistent in any way, the integrity of the analysis is vulnerable.

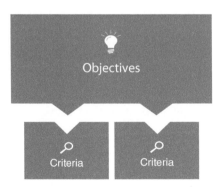

Figure 4.1 Objectives and criteria

Let's consider the differences between objectives and criteria in the context of the child support enforcement (CSE) case. The broader objective of CSE policies could be described as "reducing childhood poverty." CSE policies, in their different forms, aim to achieve this goal, but it is not their only purpose, nor is CSE the only way to reduce childhood poverty. A criterion will help the analyst assess whether or not a policy option, in the area of CSE, achieves an outcome that gets the client closer to the broader goal of poverty reduction. For example, an evaluative criterion would be *maximizing the family's receipt of child support payments from the noncustodial parent*. This criterion focuses on a measurable outcome that would demonstrate or likely lead to poverty reduction among children and their families. More contemporary objectives prioritize the "well-being of the noncustodial parent." Within this framing, an evaluative criterion would be *minimizing contact with the criminal justice system for the noncustodial parent*.

Finally, analyses may be motivated by several objectives, which could inform separate criteria. For example, the analysis could entail evaluative criteria that aim to *maximize child support payments* and *minimize contact with the criminal justice system*.

Where Do Criteria Come From?

Like defining the central problem, establishing criteria takes research and considerable tweaking to get the substance and range "just right." In addition, like the problem statement, criteria are not objectively construed. They are often imbued with normative assumptions and perspectives about what is considered "effective" or "good." Deborah Stone (2012) notably observed that even something as technical as efficiency can be subjective since it essentially "helps us attain more of the things we value," which change depending on one's point of view (p. 61). Stone argues that seemingly benign goals like equity and security can become fundamentally political and subjective. Giandomenico Majone (1988) promotes policy analysis as public deliberation, and criteria help to characterize the nature of one's argument:

> In policy analysis, as in science and in everyday reasoning, few arguments are purely rational or purely persuasive. The practical

> question, therefore, is not whether to use persuasion, but which form of persuasion to use and when.
>
> (p. 176)

Therefore, it is very challenging to establish clear and consistent evaluative standards, a reality that is not accurately reflected in the traditional rational model where criteria are assumed to be non-controversial.

However, the analyst should not aspire to rid the analysis of any subjectivity, but rather to be cognizant of it and incorporate it into the decision-making process. The formulation of criteria can come from three main sources: (i) the broader political and social context, (ii) the client, and (iii) the interests of other relevant stakeholders.

The political and social context can be considered globally or very locally. For example, criteria can be informed by broader political conversations or more general ethical ideals, such as gun violence or the "right" to health care. They can also be inspired by something as local as an organization's mission. Indeed, often equity-oriented objectives are made mainstream by the efforts of advocacy and civil rights organizations that frame issues through social justice lenses. We observe this in the child support case, as well as countless other policy areas, like voting rights and gay marriage.

Box 4.1 Getting Client Input on Objectives and Criteria

1 What is the mission of your organization or agency?
2 Why are you interested in addressing this particular problem?
3 Are there any aspects of the problem that you do not think you can reasonably address? Why?
4 What outcomes do you value? How do you describe "success" in addressing the problem?
5 Which stakeholders do you think are influential or central to the problem?
6 Is cost a contributing factor? A determining factor?

The client can play a particularly important role in constructing the criteria. One of the great challenges faced by the analyst is balancing the methodological integrity of the analysis with the client's needs (this tension will be discussed in more detail in Chapter 8). The criteria are the most obvious place where this happens. The client will have goals for the project and also particular perspectives on the issue. The client also typically possesses valuable knowledge of the issue and the stakeholders. All of this input from the client should be solicited and processed by the analyst. Questions about how the client views the goals of the project and the client's role in achieving those goals should be posed from the analyst's very first encounter. See Box 4.1 for some suggestions on how to gather input from the client on objectives and criteria.

We recommend incorporating initial and ongoing meetings with the client over the course of the project to regularly raise these questions and consult about the progress of the analytics.

See Figure 4.2 for a sample schedule.

The client's input, however, needs to be put into context and compared against other perspectives. Here is where research on and information gathering from other relevant stakeholders matter. See Figure 4.2 for a sample stakeholder chart.

Reaching out to stakeholders other than the client also helps in constructing the comprehensive range of interests that should be reflected in the criteria. Design thinking provides some useful parallels here. "Empathy," or the person-centered approach of design thinking, emphasizes a similar notion (see our discussion of design-based approaches in Chapters 1 and 3). Policies should be "designed with people and not only for them" (Allio 2014: 8), implying that the success of an option depends on how well it meets the needs and circumstances of the individuals that will use or engage with it. Criteria are in many ways the manifestation of this "design thinking" principle in policy analysis. Therefore, talking to, or researching about, the people and organizations that interact with the problem are good strategies to inform criteria.

Undoubtedly, any issue has many stakeholders. *How wide a net to cast?* The list of relevant stakeholders should be inclusive, but also informative. In an ideal world, the analyst would survey the universe of stakeholders—but in reality resources and time are limited. Instead of simply listing names and organizations, also include a brief summary of their interests in the issue, or, specifically, what each stakeholder actually has "at stake" with respect to the central problem. Which

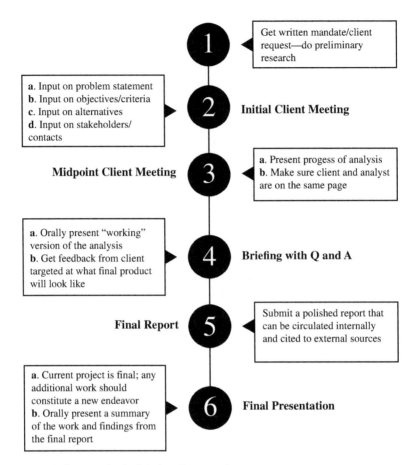

Figure 4.2 Suggested schedule for client meetings

players will be central to promoting or implementing potential policy options? Which stakeholders will be most affected by the outcomes of potential policy options? If there are stakeholders who are related, but peripheral, to the central problem, then they are not priorities for including in the criteria.

When considering the child support case, the stakeholders are varied with respect to their centrality and their power (see Figure 4.3). For example, the states, writ large, are central and influential in how policies are designed and implemented. If the analyst were examining the

Noncustodial Parents	Employers of Noncustodial Parents	Policy and Advocacy Research Organizations
Responsible for the child support obligation; financial burden is wholly on them, whether or not they can afford it; a group that is not organized and without much political voice collectively; those with meager resources are particularly vulnerable (financially, criminally, socially).	This group has been made central to the administration of CSE policies through the heavy reliance on wage garnishment; they can potentially lose their workforce if child support collection results in unpaid debt and, worst case, incarceration.	These organizations do research on and disseminate information about CSE policies and how they particularly affect families and noncustodial parents; many of these organizations have been active in raising awareness of how CSE policies disproportionately disfavor poorer men of color.

State Agencies		Children
State agencies are responsible for administering and overseeing child support policies and enforcement; therefore they have great interest in the operational and feasibility aspects of any policy or reform.	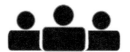	No political voice, but the most vulnerable; a lot at risk for this group (financial and social repercussions can have lasting effects).

Custodial Parents	Courts	Nonprofits Contracted out to Administer Family Interventions
Major financial stake, as their well-being (and that of their family) could depend on the child support; not well-organized either, but perhaps viewed with more sympathy than noncustodial parents (by the public).	These institutions (and the judges in particular) exercise a great deal of discretion with how CSE cases are treated; processes and culture can be notoriously ingrained at this level, but can be influenced by higher-level policy directives.	Contracted out to administer family interventions: these organizations have, perhaps, the most direct contact with the families; they provide insight on family-social implications of CSE interventions, but also are largely following directives of state and local agencies.

Figure 4.3 Sample stakeholder chart

issue for a particular state, it would make sense to identify players at the state level that have interests for or against particular policy approaches. Obviously, the noncustodial parents are key stakeholders with perhaps the most at stake: financial security, contact with the criminal justice system, and ties with their children and other family members, to name a few. These players, however, possess the least power in these situations. They are also the individuals who stand to interact most directly with the proposed policies, and therefore understanding the nature and reasons for their behavior is critical to constructing effective policy options. The centrality of their role is also compromised by their lack of availability. Where state actors can be tracked down and their decisions and actions documented, noncustodial parents can be hard to contact (because of privacy issues or logistical ones). The analyst needs to then consider surrogates who can represent their interests in formulating criteria. Community organizations or government agencies who work with these hard-to-reach populations are often informative substitutes.

The analyst now faces an important decision: **who has standing in the current analysis?** Whose interests are going to be included in the formulation of the evaluative criteria? Unfortunately, we cannot offer definitive answers to these questions; they depend on the particulars of the project, the client and the analyst. However, we can offer up two guiding principles. First, whatever decision is made, be sure that it is transparent and backed up by evidence and logic. The justification often comes out of interactions with the client and thorough research on how the range of stakeholders relate to the central problem. Second, understand how the omission of a particular dimension affects the outcome of the analysis. That is, by not considering a particular perspective or variable, how might the outcome of your analysis be biased?

For example, does the federal government have standing in an analysis that pertains to state-level policy? One could argue that the rules and regulations set forth by the federal government are more constraints or parameters for the design of possible policy options rather than interests at stake. Or put another way: all of the policy options should abide by federal regulations in order to make them minimally feasible. Therefore, the federal government's influence in the analysis becomes insignificant: it will not inform how policy options vary (and what the merits or drawbacks of those variations would be). In contrast, it would be problematic to not grant standing to the noncustodial parents, as their interaction with each policy option will undoubtedly vary and their omission could lead to inaccurately preferring one option over another.

Constructing Effective Criteria and Measures

The criteria should achieve two things: (i) **comprehensiveness** and (ii) **mutual exclusiveness**.

Comprehensiveness

We emphasized that one of the first, important steps in building criteria is assessing the universe of stakeholders; the criteria need to address this range of interests. Criteria are designed to highlight the trade-offs across options, and therefore they should capture the tension between strengths and weaknesses. It is unlikely that all interests align around a single solution, and the criteria should reflect a comprehensive picture of the pros and cons. Let's consider an issue increasingly relevant for cities all over the world: the safety of pedestrians. The attention around this issue has intensified as pedestrian deaths have reportedly reached a 40-year high (Kim 2023). The rise in pedestrian deaths has been attributed to street infrastructure and planning that creates unsafe walking environments, increasingly reckless driving, and also the growing size and weight of the vehicles themselves (Bouie 2023). Therefore, making streets safer for pedestrians requires both behavioral interventions for the drivers as well as changes to the infrastructure of the roads, or "traffic calming" measures, and the build or type of vehicle. When assessing policy options to promote pedestrian safety, a comprehensive set of criteria might look something like this:

1 Maximize pedestrian safety.
2 Minimize the harm for disadvantaged communities.
3 Minimize the burden of implementation.

The first criterion assesses the effectiveness of the policy and whether or not pedestrians are protected. The second criterion takes the distribution of impacts into account, recognizing that pedestrian deaths have disproportionately affected older adults and lower-income communities (Smart Growth America 2022; Bouie 2023). And, the last criterion considers the costs and complexities of implementation, likely for the government. The criteria address the spectrum of interests, and any tensions between them (for example, between pedestrian safety and the burden of ensuring compliance among drivers).

Mutual Exclusiveness

Criteria should also be mutually exclusive, or nonredundant. This feature is central to the methodological integrity of the analysis. It not only ensures maximum coverage of all the relevant interests, but also avoids bias in the ranking of the policy options. A good illustration of this is the overlap between two criteria for evaluating pedestrian safety:

1. Minimize the number of pedestrian deaths.
2. Maximize the safety of the walking environments.

The first criterion, focused on minimizing the number of pedestrian deaths, could be a function of the second criterion: that is, the likelihood of pedestrian harm is a function of how safe the walking options are. If an analyst were to include both criteria, the degree of pedestrian safety would be "counted" twice—once while evaluating the policy option's success in minimizing deaths and again while evaluating the option's success in maximizing the safety of the walking environment.

Deciding on a Set of Criteria

So, how can the analyst collapse all of the surveyed interests and objectives into three to five criteria? Let's consider three sample criteria for assessing policy options to promote pedestrian safety, in the context of pedestrian deaths as the safety outcome of interest:

1. Minimize the number of pedestrian deaths.
2. Minimize the risks for pedestrians on the street.
3. Maximize the safety of the walking environments.

All of these criteria assess the potential for improving pedestrian safety. The first criterion evaluates the degree to which the options curb the most extreme and observable outcome of unsafe pedestrian environments, deaths. The second criterion, however, evaluates the degree to which pedestrians are at risk (of any harm). Note that this is different than tracking the actual deaths or harm-related outcomes from proposed options. While policies could make streets and communities more or less risky for walking, they may or may not lead to fewer pedestrian deaths (if, for example, cars are getting bigger and more deadly at the same time). There also may be undesirable outcomes other than death that matter in evaluating the policies. The third criterion evaluates the general opportunity for safe walking environments. Should the analyst include all of these criteria? Are there opportunities to combine them or eliminate any?

Combining Several Criteria Into a Single Criterion

The last two criteria could be combined into a single standard that assesses to what degree the alternative minimizes the likelihood of pedestrian harm. It is useful to think about the risk to pedestrians, as it can be specified in terms of direction (e.g., it can get higher or lower) and magnitude (e.g., it can be big or small, inconsistent or pervasive). The part of the criterion that refers to the safety of the environment provides a concrete way to measure that risk. For example, there are documented features of streets and types of technologies and penalties that can affect the likelihood of pedestrian accidents. This new criterion is more comprehensive in that it provides a broad-based way to think about pedestrian safety, risk, and it provides a transparent and consistent way to determine the degree of risk for each option.

Eliminating Criteria From the Final Analysis

The analyst may also need to cut some criteria from the initial list. There are typically two reasons to eliminate a criterion from the final analysis.

First, the criterion may be **low in the order of priority** from the client's perspective. Perhaps it is a feature that is entirely outside the purview of the client or that ultimately will not have consequential impacts on the ability to move the proposed option forward. For example, prioritizing cars' ability to navigate the streets may not be viewed as important or it could be a political non-starter given recent pedestrian accidents.

A second, and common, reason is that the criterion, while important, actually **does not vary across the proposed policy options**. What this means is that when the criterion is used to differentiate the options (i.e., to help rank the options from most preferred to least preferred), it does not provide any useful information and all of the options fare about the same along the criterion's evaluative dimension. This is something that the analyst may not know until the analysis is under way (which we discuss in Chapter 6). For example, if all of the options have the same predicted effect on pedestrian deaths, then the first criterion doesn't vary. Therefore, as an evaluative criterion, it does nothing to help rank the options and can be dropped.

> **Box 4.2 Instead of Dropping a Criterion, Use a Proxy**
>
> An alternative to eliminating criteria is to instead develop proxies, which indirectly measure the outcomes of interest. For example, we could proxy for pedestrian deaths by assessing the factors that likely lead to deadly accidents (like street designs and regulations that affect pedestrian safety). There is enough research on the factors that increase the likelihood of fatalities that connecting the dots between street environments and outcomes would be credible and evidence-based. While proxies are imperfect, sometimes it is better to use them than to eliminate the criterion entirely. As we discussed in Chapter 1, analysts are working with limited information and other resource and time constraints. Rather than aiming for perfection, the analyst is working towards a defensible approximation of an ideal metric.

Using Generic Criteria as a Guideline

One useful strategy in deciding on the final set of evaluative criteria is to consult a list of general assessment standards. We propose five here:

1. Effectiveness
2. Equity (fairness)
3. Feasibility (administrative, political, and technical)
4. Cost (or financial feasibility)
5. Efficiency

Intended as points of entry for the analyst, these categories are not always mutually exclusive and need not be included in every analysis. Analyses can also include multiple criteria within each of these broader dimensions. They are suggestions for organizing the criteria and managing a comprehensive approach. Criteria should be tailored to the specific project at hand; indeed, no two analyses will have the same set of criteria. For purposes of illustration, we will return to the central problem in the child enforcement case: *how can the government reduce the debt burden for noncustodial parents?*

Effectiveness

Effectiveness is perhaps the most important category of criteria, as it evaluates how well each policy option addresses the central problem. Indeed, every analysis should have at least one criterion that captures the effectiveness of proposed alternatives. If we were to consider the central problem as *how can the government reduce the debt burden for noncustodial parents?*, then an effectiveness criterion would assess how well the options minimize or mitigate debt burdens. It should always answer the question of whether or not the proposed policy option "worked." There may be several dimensions of effectiveness, as a policy could aim to fix or improve upon multiple outcomes; all of these should be considered under the broader category of effectiveness. For example, consider two effectiveness criteria for the problem related to debt:

1. Maximize the number of noncustodial parents eligible for debt reduction.
2. Maximize the amount of debt reduction.
   - Maximize the amount of uncollectible state debt reduction[1]
   - The possibility of custodial parent debt reduction

The first criterion captures the breadth of the proposed policy's coverage, or how many noncustodial parents could potentially be affected. The second criterion captures the depth of coverage, or how much of the debt would be reduced. In addition, the second criterion differentiates between two types of debt (which are generally treated differently with respect to forgiveness; see the case description in Chapter 2 for more details). In order to motivate the effectiveness criterion, the analyst often has to do considerable research on what is considered an improvement with respect to the central problem. We will discuss strategies for researching conceptions of and metrics for effectiveness in Chapter 7.

Equity (Fairness)

The criteria in this category are often where moral or social justice obligations are met, and where the distributive burden (or benefit) from options is addressed. Equity is about "who gets what, when, and how" (Stone 2012). Achieving equity is often an important motivation for public intervention in private markets. In some cases, equity is part of the problem statement itself. However, even if equity or fairness is not explicitly stated in the central problem, we strongly encourage analysts to include it in their evaluative arsenal. This dimension is a useful counterpoint to the typical efficiency-based standards and provides both the analyst and the client with a more complete set of trade-offs.

Equity is a broad concept and can be addressed in many different ways. It usually concerns how benefits and costs from a particular policy are concentrated. Who bears the costs or reaps the benefits? Are they concentrated among those who are already disproportionately burdened or well-off? Notions of equity can be differentiated in three ways:

- Vertical versus horizontal equity: vertical equity assumes that those with more should bear a burden proportional to their position. For example, those with more income should pay higher taxes. Horizontal equity, on the other hand, assumes that everyone in similar circumstances should be treated alike, or "the equal treatment of equals" (Patton and Sawicki 1993). For example, all individuals with the same income should be subject to the same income tax rate regardless of their marital status.
- Equitable process versus equitable outcome: there are processes to achieve a particular outcome that can be inclusive and offer opportunities for equitable participation. These are distinct from equitable outcomes of the process, or "end-result justice" (Nozick 1974: 53; Stone 2012).
- Intergenerational equity: the costs and benefits of a policy can also be distributed unevenly over time. In these cases, the analyst needs to consider the fairness of making future generations pay for

contemporary benefits (or vice versa). Imposing costs on future generations can be controversial as they are not present to defend their interests while the policies are being considered.

Equity can be a challenging idea to operationalize. Is the goal of the policy to achieve more equity relative to the status quo? Or is there an ideal state of equity that the policies need to realize? Which particular sub-group(s) should the analyst prioritize in maximizing equitable outcomes? Indeed different stakeholders can look at the same issue and come to very different conclusions about equity, or as Stone (2012) calls it, the "paradox in distributive problems." Stone characterizes a distribution with three dimensions: (i) the recipients of some item or service, (ii) the item being distributed, and (iii) the process of how the distribution is decided on and carried out. These are useful parameters when considering how best to represent equity in an analysis.

History has shown how policy solutions to enforce child support payments change when considering the equity implications, and specifically the noncustodial parent's ability to pay. While the same effectiveness criterion of *maximizing the number of noncustodial parents eligible for debt reduction* could apply, the introduction of an equity-oriented criterion imposes an additional constraint on the analysis. There are policy options that might fare well under the effectiveness criterion (such as the state matching noncustodial parents' child support payments with additional funds that go towards their debt reduction), but that rank low with respect to managing the burdens being placed on individuals who cannot come up with the money to pay any support (regardless of how rich the matching incentive). In other words, notions of vertical equity would not be upheld. In this case it would make sense to include another criterion focused on how easy it is for noncustodial parents to comply with the proposed policies and therefore be eligible for debt reduction: *maximize ease of compliance by noncustodial parent*.

Feasibility (Administrative, Political, and Technical)

Feasibility criteria assess how possible it is for the policy option to actually get adopted and implemented. These criteria typically address the process-based, political, institutional or legal barriers to getting the policy done. How rigid are those barriers? How easily can they be navigated or overcome? For example, policy options that incorporate procedures for examining "ability" versus "willingness" to pay child support could come up against feasibility constraints, either due to administrative capacity of the supervising agencies or the information gaps in knowing the true motivation behind nonpayment. There might also be legal concerns. Local political environments might also make it more or less difficult to push for more flexible policies, regardless of how effective they prove to be.

Box 4.3 Thinking Ahead to Policy Implementation

1 Is there infrastructure in place to support the proposed policy changes (i.e., personnel, physical space)?
2 Are there realities or obstacles "on the ground" that could make implementation unrealistic? Lipsky (1980) documents "street level bureaucrats" in their work to provide services, and exercise discretion, in the face of policy-related, administrative, and cultural constraints.

Many of these questions can be answered by "backward mapping" (Elmore 1979): going to the source of the problem and talking to actors involved in related activities on the ground. This is akin to the stakeholder analysis discussed earlier.

Even though the implementation of any proposed policy is many months or years down the line, it is important for the analyst to consider what form it will take. The most intelligently designed policy can be a non-option if the implementation is risky or infeasible. While the minutia of policy options can be worked out over time, the analyst needs to be aware of the administrative, legal, and process-based features that could make an option more or less feasible. Here are suggestions on how to identify those features (and translate them into criteria to evaluate the implementation feasibility of the proposed policy options):

1 How many entities need to support or approve the proposed option? How many decision points are involved in getting the policy (or parts of it) in place and operational? Pressman and Wildavsky (1984), in their seminal book on implementation, determine that delays in policy implementation are a function of

---

> a the number of decision points;
> b the number of participants at each point; and
> c the intensity of their preferences.
> 2 Does the client have the authority to implement the proposed policy options? If not, who would grant that authority (and how difficult would it be)?
> 3 Are there cultural or institutional norms that would make the proposed policy changes difficult to achieve?

Feasibility criteria are often just as important as those related to effectiveness. It is not uncommon to include several criteria to capture feasibility in a single analysis, as they serve as important "reality checks" for the proposed options. A policy could be well targeted, but if political or legal hurdles are insurmountable, or if the policy's implementation is unrealistic, then the proposed solution's effectiveness is also unlikely. See Box 4.3 for a discussion of why implementation should be taken into account.

Feasibility criteria can also be used to assess how quickly an option can be adopted or implemented. Oftentimes, urgency matters. Organizations frequently rely on outside funding and must come up with strategies that produce outcomes within particular time frames set by those funders. "Policy windows" (Kingdon 2003) create political or administrative opportunities to move policies forward and their roll-out may need to be immediate. Therefore, feasibility criteria often capture "time until initiation" or "time until completion" for a project; situations where rapid policy responses are preferred will prioritize options that minimize timelines. It is important for the analyst to ask "time until what?" as there is a critical difference between minimizing the time until the policy is initiated and minimizing the time until results emerge.

Cost (or Financial Feasibility)

While cost can take different levels of priority depending on the project, rarely is it deemed completely irrelevant. Every analysis should involve some assessment of costs across the policy options, whether or not this criterion is prioritized in the final analysis. First and foremost, the analyst needs to determine the costs to *whom*? Is the criterion capturing costs to the government? To the organization providing services? To the recipient of those services? The analyst may opt to combine several different costs, but the aggregate costs could obscure variations in how those costs are distributed.

We encourage the analyst to consider cost broadly and realistically. Costs are both fixed (i.e., to set up the infrastructure for an option) and variable (i.e., to support operations over time); they can be both explicit (i.e., money outlaid to pay for materials) and implicit (i.e., opportunity costs from forgoing a competing investment); and they can be incurred at different points in time (i.e., at the start of the program or ten years out). As we will discuss later, costs do not have to be considered in quantitative terms only—and the numbers need not be precise. Typically, the costs applied to policy options are intended to indicate differences in order of magnitude. That is, it is unlikely that an option will be prioritized due to a discount of a few thousand dollars if the projects cost millions of dollars across the board. However, if one option costs several thousand dollars and another option costs several hundred thousand, the cost criterion should capture that meaningful discrepancy.

While cost always informs the viability of any strategy, it does not always make it into the final analysis. In some instances, the client may request that cost not be included, as to encourage "big thinking" about solutions. This does not mean, however, that cost should be entirely ignored. The analyst should still be prepared with cost estimates, even if they are not used to rank options. It may also be the case that the options do not vary with respect to cost. If all of the proposed alternatives are within some reasonable range of cost, it should not be used as a standard to rank them. However, again, the analyst should document the costs for each option for purposes of information.

We briefly return to the idea that costs can change over time, and that criteria should capture this variation. Costs of an option can change nominally: initial, typically large start-up costs for a social service program often take place in the first couple of years, but are not regularly incurred in the years that follow (when lower operating costs persist). Costs can also change relatively: the value of money can change over time, depending on the kinds of alternative investment options. We will go into detail on the time-value of money (or discounting) in Chapter 5.

Efficiency

Criteria related to efficiency assess the productivity, or "success," of an option relative to the cost of implementing it; essentially effectiveness and cost are collapsed into a single metric. Efficiency criteria prioritize options that maximize the number of outputs (assuming similar inputs across options). They are concerned with aggregate social welfare, rather than the distribution of the goods or services that are produced or consumed. For example, child support enforcement policies have often been evaluated based on their efficiency: how much child support debt they collect relative to the cost of implementing the collection strategy. Efficiency criteria are closely linked to cost-benefit analysis (CBA) techniques that rely on quantifying all of the benefits and costs related to an issue. Here, the desired outcome is one that maximizes net benefit ("to whom" and "of what" is open to interpretation). CBAs are most prevalent when considering major regulatory changes or large-scale capital projects (with large up-front financial investments). We discuss applications of efficiency and how they relate to CBA in more detail in Chapter 5.

While we include efficiency in the range of evaluative tools available to an analyst, we recognize that being able to convincingly quantify efficiency is difficult. In addition, even efficiency metrics can be subjectively determined, as the selection and formulation of the inputs and outputs are at the discretion of the analyst. It is important to not interpret efficiency-related criteria as more objective than other equity- or feasibility-related criteria; it is still critical to understand their context and limitations (again, these will be discussed in more detail in Chapter 5). One can also conduct a compelling analysis without including efficiency as a criterion, and instead by comparing separate measures of costs and effectiveness across the policy options.

Voting Case: Generating Criteria to Rank Alternatives

In previous chapters, we identified the central problem related to electoral participation; specifically, how to increase voter turnout. We then came up with several options to address this problem, drawing from existing programs in the United States and other countries, as well as research on what strategies are effective at getting people out to the polls:

- Mandatory voting;
- Universal or expanded vote-by-mail;
- Incentives (lottery); and
- Automatic registration.

Now, we need to develop criteria to evaluate the viability of the proposed options and to, ideally, provide a recommendation of the best one.

Who Are the Key Stakeholders and Interests to Represent?

Voters: This group includes currently registered voters, those who are registered but don't vote, and those who have not yet registered or voted. The interests of these stakeholders are key, as the policies will target their behavior and they will ultimately bear the burden or benefit of any proposed option.

State and local governments: since voter laws are designed and implemented at the level of sub-national governments, their buy-in will be critical for the success of any proposed policy. These are the entities responsible for implementing the policy and also generating political support around any proposed or adopted policy. These stakeholders, including elected officials, have financial, political, and social interests at stake

Federal government: the federal government sets laws that guide policies across the states. Therefore, any proposed option needs to abide by federal guidelines and regulations. Stakeholders at the national level, including elected officials, can also play an important role in advocating for particular policies and setting a broader political agenda that can make certain alternatives more feasible than others

Non-profit advocacy organizations: these organizations (which run the ideological gamut) can be key players in generating support around a particular policy.[2] They often have close ties to target constituencies (i.e., voters or potential voters) and also negotiate with government entities. In that sense, they can also be central to guaranteeing the effectiveness of any particular policy.

What Are the Kinds of Criteria That Matter?

Effectiveness: proposed policies should be evaluated on how well they increase voter turnout; an effective proposal would be one that increases turnout the most. Another aspect of effectiveness involves the nature of turnout. That is, should the analyst differentiate between turnout among new registrants/voters versus preexisting registrants/voters? Among older versus first-time voters? Between turnout among those who are knowledgeable and educated on the issues versus those who are not? Does this distinction matter, or can a policy be effective based solely on aggregate turnout? This decision will depend on the interests of the client.

Equity: strategies for increasing voter turnout can disproportionately affect certain parts of the population. Options that aim to increase turnout among one segment of the population can at the same time suppress turnout for others. The analyst needs to consider if and how any policy makes voting more burdensome and if the affected group is in a position to avoid or resist any suppression or disincentive. For example, there are many instances of voting laws that have disproportionate suppression effects on poorer, minority individuals.

Feasibility: many perspectives on voting reforms are rooted in ideological views on civil rights and government intervention. At least one criterion should assess the nature of support for any policy. A feasibility criterion could also relate to the technological or legal viability of an option; the analyst needs to consider whether or not proposed alternatives violate any existing laws or are not yet possible to technically implement.

Cost: there are two categories of costs in this case. First, the analyst needs to consider the costs to the government (local, state, and federal) of implementing any policy. Second, the analyst needs to consider the costs to voters of participating in any proposed policy. These could be explicit costs (like costs of traveling to the polls) or implicit costs (like the threats to privacy from making certain information public).

A Set of Comprehensive and Mutually Exclusive Criteria

Since some of the proposed options are relatively new (especially to the US context) it is difficult to come up with precise, continuous measures that can be credibly predicted for each option. Therefore, we rely on mostly categorical measures. In addition, the specifics of the measures would depend on the particular context for the policy, that is, at what level of government and at what scale.

Criterion 1: Maximize Increase in Voter Turnout
Measure: the likelihood and volume of additional voter turnout
1. Low: unlikely to increase voting among subsets of the population that are already underrepresented in registration and voting;
2. Moderate: likely to reach underrepresented populations but will not necessarily increase the volume of voters substantially;
3. High: likely to reach unrepresented populations and increase the volume of voters substantially.

Criterion 2: Minimize Cost to Government
Measure: costs to set up and administer the proposed alternative
1. Low: very high setup and operating costs;
2. Moderate: relatively modest setup costs, but high operating costs; or high setup costs but relatively low operating costs;
3. High: relatively low setup and operating costs.

Criterion 3: Maximize Political Feasibility
Measure: the likelihood of broad-based support
1. Low: likely to receive strong opposition from multiple key stakeholders that is insurmountable;
2. Moderate: objections by at most a few key stakeholders over issues that could be compensated by other aspects of the proposed option or related outcomes;
3. High: broad-based support across multiple stakeholders.

Criterion 4: Minimize Time to See Results
Measure: number of months or years until results are observable (i.e., when turnout can be documented)

Should Any One Criterion Be Weighted More Heavily?

The political feasibility of an option is paramount in the context of voting policies; much of the policy environment is driven by ideological differences and perceptions of the likelihood of voter fraud. Depending on the imminence of an election, the immediacy of a response could also be critical. It would be worth weighing either or both of these criteria more heavily than the others, especially in the case of alternatives that are otherwise similarly ranked.

Creating Labels for Criteria

As with creating an effective problem statement, words and language also matter for criteria. When constructing criteria specific to a particular analysis, the labels should reflect the specifics of the issue at hand. This is the difference between labeling the criterion *maximize effectiveness* and labeling it *maximize the number of noncustodial parents eligible for debt reduction*; clearly, the latter one makes explicit how effectiveness is being operationalized.

In addition to being context specific, the criteria labels should also help to guide the audience in their evaluative purpose. It is often useful to indicate in the criterion's label what it is trying to achieve in terms of "maximizing" or "minimizing" some objective.

Let's take a look at a set of criteria for the CSE case. We developed a set of five criteria to evaluate proposed policy options that address *how to reduce debt burden for noncustodial parents*.

1 Maximize the number of noncustodial parents eligible for debt reduction.
2 Maximize the amount of debt reduction.
3 Maximize ease of compliance by noncustodial parent.
4 Minimize cost of implementation.
5 Maximize political acceptability.

As we've discussed, the first two criteria cover *effectiveness*. The third criterion addresses issues of *equity* and *fairness*. It assesses how much burden will be placed on the noncustodial parent in pursuing options to reduce their debt. It is likely that some noncustodial parents will still be hamstrung by resource constraints and this criterion will capture that variation. The fourth criterion addresses the *cost* of implementing the proposed options, and specifically the costs to government and other partner organizations. Finally, the fifth criterion addresses *feasibility*, or, in this case, *political acceptability*. Surely there are different ideological and moral views on how to enforce child support, and this criterion should evaluate how well the policy option satisfies (or aggravates) those opposing perspectives. Altogether, the criteria are inclusive of several dimensions and are non-redundant.

It is not enough to simply list the criteria. In order for the criteria to be operational they need to be connected to *measures*. Measures are the components of criteria that facilitate the ranking of options; they articulate under what conditions a policy option will fare well with respect to a particular criterion. Some measures capture the degree to which alternatives meet some standard or goal; others capture whether or not alternatives are minimally acceptable (Bardach and Patashnik 2015). A criterion can have one or several measures, depending on how broadly it is defined.

Measures can be both *quantitative* and *categorical*, but always need to have some kind of hierarchy. By *quantitative* we mean a numerical metric that uses continuous values to count or summarize a projected outcome related to the criterion. By *categorical* we mean variables that establish classes of performance, like "high," "moderate," and "low" or "yes" and "no." Categorical measures are typically used

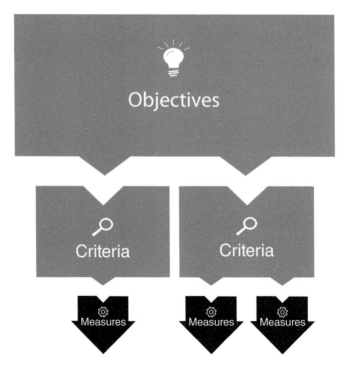

Figure 4.4 Objectives, criteria, and measures

when (i) continuous quantitative metrics are unavailable or not credible or (ii) discrete categories of performance make more conceptual sense for differentiating across the policy options. We will illustrate these points in the next two sections.

> **Box 4.4 Criteria and Measures Are Applied to Outcomes, Not Alternatives**
>
> The criteria will be applied to the *projected outcomes* of the proposed options (Bardach and Patashnik 2015). Therefore, applying criteria, and specifically their measures, is an exercise in probability. Since the proposed policy options will not have been implemented at the time of the analysis (indeed the point of the project is to assess the options *before* implementing them!), any assessment of their "success" will be an educated guess at best. The goal of the analyst is not to guarantee, but to convey a high degree of certainty in the projected outcomes. The analyst often turns to the past, using experience and research (we will discuss this process in more depth in Chapter 7), to predict how the proposed options (including the status quo) will play out in the future. The measures will assess how well the projected outcomes meet established standards of "success."

Quantitative Measures

Let us consider the criterion we created earlier, *maximize the amount of debt reduction*. Recall that we designed this criterion with two sub-criteria: (i) *maximize the amount of state debt reduction* and (ii) *possibility of custodial parent debt reduction*. In order to create a summary measure for the entire criterion, we first have to establish measures for each sub-criterion. Assuming the data are available, we propose the following measures for the sub-criteria:

1. *Maximize the amount of state debt reduction*: average share of a noncustodial parent's child support debt to the state that would be forgiven
2. *The possibility of custodial parent debt reduction*: whether or not any uncollectible custodial-parent debt would be reduced

The first measure is an example of a quantitative one. Notice that we use a measure of "share" instead of an absolute dollar amount for the first sub-criterion. This is an intentional choice to capture how well the obligation is mitigated, rather than simply how much financial value is forgiven or reduced. The latter measure obscures the effectiveness of the policy option since the absolute dollar amount says nothing about how successful the strategy is in trying to address the full debt obligation (which can vary in magnitude across noncustodial parents).

Categorical Measures

While conceptually appealing, quantitative measures could be very hard to obtain. This is the case for the second sub-criterion, *the possibility of custodial parent debt reduction*. The federal government prohibits states from unilaterally reducing debt owed to custodial parents (and many states are reluctant to even ask custodial parents if they might be willing to forgive any debt) (Heinrich et al. 2011; Pearson et al. 2012; Turetsky 2017). Most states do not address private debt in their policies and have been very reluctant to broach it. There are only a few examples, and therefore little quantitative evidence, on how this is effectively done (Ascend at the Aspen Institute & Good+Foundation 2020).

An alternative approach is to create categorical measures that still facilitate a ranking across options. For example, we can use a binary "yes" or "no" since we can project the general possibility of reducing that debt and rank options based on the readiness of that possibility.

Categorical measures can also suffice if the options diverge enough in their effectiveness. Let's reconsider the first sub-criterion, *maximize the amount of state debt reduction*. For example, if research on Alternative A projects a "90 percent" reduction and Alternative B projects a "10 percent" reduction, categorical classifications of "high" and "low" should be able to capture these stark differences. On the one hand, if the projected outcomes for the alternatives were closer (say "60 percent" and "50 percent") then the cruder classifications may not capture those differences. On the other hand, one could argue that the difference between 60 percent and 50 percent is not meaningful enough to prioritize one alternative over the other (especially if those projections are approximate); therefore, the categorical classifications would appropriately equate the alternatives with respect to this criterion.

One approach is to create three classifications: "high," "moderate," and "low." There are two ways to establish these measures. First, one category can be set to reflect the status quo. It typically makes sense to use the "low" or "moderate" classification, as the goal of the analysis is to offer up options that improve upon the status quo. If the status quo is reflected in the "moderate" classification, then there is room to convey both improvements and declines relative to the status quo. This is also a good strategy, because the analyst is the most informed about the status quo—it's the only option that has been empirically observed. Therefore, the analyst can use information on the status quo to project the likelihood of debt reduction in the context of proposed policy changes. For example, annual reports from the Office of Child Support Enforcement (renamed in 2023 as the Office of Child Support Services) documents that, nationally, public debt (i.e., Temporary Assistance for Needy Children) was reduced by about 25 percent between 2016 and 2022 (Office of Child Support Enforcement 2016, 2023).[3] We can use this statistic to set thresholds for predicted effectiveness of the proposed policy option:

1 *Maximize the amount of state debt reduction*:
   a   High: debt reduction is higher than 10 percent over a four-year period.
   b   Moderate: debt reduction is around 10 percent over a four-year period.
   c   Low: debt reduction is less than 10 percent over a four-year period.

A second approach for establishing categorical measures is to reflect different gradations in qualitative characteristics or likelihoods of outcomes. For example, experience with trying to reduce debt burdens for noncustodial parents shows that the reduction of debt owed to custodial parents is harder to achieve (Sorensen 2014; Sorensen et al. 2007). Therefore, the analyst might choose to combine the two sub-criteria to create the following measure for the umbrella criterion, *maximize the amount of debt reduction*:

a   High: debts to the government and custodial parents are reduced.
b   Moderate: only government debt is reduced.
c   Low: no change in any debt (government or custodial).

A less-nuanced metric would be a simple yes–no categorization. As we mentioned earlier, the sub-criterion *maximize the amount of debt owed to custodial parent that would be reduced* could be difficult to apply with the limited information available. Instead, a "yes" could be assigned to options that incorporate any kind of reduction of debt owed to the custodial parents (regardless of the amount). Options that don't encourage or allow for the reduction of debt to the custodial parent would get assigned a "no." This is a cruder formulation but might be preferable in cases where the analyst does not have the information to credibly predict specific reduction rates but has a good sense of the general likelihood of debt reduction taking place or not. A more nuanced distinction across rankings may also be unnecessary. For example, the reduction of private debt is so unusual in the status quo that any degree of reduction would constitute a meaningful change.

Reconciling Measures Across Sub-Criteria

How can we reconcile the measures of the sub-criteria to achieve a single ranking for the criterion overall? One strategy is to leave the two sub-criteria separate and show their measures. For the child support case, this might make sense. The two components of the criterion *maximize the amount of debt reduction* intentionally capture different aspects of the debt obligation; it could be informative for the analyst and client to see those broken out (especially if they are in tension). A second strategy is to create a summary measure, such as an average, of the two values or rankings. For this approach, the analyst needs to make a decision about how to weigh the sub-criteria. For example, if the analyst thought that *forgiving state debt* was more important than *reducing private debt*, then the former should be weighted more heavily in the summary measure (deciding on the precise weight can be challenging and often arbitrary).

Box 4.5 Using Measures to "Bound" the Analysis

"Bounding" the analysis means differentiating between measures that capture conservative and lower-bound outcomes and those that capture more aggressive and upper-bound outcomes. For example, suppose the analyst collected enough evidence to support some projected private debt reduction rates for the proposed policy options, but the research demonstrated that those numbers, based on administrative data from state agencies, likely missed informal arrangements (from parent to parent). Therefore, the analyst could still feel comfortable using the data to project debt reduction but should be clear that any numbers likely capture lower-bound estimates (that is, in reality the debt obligation rates will likely be higher). If we are convinced that this downward bias is consistently applied across all policy options, it will not interfere with the ranking of options based on this particular criterion. However, it signals to the client that any numbers should be interpreted as conservative.

Two Common Pitfalls

Confusing Criteria With Alternatives

One of the most common mistakes in constructing and applying criteria is that they too closely resemble alternatives. Criteria should not describe any particular policy strategy or prioritize a particular course of action. As we emphasized earlier, criteria set goals for particular outcomes and their measures rank options based on how well their predicted outcomes achieve the "success" standards set by the criteria. Hammond et al. (1999) differentiate "means to an end" from "ends in themselves" (p. 38). For example, one approach is to draw from other welfare program strategies and condition debt forgiveness on work requirements. However, ranking "high" on the criterion should not be contingent on using work requirements as a condition of forgiveness, as there are other ways to mitigate debt. In other words, work requirements is a "means" used to get to the "end" of reduced debt burden. Indeed, if the measure, in its rankings, prioritizes one option or mechanism over another, the analysis is inherently biased towards that approach. The analyst automatically discounts the options that have other, perhaps effective, interventions to mitigate debt.

Weighting Criteria Post-Hoc

Another common pitfall is to give more weight to certain criteria after they have been systematically applied to the alternatives. Before the criteria are applied to the alternatives, however, it is entirely legitimate (and thoughtful) to weigh one or several criteria as more (or less) important than others. The criteria are supposed to reflect the objectives and values behind the project and some may be prioritized over others. This could be informed by the client, by the reliability of the measures or by the broader political environment.

When weighting is done after the fact, it can appear as if criteria are being manipulated to make a particular policy option appear more favorable. This is in contrast to the framework's intent: to identify the optimal option based on pre-established standards of evaluation. Therefore, in order to maintain the integrity of the analysis, we recommend that analysts establish weights for criteria before applying them to the alternatives.

The Analytical Matrix

We are now ready to present a core tool for policy analysis: the analytical matrix. This is a concise and visual way for the analyst to organize policy options alongside the evaluative criteria. The policy options and criteria are arrayed along the axes, and the ranking of each option (i.e., the measure) is entered into the cells. The analytical matrix looks like this:

		CRITERIA		
ALTERNATIVES		*Criterion 1*	*Criterion 2*	*Criterion 3*
	Alternative A	Measure	Measure	Measure
	Alternative B	Measure	Measure	Measure
	Alternative C	Measure	Measure	Measure
	Alternative D	Measure	Measure	Measure

The analyst should maintain the matrix at a manageable size. For example, three or four options positioned up against three to five criteria provide space for variation and comprehensiveness but do not overwhelm the presentation. Anything much bigger becomes cumbersome.

While analysts may go through several iterations of this matrix, some quite expansive, the final version to be presented to the client or other interested audiences should be more parsed. We will go into more detail on how to use the matrix to execute the analysis in Chapter 7.

Summary

In this chapter we discussed the importance of **objectives** in framing the broader goals for the analysis and of **criteria** in systematically evaluating the merits and drawbacks of proposed policy options. Objectives indicate the moral, ideological, and political guiding principles for the project. Criteria are important methodological tools for the analysis. We consider the criteria the backbone of the analysis, and they need to be crafted with attention to the interests of central **stakeholders**, including the client. The analyst should identify who has **standing** in the analysis and construct criteria to reflect their interests. Criteria are applied to the alternatives' projected outcomes and should broadly assess the degree to which they achieve **effectiveness**, **feasibility**, **cost**, **equity**, and **efficiency**. They should be **comprehensive** and **non-redundant** in their coverage.

We discussed that criteria should be tailored to the goals and circumstances of the particular issue. **Measures** are established for each criterion, and they provide a way to rank the proposed policy options, either numerically or categorically. They need to be applied consistently to all of the proposed policy options, and they should not inherently prioritize particular alternatives. Criteria that do not differentiate across options should be dropped or used for informative purposes only. Criteria are often the source of bias in any analysis, and the analyst should work hard to maintain neutral measures. Indeed, if the criteria, and in particular their measures, are flawed, then the validity of the entire analysis could be in question.

Child Support Debt Forgiveness Case: A Recap

In Chapter 2 we settled on a central problem: *how can the government reduce the debt burden for noncustodial parents?*

In Chapter 3 we presented four policy options to reduce child support debt incurred by noncustodial parents. These alternatives were as follows:

1. Participation Incentive Program (PIP): forgive debt owed to the state after the NCP pays child support for 12 and 24 months.
2. Match Plus Outreach (MPO): for every dollar of child support paid, 50 cents of debt is forgiven; the program applies to state debt and, if the custodial parent agrees, debt owed to custodial parents; it includes outreach to custodial parents.
3. Workforce Development (WD): the state forgives debt for NCPs who enroll in a workforce development program and obtain and retain employment.
4. Automatic Forgiveness of Arrears Due to Incarceration (AFAI): the state automatically forgives arrears that noncustodial parents accrued while incarcerated in the state's prison system.

Child Support Debt Case: Criteria

We now need a mechanism for ranking those options and prioritizing the ones that are most effective and feasible. The criteria are that mechanism.

Through the course of this chapter we grappled with the process of developing criteria and have landed on six:[4]

1. *Effectiveness: Maximize the number of noncustodial parents eligible for debt reduction.*
2. *Effectiveness: Maximize the amount of state debt reduction.*
3. *Effectiveness: The possibility of custodial parent debt reduction.*
4. *Equity: Maximize ease of compliance by noncustodial parent.*
5. *Minimize cost of implementation.*
6. *Maximize political acceptability.*

The first three listed cover *effectiveness*, or how successful the option will be at reducing debt. These criteria, together, cover the breadth of coverage and the depth of reduction. The fourth criterion assesses the equity implications, or how likely the options will disproportionately burden certain noncustodial parents. The final two criteria capture feasibility. The client (the state's Department of Social Services) will undoubtedly be interested in how much the options will cost to implement (especially up against the projections of effectiveness). The client also needs to be aware of the political prospects for each option, or how feasible it will be to gain support for a proposal. Altogether, the criteria are *comprehensive*, covering a range of evaluative dimensions, and *mutually exclusive*, avoiding redundancies in terms of the dimensions they cover.

In order to make the criteria functional, we need to define measures. Let's consider each criterion, one at a time:

1 *Criterion 1: maximize the number of noncustodial parents eligible for debt reduction*
    a *Measure:* the share of low-income noncustodial parents eligible for debt reduction.
    b *Explanation:* there is a reasonable amount of research and evidence on the coverage of possible policies, and so we can feel comfortable with using a quantitative measure of eligibility. We focus on low-income noncustodial parents since they are the ones most hamstrung by debt.
2 *Criterion 2: maximize the amount of state debt reduction*
    a *Measure*: average share of a noncustodial parent's state debt that would be forgiven.
    b *Explanation*: again, there is a reasonable amount of research and evidence on the amount of debt that could be forgiven under each proposed policy.
    c *Criterion 3: the possibility of custodial parent debt reduction*
        i *Measure*: whether or not any uncollectible custodial-parent debt would be reduced.
        ii *Explanation:* the experience with reducing custodial-parent debt is very limited, and therefore it could be difficult to project any specific amount of debt reduction. However, there is some understanding of what kinds of approaches are more likely to work, and this measure will reflect a general expectation of success.
3 *Criterion 4: maximize ease of compliance by noncustodial parent*
    a *Measure:* the likelihood, or ease, of satisfying behavioral and/or other requirements (such as continuous child-support payments for a specified period of time) for debt reduction.

        i   *Low*: debt reduction is dependent on relatively long and strict terms.
        ii *Moderate*: debt reduction is conditional on terms that are relatively short (less than a year) and somewhat flexible.
        iii *High*: pretty immediate reduction of debt without onerous requirements.
   b *Explanation:* while it is difficult to capture ease of compliance with a numeric measure, we can categorize the stringency of financial conditions for becoming eligible for debt reduction. To do this, we draw on features of the proposed programs. This measure is derived from an iterative process, assessing the range of conditions from the possible options and then circling back to reflect that variation in the measures.

4 *Criterion 5: minimize cost of implementation*
   a *Measure:* payroll and other costs of implementation to state government and partner organizations (measured in dollars)
   b *Explanation:* cost estimates can usually be constructed by referencing existing programs (either similar or related), and making adjustments based on the proposed size, span, and features. Even if the cost estimates are projected with some error, as long as the error is consistent across all of the options, the rankings will still be informative. For example, if the analyst uses conservative estimates of new personnel costs, he or she must be sure to use equally conservative projections for all of the proposed options. Therefore, we can feel comfortable with projecting a quantitative measure of cost.

5 *Criterion 6: maximize political acceptability*
   a *Measure:* likelihood and intensity of opposition to proposed options from key stakeholders.
        i   *Low*: objections by several key stakeholder over issues that are likely insurmountable.
        ii *Moderate*: objections by at most a few key stakeholders over issues that could be compensated by other aspects of the proposed option or related outcomes.
        iii *High*: little or no objections by key stakeholders
   b *Explanation:* In this context, it is difficult to measure political support in a numerical way. Therefore, we opt for a categorical

measure that captures the intensity of support or feasibility based off of ideological stances and moral sentiment among the key stakeholders.

We are careful to make sure that the measures can be *consistently applied* across all options; that is, no ranking inherently favors one proposed alternative over another. As for *weighting* one of the criteria more than the others, this would typically depend on the client's preferences. For example, if the analysis were being conducted for an organization that represents the rights of noncustodial parents, the equity criterion could be weighted more heavily. In our case, where the client is a government agency, financial or political feasibility might take precedence.

Notes

1. In stressing uncollectible debt owed by low-income noncustodial parents, we assume that the state will continue to seek to collect child support arrears owed by noncustodial parents with the financial means to pay their debt.
2. For example, the American Civil Liberties Union (ACLU) is a progressive organization fighting for the expansion of voting rights, while the American Legislative Exchange Council is a conservative organization that has worked to constrain voting rights, like voter ID laws.
3. See www.acf.hhs.gov/css/resource/major-change-in-who-is-owed-child-support-arrears.
4. For simplicity, we've converted the two sub-criteria under *maximize debt reduction* to two stand-alone criteria. It is also useful to keep them separate since they capture different aspects of child support. For example, debt to the state has declined over time, while private debt has continued to grow (Sorensen 2014)—this suggests that the policy implications for each need to be assessed separately.

References

Allio, Lorenzo. 2014. *Design Thinking for Public Service Excellence*. New York, NY: UNDP Global Centre for Public Service Excellence.

Ascend at the Aspen Institute & Good+Foundation. 2020. "Implementing Sensible Debt Reduction Strategies." *Child Support Policy Fact Sheet*. https://ascend-resources.aspeninstitute.org/wp-content/uploads/2020/08/2_ChildSupport_Reducing_Arrears.pdf

Bardach, Eugene, and Eric M. Patashnik. 2015. *A Practical Guide for Policy Analysis: The Eightfold Path to More Effective Problem Solving* (5th Edition). Los Angeles, CA: CQ Press.

Bouie, Jamelle. 2023. "The Path to Reducing Pedestrian Deaths is Steep but Straight." *The New York Times* (October 21). www.nytimes.com/2023/10/21/opinion/pedestrians-cars-trucks-suvs-death.html.

Elmore, Richard F. 1979. "Backward Mapping: Implementation Research and Policy Decisions." *Political Science Quarterly 94, 4*: 601–616.

Hammond, John S., Ralph L. Keeney, and Howard Raiffa. 1999. *Smart Choices: A Practical Guide to Making Better Decisions*. Boston, MA: Harvard Business School Press.

Heinrich, Carolyn, Brett Burkhardt, Hilary Shager, and Lara Rosen. 2011. *The Families Forward Program: Final Evaluation Report*. Madison, WI: Institute for Research on Poverty, University of Wisconsin-Madison. Report Prepared for Wisconsin Department of Workforce Development (January).

Kim, Juliana. 2023. "U.S. Pedestrian Deaths Reach a 40-Year High." *NPR* (June 26). www.npr.org/2023/06/26/1184034017/us-pedestrian-deaths-high-traffic-car.

Kingdon, John W. 2003. *Agendas, Alternatives, and Public Policies* (2nd Edition). New York: Longman.

Lipsky, Michael. 1980. *Street Level Bureaucrats*. New York: Russell Sage Foundation.

Majone, Giandomenico. 1988. "Policy Analysis and Public Deliberation." In *The Power of Public Ideas*, Robert Reich (ed.). Cambridge, MA: Harvard University Press.

Nozick, Robert. 1974. *Anarchy, State and Utopia*. New York: Basic Books.

Office of Child Support Enforcement. 2016. *Preliminary Report FY2016*. Washington, DC: Author.

Office of Child Support Enforcement. 2023. *Preliminary Report FY2022*. Washington, DC: Author.

Patton, Carl V., and David S. Sawicki. 1993. *Basic Methods of Policy Analysis and Planning*. Upper Saddle River, NJ: Prentice Hall.

Pearson, Jessica, Nancy Thoennes, and Rasa Kaulnelis. 2012. *Debt Compromise Programs: Program Design and Child Support Outcomes in Five Locations*. Report Submitted by Center for Policy Research to US Office of Child Support Enforcement. https://centerforpolicyresearch.org/wp-content/uploads/Debt-Compromise-Improving-Child-Support-Outcomes-Final-Report-Nov-14-2012-1.pdf

Pressman, Jeffrey L., and Aaron Wildavsky. 1984. *Implementation: How Great Expectations in Washington are Dashed in Oakland; Or, Why It's Amazing that Federal Programs Work at All, This Being a Saga of the Economic Development Administration as Told by Two Sympathetic Observers Who Seek to Build Morals on a Foundation*. Berkeley, CA: University of California Press.

Smart Growth America. 2022. *Dangerous by Design*. https://smartgrowthamerica.org/dangerous-by-design/

Sorensen, Elaine. 2014. "Major Change in Who Is Owed Child Support Arrears." In *Child Support Fact Series* (No. 4). Washington, DC: Office of Child Support Enforcement. www.acf.hhs.gov/sites/default/files/programs/css/changes_in_who_is_owed_arrears.pdf

Sorensen, Elaine, Liliana Sousa, and Simon Schaner. 2007. *Assessing Child Support Arrears in Nine Large States and the Nation*. Washington, DC: The Urban Institute. www.urban.org/sites/default/files/publication/29736/1001242-Assessing-Child-Support-Arrears-in-Nine-Large-States-and-the-Nation.PDF

Stone, Deborah. 2012. *Policy Paradox: The Art of Political Decision Making* (3rd Edition). New York: W. W. Norton.

Turetsky, Vicki. 2017. Interview conducted in October 2017.

Weimer, David L., and Aidan R. Vining. 2011. *Policy Analysis*. Boston, MA: Longman.

5
Technical Aspects of Policy Analysis
Discounting, Cost-Benefit Analysis, and Cost-Effectiveness Analysis

Aspects of policy analysis can be quite technical, relying on the collection and management of an immense amount of quantitative information. One of the key components of policy analysis is projecting the outcomes of proposed alternatives. The technical methods discussed in this chapter address how to project and measure these outcomes in a quantitative way, and, specifically, against measures of cost. These numbers will most directly contribute to the criteria (discussed in Chapter 4), providing numerical metrics that can be compared across options. The most prominent of these methods is *cost-benefit analysis* (CBA), which has a long and controversial history in the field of policy analysis. *Cost-effectiveness analysis* (CEA), a less restrictive approach to comparing policy outcomes in terms of costs, is a popular tool across the policy spectrum. CEA underlies well-known tools, such as the environmental impact statement (EIS), which are often implemented prior to large-scale developments. Both CBA and CEA usually involve the exercise of *discounting*, a way to adjust for the time-value of money. More broadly, this concept must be applied whenever potential policies or programs involve costs or revenues that will occur over time.

We start the chapter with a discussion of discounting, as it is a central component of all of the analytical methods discussed later in the chapter. We then introduce CBA—its theoretical foundations and assumptions—and walk through how to implement it. We address the challenges of implementing a credible CBA and conclude with strategies for using it pragmatically. CEA is covered at the end of the chapter as a more flexible method for evaluating costs against benefits.

Discounting: Accounting for Time Value of Money

The intuition behind discounting is that the resources invested in any particular project are limited and could otherwise be directed into another productive activity. In other words, those resources would not sit idle were the proposed project not to take place. The analyst needs to account for this opportunity cost when assessing the economic merits of the proposed project in order to be certain that the calculation of cost is comprehensive of all potential explicit and implicit factors. This is different than estimating the risk of taking on a particular project. Discounting addresses only the cost of opting for one investment over an alternative productive use.[1]

Discounting is also important for programs and policies that incur costs at different points in time and at different frequencies. In order to be able to compare "apples to apples" the analyst needs a method for collapsing these multi-year costs into a uniform metric. Present value (PV), the product of discounting, provides this common metric. Let's consider an example in the context of child support enforcement (CSE) policies. In Chapter 2 we discussed the problem of delinquent child support payments. There is a range of perspectives on why this problem exists. One interpretation is administrative: the technologies are not in place to effectively locate and collect from the noncustodial parent. This approach dominated CSE policy reform for many years. A second interpretation is ability to pay: no matter how efficient the collection technologies, if the noncustodial parents are burdened beyond their means with obligations, they will not be able to fulfill them. These two approaches suggest two different policy solutions:

1   Improve the automation (and therefore collection) of child support collections.
2   Improve workforce development programs for noncustodial parents so that they are better able to support their children.

Table 5.1 Costs for CSE Alternatives

Year	Automatic Collection System	Targeted Workforce Development Program
0	$50,000,000	$0
1	$0	$18,000,000
2	$1,200,000	$18,540,000
3	$1,236,000	$19,096,200
4	$1,273,080	$19,669,086
5	$1,311,272	$20,259,159
Total	$55,020,352	$95,564,445

These two proposals would incur very different costs, both in the initial stages and over time. Table 5.1 illustrates these differences in a scenario for a small northeast state in the United States.

How can the analyst collapse the costs into a single, comparable metric? This is where discounting is useful. The arithmetic behind present value is fairly straightforward and summarized by the following formula:

$$\text{Present Value of Cost} = \text{PV}(\text{Cost}) = \sum_{t=0}^{k} \frac{C_t}{(1+r)^t}$$

Box 5.1 The Discount Factor

The denominator of the present value formula is also referred to as the "discount factor":

$$\frac{1}{(1+r)^t}$$

It is the amount by which the nominal value is adjusted to get the discounted amount. As the discount factor gets smaller (which happens when $(1+r)^t$ gets bigger), the present value also gets smaller.

Here, C are the costs in time t, where t ranges from 0 to k. The benefits and costs are adjusted down by the *discount rate* (r).

If the project incurs costs over five years (or $k = 5$), the formula expands in the following way:

$$\mathrm{PV}(\mathrm{Cost}) = \sum_{t=0}^{5} \frac{C_t}{(1+r)^t} = \frac{C_0}{(1+r)^0} + \frac{C_1}{(1+r)^1} + \frac{C_2}{(1+r)^2} + \frac{C_3}{(1+r)^3} + \frac{C_4}{(1+r)^4} + \frac{C_5}{(1+r)^5}$$

While it is important to understand how discounting is calculated, in practice a manually implemented formula (as earlier) is unrealistic (especially when a project extends over many years). Nowadays applications as basic as Microsoft Excel contain pre-programmed commands that calculate present value in one step.

Box 5.2 Using Microsoft Excel to Calculate Present Value

While walking through the underlying formulae is important to understand how discounting works, it is not necessary to manually calculate present values. Discounting is a widely used tool that is standardized into every data management and statistical package these days. Even the most rudimentary data management tools, like Excel, contain pre-programmed procedures for calculating present value. To calculate present values in Excel, the analyst needs to input the following information:

- Time: a row for each year in the analysis
- Nominal monetary values: costs, for example, for each year in the analysis
- Discount rate

Then, present value can be calculated in a single cell, referencing the earlier information in the pre-programmed formula in Excel:

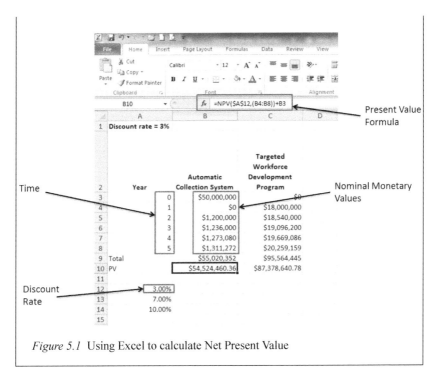

Figure 5.1 Using Excel to calculate Net Present Value

What is the discount rate? Where does it come from? The discount rate is best understood as a "reverse interest rate," or the rate at which the resources would be otherwise productively invested. This goes back to the idea that those monies would not be sitting idle but would be earning some return in another use. For example, if you had $100 today, you could spend it or put it in a savings account where it earns 5 percent. If you parked that money in the savings account, that $100 would be worth $105 in one year. If you spend the $100 now, you are forgoing the earned interest of $5 (or 5 percent of $100). Put differently, assuming a discount rate of 5 percent, if you spent $100 one year from now, that would be the equivalent of spending about $95.24 today. This means $95.24 is the present value of $100 one year from now, using a discount rate of 5 percent. This opportunity cost needs to be captured in the valuation of any option that has costs and benefits over time.

In practice, the discount rate is usually standardized by industry or sector. There is typically some rate that captures the prevailing return and projects use these accepted rates. For example, the Congressional Budget Office (CBO) and the Office of Management and Budget (OMB) are the two US government agencies that most commonly employ discounting in the context of CBA. The CBO uses a rate that is based on its estimate of the long-term cost of borrowing for the federal government (which is generally considered conservative, or less than 3 percent). The OMB has historically recommended a discount rate that is based on the rate of return to private investment (which is generally considered to be an upper-bound for government projects, since the rate of return in the private sector is typically higher than that in the public sector). Until recently, when the rates were adjusted down, it recommended running analyses with discount rates up to 7 percent (Henrichson and Rinaldi 2014; Office of Management and Budget 2023). The Vera Institute for Justice does research and analysis on criminal justice policy; it typically uses a discount rate closer to 3 percent, which is on the lower end (Henrichson and Rinaldi 2014). It might also be safer to use a lower discount rate when projecting costs and benefits over long time horizons, as those values inevitably get more uncertain as the projections extend further out into the future (Livermore and Revesz 2020). Projects can also have very particular circumstances: if funding for a housing project would otherwise be sitting in an endowment fund earning 8 percent return, this could also be a reasonable discount rate for that project. Stokey and Zeckhauser (1978) designate the appropriate discount rate as the "weighted average of the rates of return for all of the displaced uses of funds" (p. 171). Therefore, it could be a summative value of several alternative investment mechanisms. An alternative perspective is that the discount rate should be more normative, or a "conscious value judgment as to the rate at which society wishes to trade-off future for present resources" (Stokey and Zeckhauser 1978: 173). For example, in guidelines from the Obama administration for calculating the social cost of carbon, a 3 percent discount rate was recommended to account for burdens placed on future generations (Livermore and Revesz 2020). This determination is likely dependent on the context or issue of concern (e.g., there will be different social trade-offs for protecting the environment than for preserving affordable housing). *Ultimately, if the net present value (NPV) is positive, the project is performing better than the alternative uses off of which the discount rate was based.*

Table 5.2 Applying the Discount Rate to Get Present Values

Year	Automatic Collection System	Targeted Workforce Development Program	Year	Automatic Collection System	Targeted Workforce Development Program
Discount rate: 3%			Discount rate: 7%		
0	$50,000,000	$0	0	$50,000,000	$0
1	$0	$18,000,000	1	$0	$18,000,000
2	$1,200,000	$18,540,000	2	$1,200,000	$18,540,000
3	$1,236,000	$19,096,200	3	$1,236,000	$19,096,200
4	$1,273,080	$19,669,086	4	$1,273,080	$19,669,086
5	$1,311,272	$20,259,159	5	$1,311,272	$20,259,159
Total	$55,020,352	$95,564,445	Total	$55,020,352	$95,564,445
PV	$54,524,460	$87,378,641	PV	$53,963,216	$78,054,123

Let us consider the present values for the two policy options when we apply two different discount rates.

We want to highlight three implications from the illustration. First, values itemized in year $t = 0$ are not discounted. Since these monies are expended or earned in the present, there is no need to adjust their time-value. The formula supports this: the denominator, $(1 + r)^0$, is equal to 1 (since anything raised to the "0" power is 1) and therefore does not impact the numerator, C_0.

Second, a higher discount rate means smaller present values. Table 5.3 is an example of a summary table that succinctly shows how PVs change across a wider range of discount rates.

The third implication is that as the analysis extends out in time (as t approaches k), the denominator grows. This means that costs, for example, included in later years are discounted more than earlier entries. Therefore, it is important to pay attention to the point at which costs are entered into the calculation of present value; it is not uncommon to "backload" big costs to shrink the present value of cost (since costs in later years are discounted more than those included in a year closer to $t = 0$). For example, Table 5.3 shows how increasing the discount rate changes the NPV differently across the two options. For the Automatic Collection System, the NPV goes down as the discount rate increases, but marginally so. In contrast, the decrease in NPV is much

Table 5.3 Summary Table of Present Values Across a Range of Discount Rates

Discount Rate	Automatic Collection System	Targeted Workforce Development Program
2%	$54,681,902	$89,982,443
3%	$54,524,460	$87,378,641
7%	$53,963,216	$78,054,123
10%	$53,604,088	$72,046,802

Table 5.4 Deferring Costs to Later Year

Year	Costs Up Front	Costs Deferred
	Automatic Collection System	Automatic Collection System
0	$50,000,000	$0
1	$0	$0
2	$1,200,000	$1,200,000
3	$1,236,000	$1,236,000
4	$1,273,080	$1,273,080
5	$1,311,272	$51,311,272
Total	$55,020,352	$55,020,352
PV	$54,524,460	$47,654,900

more dramatic for the Workforce Development option. This is due to the fact that the second option has bigger costs later on in time; therefore, those bigger values are discounted more when the discount rate increases. The Collection System option has costs later on, but they are much smaller in magnitude.

In addition, Table 5.4 illustrates, for the Automatic Collection System, the difference between (i) including a lot of costs up front and (ii) deferring those large up-front costs to $t = 5$. A discount rate of 3 percent is used.

We see that the present value of the costs decreases from nearly $55 million when there are large up-front costs at the outset to less than $48 million when they are delayed to Year 5. Ultimately, most important is that the timing of the costs in the expense schedule corresponds with the timing of when they actually take place in practice.

Voting Case: How to Value the Benefits of Voting

How Does One Value the Benefits of Voting?

Projecting the monetized costs of a voting intervention is relatively straightforward, compared with projecting the monetized benefits. How does one classify and then assign dollar values to the benefits of voting interventions, and voting more broadly? We consider here one particular area for increasing turnout: voter registration. See examples of monetizing costs and benefits in Tables 5.5 and 5.6.

What Is the Motivation for Voter Registration Policies?

The logic is simple: if more people are registered, then more people are likely to vote. Registration is the first hurdle in becoming an active participant in the electoral process, and if it cannot be overcome (or if there are large costs to overcoming it), then the opportunities to vote are diminished.

What Are the Ways to Affect Voter Registration?

Policies that address voter registration tend to focus on three aspects:

1 Refining and "cleaning" voter registration rolls
2 Growing registration rolls
3 Restricting registration rolls

While at least two of these strategies can be used to suppress voter participation, we will focus on one particular policy that aims to expand access to voting: online registration. Online voter registration allows individuals to register to vote via Internet-based systems. Advocates claim that it "saves taxpayer dollars, increases the accuracy of voter rolls, and provides a convenient option for Americans who wish to register or update their information" (The Pew Charitable Trusts 2014). Most systems, however, require some form of state government ID, since the electronic form is verified by state officials (MIT Election Lab 2023). Those skeptical of online registration are concerned about fraud and security threats. As of 2021, 40 states had or were in the process of building online registration systems (Brennan Center for Justice 2023); all had features to protect the information submitted and to verify the identity of the registrant (see The Pew Charitable Trusts' 2014 brief for more detail on typical system features).

What Costs Are Involved?

The costs of building and running online voter registration systems largely fall on state and local governments. There are all usually easy to monetize. They tend to involve the following (Choi et al. 2013):

- Setting up the online infrastructure: this includes the material (i.e., software), labor, and training costs of building the Internet-based system. These costs can be large but are one-time, initial expenditures.
- Maintaining the system: these costs are ongoing and variable, depending on the amount of labor required (i.e., number of personnel or hours logged) and the amount of other material inputs (like printing and software).
- Advertising and outreach: these costs are typically incurred over the initial year of the system's roll-out. The costs will be a function of the inputs (i.e., labor, materials) needed to reach the population of existing and potential registrants.

There could also be costs to users, in terms of learning about how to use the online system. These are not typically monetized in CBAs for these kinds of systems.

How Does One Value the Benefits of Voting?

What Are the Benefits?

The benefits accrued from Internet-based registration systems are typically valued as monetary savings, in terms of personnel, materials, and time, as follows:

- The government benefits from reduced printing costs (since much fewer paper registration forms are needed), savings in personnel's time spent on deciphering, entering, and correcting manually produced registration forms and a lower number of poll workers needed to address election-day registration issues.
- Individual registrants benefit from savings from not registering in person or via mail, both of which incur material and time costs.

What Is Missing?

As is the case with most CBAs, the monetized costs and benefits described earlier are incomplete. They cannot capture the full range of social costs and benefits associated with an online registration system. For example, it is difficult to assign dollar values to the following:

- The potential cost of fraudulent registrations;
- The potential costs from security breaches that compromise personal information;

- The benefits from enfranchisement and access to the electoral process; and
- The benefits from a more politically engaged electorate more broadly.

The analyst has several options for addressing these omissions:

- Capture them in more qualitative criteria.
- Consider the possibility that some or all of the monetized components of the CBA capture some of these social costs or benefits.
- Evaluate whether or not these social costs and benefits actually vary across the options being considered.

Table 5.5 Costs for Online Registration System

Infrastructure Set-up (Year 0)	Outreach (Year 1)	Maintenance (Annual, Decreases 5% per Year)	Infrastructure Update (Year 5)
$580,000	$650,000	Starting at $90,000	$200,000

Table 5.6 Calculating Present Value for Online Registration System

Year	Online Registration Costs	Year	Online Registration Costs	Year	Online Registration Costs
Discount rate: 1.5%		Discount rate: 4%		Discount rate: 6.5%	
0	$580,000	0	$580,000	0	$580,000
1	$740,000	1	$740,000	1	$740,000
2	$85,500	2	$85,500	2	$85,500
3	$81,225	3	$81,225	3	$81,225
4	$77,164	4	$77,164	4	$77,164
5	$273,306	5	$273,306	5	$273,306
Total	$1,837,194	Total	$1,837,194	Total	$1,837,194
PV	$1,796,134	PV	$1,733,394	PV	$1,676,921

CBA Introduced

It is rarely the case that governments or organizations are working with unlimited resources and timetables. They have to make choices about how to dedicate resources across policy options and over time. One of the most well-known tools to guide such decisions is CBA. CBA involves monetizing the costs and benefits of a project or endeavor and then comparing those values to see if the latter exceeds the former. CBA has become widespread since World War II (Stokey and Zeckhauser 1978). The use of CBA has been mandated by the US federal government, in one form or another, since the early 1980s.[2] Guidelines for US federal agencies conducting cost-benefit-analysis are promulgated in Circular A-4, which is updated periodically to reflect new priorities and practices in "standardizing the way benefits and costs of Federal regulatory actions are measured and reported" (Office of Management Budget 2023: 2).[3] A similar practice is present in most Western industrialized nations (Boardman et al. 2018). These days, CBA is used in and for a wide range of contexts and issues, including the following:

- motivating the adoption of regulatory policies;
- assessing the merits of criminal justice interventions; and
- investing in large-scale infrastructure and military defense projects.

CBA-like methods are embraced across the political and institutional spectrum: social return on investment (SROI) is a similar approach that has been applied to social impact investing. The Obama administration is known for implementing "cost-benefit progressivism"—applying cost-benefit principles and techniques to evaluating and furthering progressive policies and regulations (Livermore and Revesz 2020). Regardless of its orientation, CBA tends to lend itself to projects that require large up-front financial investments, have cost and revenue flows over a number of years (often decades), and involve both individual and social costs and benefits.

Conducting CBA is not a simple or straightforward task. We only scratch the surface in this chapter. CBA requires considerable technical and analytical expertise to carry it out in a comprehensive way. In the context of policy analysis, CBA is often used *ex ante*, or before any policies have actually been implemented, and therefore requires methods to deal with prediction and uncertainty. Program evaluation methods can sometimes use CBA in an *ex post* fashion, to assess how well a particular policy or intervention has performed in the past.

The fundamental model of CBA is intuitive and used widely. Indeed, policies that can be shown to achieve *both* efficiency and equity goals are often more viable (Vining and Weimer 2009). CBA is an important part of making the efficiency case. This chapter will provide enough guidance for creating basic CBAs, including how to discount and conduct CEAs. More importantly, this chapter will equip the analyst to understand and critique CBAs, such that he or she can be an informed *consumer* of the widely used tool.

In addition to covering the fundamentals of CBA, we consider its technical and ethical limitations and the challenges with applying it in a realistic way. We offer strategies for using CBA in the context of social justice issues and, more generally, for applying it flexibly. CBA is one of several evaluative components in an analysis, and we expect that it will be used to supplement, not replace, other criteria. We repeatedly return to the notion that "CBA is a 'decision tool, not a decision rule'" (Henrichson and Rinaldi 2014).

What Is CBA?

CBA is what the name implies: an assessment of the costs and benefits of a project. The costs are understood as resources employed and the benefits are the opposite, cost savings (or negative costs) (Patton et al. 2013: 194–195). Once the costs and benefits for a project have been determined (this process will be discussed in more detail later), the overall merits for the project are captured in the difference between those costs and benefits. CBA relies on a very intuitive formula:

Net Benefit = *Benefits* − *Costs*, or
$NB = B - C$

Comparing costs to benefits is not a novel idea; indeed, the stagist method that we have presented thus far essentially weighs the costs against the benefits for proposed policy options. The innovation of

CBA is that it relies entirely on monetizing the costs and benefits, or expressing everything in dollar terms. In monetizing costs and benefits, it collapses multiple criteria (like cost, effectiveness, and time) into a single metric, the net benefit. Therefore, the working equation for a CBA is this:

$$\$NB = \$B - \$C$$

We would then use the $\$NB$ to measure efficiency across the proposed policy options and, holding all else constant, select the option that maximizes the net benefit. This equation sets up a basic decision rule: proceed with the project if the net benefit is greater than zero. This indicates that, overall, the benefits of the option exceed the costs and that social welfare is improved compared to the status quo. If the net benefit is negative, then the costs exceed the benefits, and, using this decision criterion alone, the project is not worth pursuing. If the net benefit is zero, and all of the social costs and benefits are indeed included in the analysis, then there is no economic reason to move away from the status quo. There may be other non-economic reasons, though, and these are addressed later on in the chapter.

CBA has its roots in neoclassical economics. It builds on the assumption that governments have limited resources and they must make choices (about services, investments, policies) within these constraints. They must decide on how to allocate these limited resources across a multitude of policy and spending options. CBA is used to make sure this allocation is done as efficiently as possible (Boardman et al. 2018). As such, CBAs are often included in policy analysis as the key indicator of efficiency. Enthusiasts of CBA assert that it converts complex policies into an outcome (namely, money) that is universally understood and that facilitates the comparison of otherwise discrete options by using a common unit of analysis (i.e., dollars). Livermore and Revesz (2020) add that when regulations are justified by robust cost-benefit-analyses, it makes them harder to undo. Some also argue that CBA promotes democratic decision making, as it minimizes the "vagaries" of the political process (Boardman et al. 2018) and can be used to capture diffuse interests (Boardman et al. 2018: 43).

To understand the rationale behind CBA, one first needs to understand the concept of *Pareto efficiency*. An allocation of goods is *Pareto efficient* if there is no other alternative that would make at least one person better off without making anyone else worse off. Boardman et al. (2018) makes the point that theoretically this is a noble goal: "One would have to be malevolent not to want to achieve Pareto efficiency—why forgo gains to persons that would not inflict losses on other?" (p. 29). It turns out that this is an incredibly difficult condition to uphold. Indeed, Stiglitz (1998) talks about "near-Pareto" improvements, which bring benefits to a large group and costs to a narrowly defined group. Many policies achieve this less restrictive standard (but nevertheless are unachievable due to other government and political failures).

A less restrictive requirement, known as the *Kaldor Hicks criterion*, establishes the *potential* for compensating any losses. That is, an allocation can be efficient if those made worse off could be fully compensated for their losses. The key is that the compensation need not be expended but merely that the option to compensate exists (Stokey and Zeckhauser 1978). This criterion constitutes a core tenet of CBA and its suitability for assessing a project's efficient allocation of resources. In sum, as long as all inputs into the CBA are valued monetarily and include opportunity costs (or what is economically forgone in pursuing a particular option), a positive net benefit should indicate that the alternative is potentially *Pareto improving*.

CBA is an assessment of how an intervention affects aggregate social welfare. That is, it does not tell us anything about how resources are distributed or transferred across sub-groups, but only the overall allocative efficiency of the option. If the analysis produces a positive net benefit, then society overall is better off. However, the net benefit, in and of itself, does not show how resources were allocated to get to that outcome. We will address issues of distribution later in this chapter.

Executing a CBA follows a relatively consistent set of steps (Boardman et al. 2018):

1. Determine who or what has standing.
2. Identify which costs and benefits to include (and how they will be measured).

3 Assign monetary values to the costs and benefits.
4 Apply time value of money methods.
5 Use a decision criterion for moving forward.

Step 1: Determine Who or What Has Standing

We have mentioned the concept of standing before. When considering which criteria to include in the analysis in Chapter 4, the analyst first needed to assess which stakeholders or interests should be reflected. The same logic applies in the context of CBA. Before isolating which particular costs and benefits are included, the analyst needs to determine which individuals or entities "count" in the CBA. Whose benefits and costs will be counted when calculating the net benefit? Whose preferences should be included? Should the interests of future generations be counted? Should those of other countries, states, or cities be considered? For example, we distinguished between the federal government and the noncustodial parent, and how the former might not be directly relevant when assessing state-level policy solutions. In calculating the costs and benefits of a policy, should the children themselves be included as separate interests?

These are not trivial decisions. The omission (or inclusion) of particular stakeholders can dramatically change the magnitude and sign of the net benefit calculation. However, a clear delineation of who or what is counted is necessary mathematically, as the analyst needs to know which values to include or exclude. The determination of standing also makes a statement about which interests are most directly affected by the central problem (and, in turn, the proposed policies to address it) (Trumbell 1990). Whittington and MacRae (1986) argue that the determination of standing is a political and philosophical exercise, while others, like Zerbe (1991) and Sen (2001), say it entirely depends on legally enshrined rights. As we discuss in more detail, it is possible for a stakeholder to have standing in the overall analysis, but not in the CBA. There are myriad reasons why certain interests are better captured as non-monetized values.

Step 2: Identify Which Costs and Benefits to Include (and How They Will Be Measured)

Once standing has been established, the analyst needs to determine which costs and benefits to include for each relevant stakeholder. Who bears the costs and what forms do they take? Similarly, who reaps the benefits and through what means? It is likely that stakeholders face myriad costs and benefits: the key is to identify those with a connection to the problem at hand and the proposed solutions. Let us consider, again, the child support enforcement case. For alternatives that minimize the nonpayment of child support, the costs, for example, are borne by the government as the administrator and also by the noncustodial parent. Administrative costs include the very explicit outlays of material and personnel expenses. At the same time, the federal government could be saving costs from incarceration, should the noncustodial parent be able to successfully pay the child support. Are these included in the CBA? The noncustodial parent bears the explicit cost of the child support payment itself. However, these costs are also potentially benefits to the custodial parent and/or state government. So, are they included as costs or benefits, or both? We next present some things to consider when approaching these questions.

When determining costs and benefits, the analyst should keep three things in mind.

1 Costs and Benefits Can Be Both Internal and External to the Stakeholder

This idea is closely related to the concept of externalities. Costs can be borne solely by the individual engaging in some behavior, like someone who smokes cigarettes. Those individual actions, however, can also induce costs on people or places external to that person. The clearest example here is second-hand smoke. These are negative externalities, which have economic and social implications for overall welfare, and should be priced in addition to the internal costs. For these reasons, it is common to include both the internal (individually borne) and external costs in the CBA. For example, nonpayment of child support not only results in loss of income for the custodial family, but also costs to society and taxpayers in the form of incarceration for the noncustodial parent or social services to support children who have an absentee parent.

2 Costs and Benefits Can Be Both Primary and Secondary

The nature of the problem, and the proposed solutions, will never exist in a vacuum. Therefore, many costs and benefits will come directly out of the proposed intervention. For example, potential earnings (and increased ability to pay child support) from an option that supports employment prospects for noncustodial parents are primary effects. Still, there are myriad markets and stakeholders that are indirectly related to the central problem (and the proposed solutions). They too might experience *spillover* costs or benefits (sometimes referred to as "co-benefits") from the intervention under consideration (Boardman et al. 2018).

For example, the labor market (and economy) more broadly could reap benefits from investments in human capital or employment matching for unemployed noncustodial parents. These new participants in the labor market may make productive contributions, but how much? And how much of these contributions would have taken place in the absence of such an intervention? Another example is found at the U.S. Environmental Protection Agency (EPA). For decades, under both Republican and Democrat presidents, the EPA has accounted for co-benefits in their CBAs (with the exception of politically motivated lapses during the Trump administration). For example, Obama-era analyses of regulations to establish mercury and air toxicity standards found that the technologies in place to control mercury and toxic emissions would also meaningfully reduce other unhealthy particulates in the air. The EPA estimated that these co-benefits would save thousands of lives per year (Livermore and Revesz 2020). These are all secondary effects, since they are related to but distinct from the immediate focus of the emissions regulation under consideration.

There is no consensus on how to deal with secondary effects, as they are real but can be difficult to distinguish from primary effects. If the secondary effects cannot be convincingly separated from the primary ones, then the analysis is subject to *double counting* some of these overlapping costs and benefits. This is when the same cost or benefit is included more than once. This is an important concern, as double counting can significantly push the net benefit up or down (depending on whether the costs or benefits are being double-counted). The tendency is to double-count benefits, as to inflate the upside of the analysis. For this reason, analysts need to take care when including secondary effects, especially benefits. One pragmatic way to present the benefits is to bound the estimates with and without secondary effects, and to be transparent about which values might be unrealistically conservative or optimistically high.

3 Costs and Benefits Can Be Explicit and Implicit (Opportunity Cost)

Costs and benefits can be thought of in terms of explicit outlays or gains. These are consistent with the examples given thus far. Costs and benefits can also be expressed in terms of what is forgone, in the case of costs, or what is saved, in the case of benefits. Inevitably, when the government or the client decides to invest in one option, another option is forgone. There are costs to *not* doing something, and those are known as *opportunity costs*. For example, developing a piece of land into housing incurs an opportunity cost of forgoing any benefits associated with selling that piece of land. Likewise, moving forward with a new option can mean savings from discontinuing a current activity. As we mentioned earlier, policies that increase the likelihood of child support payment could reduce the likelihood of incarceration for the noncustodial parent and induce savings from reduced incarceration rates. Here the challenge is to determine which—of many—forgone options are included. In addition, the analysis itself is often comparing outcomes across a range of possible alternatives; therefore, the opportunity costs or savings of not doing one of the competing alternatives need not be included in the CBA of each alternative (as these relative costs and benefits will inherently be considered when comparing explicit costs or benefits across the proposed options).

As a general approach, we recommend first doing a thorough assessment of costs and benefits as they pertain to the status quo. What are the costs and benefits (and how are they distributed) without any proposed intervention? This creates a workable baseline off of which changes in costs and benefits can be estimated. In other words, the net benefit would be $0 for the status quo, since it does not involve any intervention or change in action. For each proposed policy, the analyst should take the same set of costs and benefits and determine if and how they change relative to current conditions. For example, there are already costs in place for administering child support compliance and collection—what *new* administrative costs would the alternative introduce?

Step 3: Assign Monetary Values to the Costs and Benefits

As we stated earlier, the crux of CBA is the monetization of costs and benefits. It converts otherwise irreconcilable inputs into a single denomination, allowing for consistent comparisons across the status quo and proposed policy options. Once the costs and benefits have been itemized, the next step is to assign dollar values to each of those inputs. The method assumes that individuals have well-defined preferences over policies (and their potential impacts) (Kornhauser 2001). This is perhaps the most controversial part of CBA, and the challenges with credibly and ethically monetizing costs and benefits will be discussed later in the chapter. Here we focus on the various strategies for assigning dollar values.

Box 5.3 Marginal Valuation

When valuing costs, it is important to distinguish between fixed and variable costs. Fixed costs are lump sums that do not vary with the amount of input (or in the case of benefits, output). Variable costs, however, change over the volume of inputs. For example, there is a variable cost associated with each child support case, and the total cost of the program would vary with the number of cases handled.

Therefore, in valuing costs and benefits, what is most relevant for the analyst is the *marginal* cost (benefit) for the input (output) of interest. To obtain the total cost, the *marginal* dollar amount is multiplied by the quantity or volume of the input/output of interest. For example, let's consider the proposed program in employment support services. First, the analyst knows that it costs $2,500 per year to provide those services to a single noncustodial parent. It is also projected that the proposed program will reach 6,000 noncustodial parents. Therefore, the projected cost is $2,500 * 6,000, or $15,000,000.

There are three main approaches to assigning dollar values to costs and benefits:

1. *Market prices*: if the cost or benefit is represented by a good or service that is actually transacted on the market, then the prices from actual transactions can be used. For example, purchase prices of healthy food could be used to value healthy eating. The assumption

here is that prices are revealed preferences and therefore the most direct representation of how a good or service is valued. There are two main drawbacks to this approach. First, finding market prices for inputs can be challenging, especially when working with services or goods that are not typically traded in a market (how do you monetarily value the time spent between a child and his or her parent?). Second, market prices will often not reflect social costs or benefits; indeed, government intervention is often motivated as a way to solve these "market failures."

2 *Shadow prices*: when there is no market for a good or service, analysts can proxy for this price with *shadow prices*. Specifically, analogous markets can be used to estimate monetary values for the good or service of interest. For example, if there is a public good or service that needs to be valued, there could be an analogous good or service that is transacted on the private market. If the government wanted to monetize the value of time saved in commuting from improved transportation investments, it could use wages from private sector jobs to capture gains in productivity. Or it could look at the difference in ticket costs of riding express versus local transportation. If a hospital wanted to monetize the value of patients living safely in their communities, it could use per diem costs of treatment that are avoided (what Weimer and Vining refer to as the "avoided cost method") (2009).

This approach is limiting in a number of ways. In order to implement shadow prices, the analyst usually has to make generalizations about how the prices apply to different subsets of affected individuals. For example, using wages to value time saved assumes that the trade-off between work and leisure is absolute (i.e., can people travel and work at the same time?) and that it is uniform across all wage levels and types of non-work activity. The marginal utility of that extra dollar earned could vary dramatically across classes of transportation users; that is, earning an additional dollar might matter more to someone earning a base rate of $10 per hour than someone earning $500 per hour. This discrepancy would not be reflected in a single wage number.

> **Box 5.4 Hedonic Price Models**
>
> Hedonic modeling (or regression analysis) is a method for valuing a good by breaking it down into its constituent characteristics.[4] It relies on revealed preferences to infer valuations of goods or services that are not typically transacted on the market (and therefore without prices attached). For example, it is commonly used for estimating the price of housing, and valuing the individual structural and locational characteristics of the home. The price of a home is dependent on structural features, like its size, number of bedrooms, age, and location, such as how close it is to neighborhood amenities or whether it is on a noisy block. If the analyst has information on the price of the home and the presence and nature of the structural and locational features, then the regression analysis will estimate the contributing price of each structural and locational feature into the aggregate price. An analogous approach is also used in other contexts (Weimer and Vining 2011), such as the following:
>
> - valuing life using risk-wage trade-offs;
> - valuing the quality of public schools; and
> - valuing inter-city salary discrepancies due to differences in quality of life.
>
> The data and computational demands for a credible hedonic analysis are substantial, as the analyst needs the previous information over a reasonably sized sample. It also assumes that individuals are aware of the value of the component characteristics and incorporate them into the aggregate pricing of the good. It does, however, offer a useful conceptual framework for thinking about how to value both tangible characteristics (like the square footage of a home) and intangible characteristics (like proximity to public transit).

3. *Contingent valuation.* Contingent prices are actually a kind of shadow price, in that they are used when market prices are not available. Instead of observing valuations through the market, contingent prices are obtained through surveys. The surveys set up hypothetical situations and respondents have to answer questions to reveal their willingness-to-pay (WTP). For example, a scenario would be described—such as the possibility of having trash picked up twice a week (instead of once a week)—and then the survey

would ask something like: *if the increase in taxes would be $100 per year, would you support this change in service?* The survey would, in different versions, ask about different tax increases to see how responses vary.

These surveys are usually used as a final resort, when there is no credible information from the market to inform valuation. The surveys are designed to elicit people's WTP under certain scenarios, and particularly under circumstances of changing quality or quantity (Boardman et al. 2018). These WTPs are collected and then extrapolated to represent valuations across the broader population.

There are a number of limitations with the contingent valuation approach. First and foremost, the accuracy of the values depends on the accuracy of the respondents in estimating their WTP under hypothetical circumstances. Any error in the response could be due to a number of factors, including, but not limited to, how the question is framed, how the respondent personally interprets the hypothetical scenario, an unwitting tendency to overestimate WTP in the context of theoretical options, or a strategic underestimation of WTP to avoid potential burdens in the future. Posner (2001) summarizes Amartya Sen's apt description of the challenge in this way:

> [W]e do not buy endangered species the way we buy toothpaste, and so while asking a person what he would pay for a tube of toothpaste will elicit a meaningful answer, asking him what an endangered species is worth to him will not.
>
> (p. 341)

Second, WTP could be different than willingness-to-accept (WTA) the loss of something or the willingness-to-sell (WTS) (Boardman et al. 2018; Kelman 1992). For example, the WTP to live in a particular neighborhood could be very different than the WTS for a long-standing home in that same neighborhood. The former valuation is unlikely to capture the intangible value of community ties that is embodied in the latter valuation. This is consistent with a body of evidence from behavioral economics that shows that the same item tends to be valued more highly when presented as a loss than when it is framed as a gain (Sunstein 2014).

Finally, if the project under consideration has an extended lifespan, then the analyst has to also consider how these values might change over time. For example, if the CBA is assessing the economic viability of building a bridge or a housing project, both the costs and benefits can change over time. Maintenance costs could increase over time as the structure ages. If the project earns income, say from tolls or rents, then those rates could change over time as well, as the demand for and use of the infrastructure increases. Projecting these changes into the future is subject to great uncertainty. Therefore, it is wise to implement *sensitivity analyses* (discussed in more detail next) to test how the NPV changes in the context of more modest or dramatic changes over time.

Step 4: Apply Time Value of Money Methods

The goal of CBA is to collapse flows of monetized costs and benefits into a single value (NPV) that can be compared across options. The value of money, however, is not constant over time, and this variation needs to be accounted for in the collapsed calculation of NPV. This concept, discussed at the beginning of this chapter, is known as *time value of money*, and the method for accounting for it is known as *discounting*. This correction is even more important for projects that have different lifespans—it facilitates the comparison between a 10-year project and a 25-year project.

To convert the inputs of CBA to present values, we build off of the cost-benefit formula presented earlier:

$$\$NB = \$B - \$C$$

In order to account for time value of money, we augment the formula for net benefit in the following way:

$$\$NPV = \text{PV}(\text{Benefits}) - \text{PV}(\text{Costs}) = \text{PV}(B) - \text{PV}(C)$$

where

$$PV(B) = \sum_{t=0}^{k} \frac{B_t}{(1+r)^t}$$

$$PV(C) = \sum_{t=0}^{k} \frac{C_t}{(1+r)^t}$$

Here, B are the benefits in time t and C are the costs in time t, where t ranges from 0 to k. The benefits and costs are adjusted down by the *discount rate* (r). *NPV* is the discounted version of the unadjusted net benefit. As with net benefit, if *NPV* is positive, then the discounted benefits exceed the discounted costs; if *NPV* is negative, then the costs exceed the benefits.

Let's consider again the following policy options and their respective costs (the discount rate is still 3 percent). Table 5.7 presents the program costs again.

CSE policies often undergo CBAs, and the primary benefit of interest is typically the child support collections themselves. In the case of improved automated collection, increased collections occur primarily through efficiencies in processing times, which result in more rapid collections (and higher collection amounts accrued over time). In the case of workforce development programs, increased collections occur primarily through improvements in the noncustodial parent's ability to pay (and the collection of payments that were previously delinquent).

Table 5.7 Costs for Child Support Enforcement Alternatives

Year	Automatic Collection System	Targeted Workforce Development Program
0	$50,000,000	$0
1	$0	$18,000,000
2	$1,200,000	$16,200,000
3	$1,236,000	$14,580,000
4	$1,273,080	$13,122,000
5	$1,311,272	$11,809,800
Total	$55,020,352	$73,711,800
PV	$54,524,460	$67,934,512

Table 5.8 Costs and Benefits for Child Support Enforcement Alternatives

Year	Costs (i.e., administrative)		Benefits (i.e., child support collection)	
	Automatic Collection System	Targeted Workforce Development Program	Automatic Collection System	Targeted Workforce Development Program
0	$50,000,000	$0	$0	$0
1	$0	$18,000,000	$13,000,000	$15,000,000
2	$1,200,000	$16,200,000	$13,130,000	$13,500,000
3	$1,236,000	$14,580,000	$13,261,300	$12,150,000
4	$1,273,080	$13,122,000	$13,393,913	$10,935,000
5	$1,311,272	$11,809,800	$52,785,213	$9,841,500
Total	$55,020,352	$73,711,800	$105,570,426	$61,426,500
PV	$54,524,460	$67,934,512	$94,566,918	$56,612,093

These collections are monetary benefits directly accrued by the state but also, indirectly, by the noncustodial parent and child. Like the costs, these benefits can fluctuate over time. Table 5.8 is an example of how those benefits might be projected in the proposed policy options.

Table 5.9 adds in a column for net benefit and calculates the NPV for each option. First, you can see that while the total net benefit is negative for the Automatic Collection System, the discounted net present value is positive due to enough benefits in the early years that do not get discounted by much. The net present value of the Workforce Development program, however, is still negative even after discounting, given the persistent negative net benefits over time.

Recall two important features of discounting. First, a higher discount rate means smaller present values. Therefore, assuming that benefits and costs are distributed evenly across the lifetime of the project, higher discount rates will make it harder to achieve positive NPVs (which, holding all else constant, indicate a more beneficial policy option). Second, as the analysis extends out in time (as t approaches k), the denominator grows. This means that benefits and costs included in later years are discounted more than earlier entries. Therefore, it is important to pay attention to the point at which benefit and costs are entered into the CBA; it is not uncommon to "backload" costs and "frontload" benefits in order to inflate the NPV (since the former would be discounted more

Table 5.9 Net Benefits for CSE Alternatives

Year	Costs		Benefits		Net Benefit	
	Automatic Collection System	Targeted Workforce Development Program	Automatic Collection System	Targeted Workforce Development Program	Automatic Collection System	Targeted Workforce Development Program
0	$50,000,000	$0	$0	$0	—$50,000,000	$0
1	$0	$18,000,000	$13,000,000	$15,000,000	$13,000,000	—$3,000,000
2	$1,200,000	$16,200,000	$13,130,000	$13,500,000	$11,930,000	—$2,700,000
3	$1,236,000	$14,580,000	$13,261,300	$12,150,000	$12,025,300	—$2,430,000
4	$1,273,080	$13,122,000	$13,393,913	$10,935,000	$12,120,833	—$2,187,000
5	$1,311,272	$11,809,800	$52,785,213	$9,841,500	$51,473,941	—$1,968,300
Total	$55,020,352	$73,711,800	$52,785,213	$61,426,500	—$2,235,139	—$12,285,300
PV	$54,524,460	$67,934,512	$94,566,918	$56,612,093	$40,042,458	—$11,322,419

Table 5.10 Delayed Costs and Up-Front Benefits

Year	Costs Targeted Workforce Development Program	Benefits Targeted Workforce Development Program	Net Benefit Targeted Workforce Development Program
0	$0	$0	$0
1	$0	$38,085,000	$38,085,000
2	$0	$23,341,500	$23,341,500
3	$0	$0	$0
4	$47,322,000	$0	—$47,322,000
5	$26,389,800	$0	—$26,389,800
Total	$73,711,800	$61,426,500	—$12,285,300
PV	$64,809,057	$58,977,331	—$5,831,727

than the latter). For example, consider what happens to the NPV for the workforce development option when costs are delayed to Years 4 and 5 and benefits are moved up to Years 2 and 3. See Table 5.10.

The net benefit is still negative but half the magnitude (indicating it is more favorable than it was before).

Discounting in the Context of CBA Raises Some Questions

1. Should all inputs into the CBA be subject to the same discount rate? For example, should costs and benefits be discounted in the same way? Should costs and benefits to the public and private sectors be discounted in the same way?
2. Should the discount rate be applied to goods and services not traded in a market? For example, how does one discount the value of good health or risk of death? Are the preferences of future generations accurately represented in today's market-based discount rates?
3. How far out in time can the analyst realistically predict (and discount)? How robust are discount rates over time? Is it right to discount costs and benefits further out in time more than more immediate costs?

These are not easy questions to answer but should be considered up against the popularity of the tool. Many of these questions raise normative issues, rather than technical ones. This is another reason why CBA should not be misrepresented as an impartial scientific method.

Sensitivity Analyses

The CBA is only as good as the assumptions behind it. The analyst will inevitably need to make decisions about which inputs to include, and consensus on these assumptions across all parties involved is unlikely. Rather than relying on a single set of assumptions and inputs as absolute, we recommend that the analyst employ sensitivity analyses to *bound* the results of the CBA. The resulting NPV will therefore be a range of values, reflecting various sets of assumptions and inputs, rather than a single "truth."

Sensitivity analyses entail running CBAs for various scenarios, where the analyst changes one or more variables. It is unwise to vary more than one input at a time for sensitivity analyses, so that any resulting change in the NPV is clearly linked to the adjusted input. Based on the formula presented earlier, there are four variables that can change in the analysis: benefits (B), costs (C), time (or t, the number of years over which the analysis is projected), and the discount rate (r).

Changing the benefits or costs could involve running versions where certain benefits or costs are included or excluded or where different rates of change over time are tested. Since NPV is a function of money flows over time, changing the time period over which the analysis is conducted can also produce different results. Finally, testing the sensitivity of the analysis to various discount rates can be important in demonstrating how vulnerable the outcome is to fluctuations in conditions external to the project itself.

Box 5.5 Internal Rate of Return

Internal rate of return (IRR) is a metric often used to capture the yield of an investment. Specifically, it is the discount rate at which the investment breaks even, or where the discounted value of the costs equals the discounted value of the benefits (i.e., NPV = 0). When there is only one option under consideration other than the status quo, the IRR can be used as a decision criterion: the proposed project should proceed if the IRR is less than the designated discount rate. Why? Because the project should only be pursued if it offers a rate of return that is greater than what would be produced by investing the same

> money in some other productive venture (as captured by the discount rate). It is not recommended that the IRR be used as a stand-alone criterion, but it can be a useful benchmark for considering how sensitive the results are to the discount rate (Boardman et al. 2018; Stokey and Zeckhauser 1978).

How can the analyst decide on which factors to vary for the sensitivity analyses? It is usually most prudent to test different scenarios for the inputs that are most controversial or tenuous. This is almost always the case with the discount rate, since it is usually based off of some expectation about the future performance of an investment or market. Does the project become infeasible if market conditions change and push the discount rate down? How favorable would conditions need to be (i.e., how high would the discount rate need to be) to see a positive NPV? Sensitivity analyses are a way to answer these questions. For example, if a project's CBA produces a very negative NPV, it is a useful exercise to determine the discount rate at which the analyses would break even (or produce an NPV = 0). This rate, also known as the internal rate of return (IRR), is a useful benchmark for the client to understand what kinds of assumptions would need to be made in order to make the project economically efficient. For example, if a CBA produces an IRR of 15 percent, then the project is likely infeasible: it would reach a break-even point only if 15 percent were a credible return for alternative investments.

Sensitivity analyses are most succinctly displayed in matrices that show a range of NPVs for different values of the inputs being varied. Table 5.11 shows different NPVs for a range of discount rates:

Table 5.11 NPVs for a Range of Discount Rates

Discount Rate	Automatic Collection System	Targeted Workforce Development Program
2%	$43,362,860	-$11,629,375
3%	$40,042,458	-$11,322,419
7%	$28,333,017	-$10,217,449
10%	$20,952,431	-$9,500,283

Table 5.12 NPVs for a Range of Growth Rates

Cost Growth Rate	Automatic Collection System
0%	$40,236,318
3%	$40,042,458
5%	$39,908,963

Another point of contention might be the rate at which any input changes over time. For example, thus far we have assumed an annual growth in collection benefits of 1 percent in the automated collection option. What happens when we assume no growth—or more growth? For example, if costs actually grow at 5 percent per year instead of 3 percent, the NPV is only marginally lower (see Table 5.12). Similarly, a no-growth assumption yields a marginally higher NPV. This suggests that the outcome of the CBA is not highly sensitive to these growth assumptions, mostly because the benefits so far exceed the costs.

Certain benefits or costs could also be subject to criticism, and the analyst would be wise to run CBAs with and without those controversial inputs. For example, what happens to the NPVs when benefits accrued to other government agencies are included? In the end, the goal is not a definitive, singular NPV. Rather, the analyst should aim to gain an understanding of how the NPV fluctuates should central assumptions or conditions change, and especially, should they become less favorable.

Step 5: Use a Decision Criterion for Moving Forward

The results of the CBA can be applied in two ways. Oftentimes, the client comes to the table with pre-determined thresholds beyond which the project is not economically feasible. That is, the goal of the CBA is to determine whether or not the flow of revenues (benefits) over time justify the up-front investment that is being offered by the client (or some other investor). Therefore, the first way to apply CBA is to require that the NPV be positive, regardless of how it compares to the NPV of competing options, in order to move forward. In other words, the discounted flow of revenues needs to exceed the up-front costs. All else equal, the analyst would recommend options with a positive NPV.

Box 5.6 What is a Benefit-Cost Ratio?

A benefit-cost ratio (BCR) is another way to represent the NPV for a project. It is calculated as

$PV(B)/PV(C)$

Like NPV, it is a numerical expression of whether or not benefits exceed the costs. When benefits are greater than costs, the ratio will exceed 1. When the costs and benefits are equal, the ratio will be equal to 1. And when the benefits are smaller than the costs, the ratio will be less than 1. It is an accessible, succinct indicator for assessing the economic viability of a project. However, the BCR can obscure the absolute magnitude of the net benefit, which can have important practical implications.

Consider two scenarios.

In **Scenario A**, $PV(B) = \$300$ and $PV(C) = \$50$.

Therefore:

$BCR = PV(B)/PV(C) = \$300/\$50 = 6$
$NPV = PV(B) - PV(C) = \$300 - \$50 = \$250$

In **Scenario B**, $PV(B) = \$50,000$ and $PV(C) = \$25,000$. Therefore:

$BCR = PV(B)/PV(C) = \$50,000/\$25,000 = 2$
$NPV = PV(B) - PV(C) = \$50,000 - \$25,000 = \$25,000$

If we rely on the BCR alone, we would opt to move forward with Scenario A, which has the bigger BCR. However, the NPV for Scenario B is 100 times bigger. The larger NPV could mean that we should move forward with Scenario B.

Return on investment (ROI) is an alternative to the BCR that compares *net benefit* to the total amount invested in the project. It is calculated as a ratio between the two ($NPV/PV(C)$), and is typically expressed as a percentage.

For example, the ROI for Scenario A would be

$\$250/\$50 = 6$, or 600%.

Like the BCR, if the ROI is positive, then the project should be considered.

A second way to view the CBA is as one of several criteria in the analytical matrix we established in Chapter 4. This means that the NPV is a measure to be calculated and then compared across the proposed policy options. Therefore, the preferred policy option is not necessarily based on a positive NPV, but rather the highest NPV among all of the options. This is an important distinction, because a project could produce a negative NPV but still possess the highest NPV relative to the other competing options (if all of them produce negative NPVs). When CBA is used as one of several decision criteria, a positive NPV may not be necessary or sufficient; other, qualitative criteria may capture aspects (especially benefits) that are not monetized in the CBA, making the negative NPV less deterministic.

Why CBA Is Hard to Do in Practice

Like other economistic decision-making models that we've already discussed, the rationale and structure of CBA is straightforward and appealing in how it collapses benefits and costs into succinct dollar values. It turns out, however, that implementing CBA in practice is quite challenging. The technical aspects of assigning dollar amounts are often extremely complex and the assumptions that undergird the CBA are often unrealistic and questionable in their fairness. In addition, when faced with tight timelines, analysts often cannot access the information or resources necessary to complete robust CBAs. CBAs can take a long time and can be very expensive to complete. Here we discuss the main reasons why CBA is difficult to put into practice. Our goal is not to discourage, wholesale, the use of CBA. Rather, we aim to bring to the forefront the limitations so that CBAs can be implemented and consumed with the right degree of skepticism. At the very least, analysts should be prepared to critically assess and apply CBAs produced by others.

Justifying the Assumptions

In their book on policy analysis, Stokey and Zeckhauser (1978) state that CBAs can be "no more precise than the valuations and assumptions that they employ" (p. 135). Therefore, the credibility of the CBA will depend entirely on how convincingly inputs are motivated and calculated. By "assumption," we mean the parameters of the analysis that are set at the get-go, that are taken as given. For example, the discount rate is a critical assumption, as is the time period over which the analysis is conducted. We've discussed how changes in the discount rate can alter the NPV significantly. Discounting in general also trivializes long-term impacts and ignores the possibility of irreversible, permanent harm (for example, to the environment) (Ackerman and Heinzerling 2004). Decisions about how inputs vary (or don't vary) over time are also assumptions. Moreover, *when* in the timeline benefits and costs are included is a critical component, and one that is often unpredictable as the time period extends farther and farther out.

The credibility of the CBA's assumptions is further complicated by the fact that "credible" and "reasonable" can mean different things to different people. CBA is often presented as an objective approach to valuing costs and benefits. CBA is actually subjective to the orientation of the analyst (and the client for whom the analysis is being conducted). Stone (2012), in her critique of the rational decision-making framework, relies heavily on this point. According to her, efficiency is a "contestable concept" where the underlying assumptions are typically political moves rather than technical claims. Livermore and Revesz (2020) provide a contemporary example of this by documenting the manipulation of CBA assumptions during the Trump administration in order to weaken environmental regulations to benefit certain political and industry interests. In the polis (Stone's political counterpoint to the economic market), information is manipulated and deliberately obscured and no exchange is voluntary—coercion is pervasive. Therefore, assumptions entirely depend on who is making them and to what end.

Therefore, informed consumers and purveyors of CBAs have a responsibility to interrogate the assumptions and interpret the results in light of how realistic they are.

Is It Possible to Put a Dollar Amount on Priceless Things?

As we discussed earlier, the central tenet of CBA is the assignment of dollar values to the benefits and costs. When the CBA involves valuing items or services that are commonly traded on the market, the valuation is more straightforward. However, when projects require the valuation of costs and benefits that are not typically transacted, the numbers become more tenuous. Indeed, CBA systematically disfavors inputs, typically benefits, that cannot be accurately priced (Ackerman and Heinzerling 2004). For example, in the case of interventions to increase voter turnout, how does one value the benefits associated with going to the polls?

Perhaps even more controversial is the valuation of things that are inherently *priceless*. In these cases, putting a dollar amount on something, like a human life, is so often farfetched that any value, however well-reasoned it may be, is without credibility. It also challenges what is ethically and philosophically acceptable (Nussbaum 2001; Kelman 1992). Similarly, Nussbaum argues that there are certain "tragic" costs, like constitutional violations, that no one should ever be expected to bear—these cannot be offset by any valuation of benefits.

Box 5.7 Valuing Human Life

One of the most controversial aspects of CBA is how to monetize the value of human life. How does one put a dollar amount on a person's worth? Not only is the question morally uncomfortable, but it is also very difficult to answer empirically. There is great variation in how individuals live their lives, both professionally and personally. The latter is particularly difficult to capture monetarily. However, many policies and regulations are designed to save lives and therefore rely on their valuation.

Actual lives versus statistical lives: in the context of CBA, the value of life itself is different than the value of what is known as "statistical life" (Ackerman and Heinzerling 2004; Sunstein 2014). The valuation of "statistical life" is based on the WTP to avoid particular risks. Therefore, in theory, the valuation of "statistical life" should vary in two ways: across risks and then across individuals, who will be willing to pay different amounts to avoid similarly risky situations.

How does one go about valuing life? There are several approaches to assigning a dollar amount to a human life, all flawed in some way (Ackerman and Heinzerling 2004).

- Surveys on attitudes towards risks: these are usually asked with respect to risks for the individual being surveyed and not to risks for others.

- Future earnings: this approach implies that those with the potential to earn more should be worth more.
- Wage-risk analysis: this approach infers value of life from the extra earnings acquired through riskier jobs (and assumes job choices accurately reflect the valuation of life).
- Contingent valuation: individuals are asked to place a dollar value on the risk of dying (usually under hypothetical scenarios). This approach is vulnerable to the criticisms of contingent valuation discussed earlier.

According to Sunstein (2014), contemporary US regulatory policy largely relies on the first strategy (risk valuation) and uses a single valuation for life, regardless of the individual's age, race, gender, socioeconomic class, or any other defining feature.

In their book titled *Priceless*, Frank Ackerman and Lisa Heinzerling (2004) describe this scenario in the following way:

> When the question is whether to allow one person to hurt another, or to destroy a natural resource; when a life or landscape cannot be replaced; when harms stretch out over decades or even generations; when outcomes are uncertain; when risks are shared or resources are used in common; when the people "buying" harms have no relationship with the people actually harmed—then we are in realm of the priceless, where market values tell us little about the social values at stake.
>
> (pp. 8–9)

The term "nonuse value" is used to describe entities that cannot be monetized, for their mere being is the benefit (or potential loss) to be assigned a dollar value rather than any direct use. Indeed, people may be willing to pay for the existence of some things, but won't ever actually "consume" or experience them (Boardman et al. 2018: 339). Types of "nonuse values" include (Ackerman and Heinzerling 2004) the following.

- Existence value: the value of knowing that a special place or resource exists, even if no one uses it;

- Option value: the value of knowing that the opportunity, or option, exists to use a resource in the future;
- Bequest value: the value of being able to pass natural resources to future generations.

Therefore, gleaning prices from market transactions, or even behavioral responses more generally, is difficult. Complicating the valuation of these kinds of goods is the fact that people *can* actively consume them while at the same time passively valuing the preservation of the good for future generations (Boardman et al. 2018: 340). The environment, broadly, is a perfect example of something that cannot be priced, but yet possesses great value to society at large. Similarly, how can the analyst value the presence of and love from a parent for a child? True, one could use "avoided" health care costs for psychological trauma or educational costs for behavioral counseling, but it is more likely than not that these grossly underestimate the "existence value" of family connection and support.

Who Gets Counted?

Before implementing a CBA, the analyst needs to identify *which* costs and benefits are included in the analysis. This is not a simple decision and can have significant implications for the outcome of the CBA. In addition, costs and benefits may entirely depend on who is included—that is, what is considered a cost to one stakeholder could be a benefit to another. If both are included, how should those tensions be treated? Whose interests are reflected in the analysis? Do they perfectly balance one another out, or is one stakeholder's experience of an item's cost valued differently than another stakeholder's experience of the same item as a benefit? For example, should child support collections be included as a benefit to the state (or custodial parent) or as a cost to the noncustodial parent?

Uncertainty in Forward-Looking CBAs

In policy analysis, CBA is usually conducted *ex ante*, or before any project or policy has actually been implemented. Therefore, valuations are predicted, with some degree of uncertainty—and the uncertainty likely increases as the time horizon extends farther and farther out. Some level of uncertainty is unavoidable in the context of CBAs, since the analyst is essentially predicting the future based on information from past events. Furthermore, oftentimes predictions are based on past experiences with similar, but not identical, circumstances or technologies.

In their book *Cost-Benefit Analysis*, Boardman et al. (2018) identify four main types of errors that emerge out of CBA studies. The common thread through these categories of error is that the direction of the bias is unclear. As we've discussed in the context of criteria in Chapter 4, when there is error in the analysis (which there inevitably will be), the best that the analyst can do is understand the direction (and magnitude) of that error so that the options can still be ranked relative to one another. If the direction and severity of the error are unclear, then the outcome of the CBA is more vulnerable to criticism.

1 Omission error: this occurs when the analyst leaves out a cost or benefit because it is too unlikely to occur or its potential impact is under dispute. Not only is the item omitted, but it is unclear how the omission would affect the final NPV—that is, does it bias it up or down? It is expected that these kinds of errors are more prevalent for cost and benefit estimates further out.
2 Forecasting error: this kind of error usually results from complexity or changes in technologies and behavioral responses over time. In these cases it is difficult to credibly predict responses to interventions beyond a short time horizon, because the "cause-and-effect" mechanism gets increasingly intricate. Boardman et al. (2018: 183) warn that analysts often deal with such uncertainties by relying on cognitive biases that influence them to weigh low probability "good" events more than low probability "bad" events. These kinds of calculations can make a project very vulnerable should unlikely, but consequential, events overwhelm the predicted flow of benefits.
3 Valuation error: even when there are prices to value costs or benefits, the estimates of such prices can vary tremendously. Picking one value, or reconciling several, can introduce error into the calculation (and, again, the direction of the error is unclear).
4 Measurement error: in many instances, costs and benefits are relatively easier to extrapolate from other projects or interventions

(especially those that induce similar impacts). However, even when impacts from other scenarios have been estimated and valued, they can often be measured with error. For example, continued increases in child support collection rates have been accompanied by persistent declines in the welfare rolls. It is possible that the two are related: in other words, those leaving the welfare rolls could have been those least likely to pay.

Using CBA Flexibly and Pragmatically

It is clear that CBA can be controversial. Even though it is presented as an objective tool to facilitate the weighing of costs and benefits across policy options, it can easily be influenced by rigid and unrealistic assumptions and can be vulnerable to the analysts' biases as well as unintended measurement error. We discuss in this section approaches for using CBA flexibly and pragmatically. Livermore and Revesz (2020) aptly describe CBA as a set of "guardrails." CBA doesn't eliminate policy discretion, but rather it provides standards and value benchmarks to make sure it doesn't get bent towards certain political pressures or interests. It can be an informative part of a broader, multi-faceted analysis, but it should rarely be the only tool. Indeed, there are usually costs and benefits that cannot be credibly monetized, and these should be accounted for in other ways.

It is important to keep in mind that, in the world of policy, many people think in terms of dollars and cents; therefore it is often compelling to be able to convey the benefits and costs in that way. Governments, like private companies, want to know about a program's return on investment. Cass Sunstein, who is famous for applying behavioral economics and psychological frames to regulatory policy design and evaluation, promotes a "humanized" version of CBA. He argues that CBA is an effective method for "putting 'on screen' important social facts that might otherwise escape public and private attention." He asserts that CBA can facilitate "priority-setting," to "ensure sensible balancing and not to efface qualitative differences" across options (Sunstein 2001: 224; Sunstein 2014: 173). Sunstein (2014) stresses the importance of understanding the *human* response to policies (as opposed to the rational actor's response), which involves capturing the non-quantifiable things and learning from the individuals whom the policy intends to serve. As an approach, CBA should not be ruled out. However, it should be used with care and context.

Dealing With Uncertainty by Bounding the CBA Outcomes

The analyst's goal should be twofold with respect to uncertainty: minimize it as best possible, and be transparent about it. One strategy for achieving these two goals is the *bounding* of NPV. Bounding involves projecting NPV under various conditions and then using the different values produced to construct a range of NPVs (instead of a single estimate). Specifically, if a particular assumption about one of the costs is knowingly conservative, the resulting NPV would be considered an *upper bound*: if costs turn out to be higher than assumed, the NPV would actually be lower. Likewise, if a particular assumption is aggressive, the resulting NPV would be considered a *lower bound*: if costs turn out to be lower than assumed, the NPV would actually be higher. For example, if the potential growth of collections is uncertain, the analyst could bound the collection benefits between amounts based on no growth ($PV(B) = \$59,500,000$) and 3 percent growth ($PV(B) = \$63,100,000$).

Another version of a bounding exercise is "break-even analysis." This tool is often used when certain benefits cannot be quantified and included in the CBA. Instead, given the monetized costs, it is possible to put a number on the benefits that would be needed to justify those costs of the proposed regulation or policy. For example, if it is known that it would cost $10 million to save 50 acres of marshland, then the benefit of an acre of preserved marshland would need to be at least $200,000 (adapted from Livermore and Revesz 2020). At a minimum, this provides a magnitude of benefit that may be easier to comprehend and assess as achievable than a precise dollar valuation.

Bounding is a pragmatic and transparent way to deal with inputs that are difficult to quantify or that are subject to controversy (Sunstein 2014: 173). If clients are provided with a range of values, and the assumptions that undergird them, then they can proceed with the number with which they feel most comfortable. These "conditional justifications," as Sunstein (2014) labels them (p. 81), are meant to promote accountability about what information is missing.

Testing for Distributive Effects

One of the most pervasive critiques of CBA is that it leaves out "distributive justice" (Posner 2001)—that certain individuals or groups may disproportionately bear the burdens (or enjoy the benefits) more than others. Moreover, individuals and groups may value risk and opportunity differently (compared to each other and compared to the analyst conducting the CBA) (Ackerman and Heinzerling 2004; Richardson 2001). Indeed, Ackerman and Heinzerling (2004) observe that "[i]f decisions were based strictly on cost-benefit analysis and willingness to pay, most environmental burdens would end up being imposed on the countries, communities, and individuals with the least resources" (p. 151). CBA is not traditionally used for assessing fairness or equity.

Sunstein (2014), in reference to distributive CBAs, affirms that "[t]he virtue of this formulation is that it is uncontentious; the vice is that it is vacuous" (p. 253). CBAs can be constructed to account for distributive effects, but, as Sunstein and others suggest (Stokey and Zeckhauser 1978; Boardman et al. 2018), it is a tricky proposition. Two of the most common ways to technically implement this are (i) to stratify the CBAs along some dimension that captures group differences and then run the CBAs separately for each group or (ii) to assign weights to certain inputs depending on the group to which they are attributed. Economists argue that any weights or stratification should link back to differences in income or wealth, since these factors will track disparities in how different groups value the goods and services that are included in the CBA.

While these approaches make sense in theory, they are controversial to implement. Most significantly, choices about the strata or weights are arbitrary at best or distortionary at worst. For example, if weights were based on WTP, then more affluent individuals or groups would be weighted more (Sunstein 2014). This is certainly not a more equitable outcome. Therefore, Sunstein makes the case that unweighted CBAs could reasonably be used if uniform calculations (i.e., those without any weights) would benefit the poor. Weights may also be hard to justify given the existing evidence on the topic, or they may just be too administratively burdensome to include (Sunstein 2014: 109). Moreover, how are projects evaluated if distributional outcomes point towards a different policy solution that those that are efficiency oriented? Which goal takes priority? A more agnostic, and illustrative, approach is to simply present the CBAs across the different groups without any attempt to reconcile them. As a piece of information, understanding how net benefits might vary across groups could be very valuable for the client. For example, the analyst may be concerned with the distribution of benefits and costs across families by race or ethnicity, or across geographic locations (i.e., rural versus urban). In sum, within the CBA framework it *is* possible to model distributive effects, but the methods and assumptions are often tenuous and subjective.

An Alternative to CBA: Cost-Effectiveness Analysis

An alternative, less restrictive method for assessing costs against benefits is cost-effectiveness analysis (CEA). Instead of monetizing both benefits and costs, this method monetizes costs and tracks benefits only in terms of metrics of "success." Most directly, this approach addresses the inherent difficulty with putting a dollar amount on benefits. CEA is still a means of assessing efficiency, but it captures "technical efficiency," or how productive each dollar of investment can be, rather than "allocative efficiency," which assesses marginal costs against benefits and is better captured in a CBA (Boardman et al. 2018: 511). Therefore, CEA can be used to rank options in terms of how outcomes are achieved relative to the costs invested; however, it cannot, like CBA, determine whether something is economically "worth" doing. CEA also focuses on one benefit at a time, rather than bundling multiple benefits into a single metric as is done in CBA.

In order to execute CEA, the metrics of "success" or "effectiveness" have to be identified. For example, what if the outcome of interest was not necessarily the amount of money collected, but rather the number of child support cases resolved? Since child support cases can involve many dimensions (financial, psychological, and social), the number of cases may be more relevant. Even more likely is the fact that statistics on the number of cases may be easier to obtain and project. As in a CBA analysis, the potential change in these outcomes in the context of each policy option still has to be projected—however, the next step of assigning a dollar value is not taken. CEAs project outcomes for "every dollar spent" and therefore facilitate a comparison of return on investment across options.

There are two approaches to CEA (Weimer and Vining 2011):

1 *The fixed budget approach*: a given level of spending is set and the analyst identifies the option that produces the greatest benefit (or the best outcome related to effectiveness) within the set budget. For example, if an organization spends $500,000 on a healthy eating initiative, how many participants will lose weight in the first year after completing the program? Or, for every dollar spent on the program, what is the likelihood of losing weight? This approach is particularly useful when clients have a set budget or spending item that needs to be allocated to a single project. The question is then, which one gets the client the "biggest bang for the buck"?
2 *The fixed effectiveness approach*: a specific level of benefit (or effectiveness) is set and the analyst identifies the option that achieves that benefit at the lowest cost. For example, if the organization running a healthy eating initiative knows that it wants to see weight losses of 10 percent, what option spends the least to achieve that goal? This approach is useful when the client has concrete goals for the outcome that needs to be achieved, and the spending to achieve them is either unknown or more flexible.

Let's consider CEA in the context of the two CSE policy options presented earlier. Refer to Table 5.13 for the numbers.

The CEA indicates that automatic collection policy is only slightly more cost effective: for every $10,000 dollars spent, just over four cases are resolved as compared to just under four cases for the workforce development policy. While the same option comes out on top (compared to the CBA), the margin of superiority is much smaller (and perhaps not even that meaningful).

Even though CEAs do not generally address allocative efficiency, they can still satisfy clients' desires to see a criterion that captures how well resources or investments achieve certain goals. CEAs are usually easier to implement since they do not require assigning a dollar amount to outcomes that are not easily assigned a market price (and therefore omitted or inaccurately valued in a CBA).

Table 5.13 Cost-Effectiveness Analysis

	Automatic Collection System	Targeted Workforce Development Program
Cost ($PV)	$54,524,460	$67,934,512
Effectiveness (# Cases resolved)	24,073	24,571
# Cases resolved per $1	0.0004	0.0004
# Cases resolved per $10k	4.4	3.6

Supplementing the Analysis With Other Criteria

Given the limitations of CBA as a stand-alone evaluation tool, the best strategy for ensuring a comprehensive analysis is to supplement it with other, non-monetized criteria. CBA, and the WTP metrics that constitute it, is a reliable way to "raise red flags" about a project (Richardson 2001), but it is incomplete. For example, it is often possible to monetize costs, but not benefits. Therefore, other criteria could capture various aspects of the benefits. Other criteria are also useful in assessing the political or administrative feasibility of a project, or how the costs and benefits are distributed (rather than their aggregate value alone). For example, while it may be possible to monetize tourism revenues from visitors to parks and natural resources, it is difficult to assign a dollar amount that accurately values the existence (or degradation) of the park. A more qualitative criterion would perhaps differentiate policy options in terms of their potential to destroy or harm the natural resource—while the magnitude of harm is identifiable, its dollar value less so.

Our proposal is consistent with "multiple criterion analysis" or a "multi-attribute trade-off" approach put forth by Ackerman and Heinzerling (2004: 208). They suggest four principles for achieving a multi-faceted approach:

1 Use holistic, rather than atomistic, methods of evaluating costs and benefits: costs and benefits considered together, but not forced to be in the same units.
2 Moral imperatives are more powerful than cost comparisons: lead with value-based priorities and consider costs later in the decision process.

3 Adopt a precautionary approach to uncertain, potentially dangerous risks: tilt towards protecting current and future generations (even if costs are high).
4 Promote fairness towards the poor and powerless today, and toward future generations: ethical questions should be answered prior to CBA, and the analyst will likely need to look beyond the "market" to address distributional issues.

These principles echo the general approach to evaluative criteria presented in Chapter 4. CBA, like other forms of criteria, is best viewed as an evaluative method rather than a decision rule (Posner 2001). In practice, CBA will be one of several criteria used to rank proposed policy options.

Summary

Policy analysts often have to marshal or implement technical analyses in the design and comparison of policy options. In this chapter we reviewed the most widely used technical methods: **discounting**, **CBA**, and **CEA**. These are all quantitative methods that rely on **monetizing** costs and benefits, rather than using qualitative or non-monetized metrics to assess the merits and drawbacks of a policy alternative. **Discounting** takes the time-value of money into account by factoring in the opportunity costs of alternative investments. **CBA** assigns dollar values to costs and benefits and calculates the net benefit to measure the overall welfare effects from an alternative. **CEA** assigns dollar amounts only to the costs and compares them to non-monetized metrics of "success."

These approaches are popular: they simplify otherwise complex issues into a concept that everyone can understand—money. Some argue that they also bring to bear the interests that are not necessarily at the policy-making "table"; benefits and costs can, and should, be construed broadly. These technical approaches also raise a host of methodological and philosophical issues. CBA, in particular, is a complicated technique to implement, requiring impressive amounts of information and data. The outcomes of a CBA entirely depend on the analyst's **assumptions** about who or what counts in the analysis, how values change over time and how values are assigned in the first place.

Variation in any one of these features can dramatically change the NPV and can therefore have consequential implications for which policies are promoted and adopted.

Many of the limitations of CBAs, and related techniques, can be addressed by including them as one of several evaluative components in the analysis. If there is **uncertainty** in monetizing key inputs, then they should be captured or supplemented by non-monetized metrics. **Cost-effectiveness** is a useful compromise, since costs are usually easier to value in dollar terms. It is important that the analyst not extend a CBA, for example, beyond its reasonable limits. In addition, the goal of any CBA should not be a singular estimate of NPV, but rather a **bounded projection** of net benefits that shows the "best" and "worst" case scenarios, depending on how aggressive or conservative the underlying assumptions may be.

We encourage the analyst to become an informed consumer of these techniques and consider them one of several tools to assess trade-offs across proposed policy options. Policy analysis should rely on a holistic framework, drawing from economistic methods, such as those presented in this chapter, and more interdisciplinary approaches to information collection and inquiry.

Notes

1. This is also different from adjusting for inflation or for purchasing power over time. It is very difficult to project inflation rates into the future, and the discount rates (or alternative returns on investment) usually factor in expectations about changes in purchasing power (Weimer and Vining 2011). Therefore, the discounting conducted here will be applied to nominal, or unadjusted, values.
2. President Ronald Reagan issued Executive Order 12291 in 1981 (available at www.archives.gov/federal-register/codification/executive-order/12291.html), which mandated that "Regulatory action shall not be undertaken unless the potential benefits to society from the regulation outweigh the potential costs to society."
3. Available at: chrome-extension://efaidnbmnnnibpcajpcglclefindmkaj/www.whitehouse.gov/wp-content/uploads/2023/11/CircularA-4.pdf
4. For an excellent description of the theoretical and empirical aspects of hedonic modeling, see Sheppard (1999).

References

Ackerman, Frank, and Lisa Heinzerling. 2004. *Priceless: On Knowing the Price of Everything and the Value of Nothing.* New York: The New Press.

Boardman, A.E., D.H. Greenberg, A.R. Vining, and D.L. Weimer. 2018. *Cost-Benefit Analysis: Concepts and Practice* (5th Edition). New York: Cambridge University Press.

Brennan Center for Justice. 2023. *Automatic Voter Registration, a Summary*. www.brennancenter.org/our-work/research-reports/automatic-voter-registration-summary

Choi, Iseul, Josef Dvorak, Steven Kulig, Katie Lorenze, and Amanda Wilmarth. 2013. *Cost-Benefit Analysis of Implementing an Online Voter Registration System in Wisconsin*. Madison: Wisconsin Government Accountability Board.

Henrichson, Christian, and Joshua Rinaldi. 2014. *Cost-Benefit Analysis and Justice Policy Toolkit*. New York: Vera Institute of Justice.

Kelman, Steven. 1992. "Cost-Benefit Analysis: An Ethical Critique." In *The Moral Dimension of Public Policy Choice*, John Martin Gilroy, and Maurice Wade (eds.). Pittsburgh: University of Pittsburgh Press.

Kornhauser, Lewis A. 2001. "On Justifying Cost-Benefit Analysis." In *Cost-Benefit Analysis: Legal, Economic and Philosophical Perspectives*, Matthew D. Adler, and Eric A. Posner (eds.). Chicago: University of Chicago Press.

Livermore, Michael A., and Richard L. Revesz. 2020. *Reviving Rationality: Saving Cost-benefit Analysis for the Sake of the Environment and Our Health*. New York: Oxford University Press.

MIT Election Lab. 2023. *Automatic Voter Registration Explainer* (February 16). https://electionlab.mit.edu/research/automatic-voter-registration

Nussbaum, Martha. 2001. "The Costs of Tragedy: Some Moral Limits of Cost-Benefit Analysis." In *Cost-Benefit Analysis: Legal, Economic and Philosophical Perspectives*, Matthew D. Adler, and Eric A. Posner (eds.). Chicago: University of Chicago Press.

Office of Management and Budget. 2023. *Circular No. A-4* (November). chrome-extension://efaidnbmnnnibpcajpcglclefindmkaj/www.whitehouse.gov/wp-content/uploads/2023/11/CircularA-4.pdf

Patton, Carl V., David S. Sawicki, and Jennifer J. Clark. 2013. *Basic Methods of Policy Analysis and Planning* (3rd Edition). Boston, MA: Pearson.

The Pew Charitable Trusts. 2014. *Understanding Online Voter Registration*. www.pewtrusts.org/en/projects/archived-projects/election-initiatives/about/upgrading-voter-registration/online-voter-registration

Posner, Richard A. 2001. "Cost-Benefit Analysis: Definition, Justification, and Comment on Conference Papers." In *Cost-Benefit Analysis: Legal, Economic and Philosophical Perspectives*, Matthew D. Adler, and Eric A. Posner (eds.). Chicago: University of Chicago Press.

Richardson, Henry S. 2001. "The Stupidity of the Cost-Benefit Standard." In *Cost-Benefit Analysis: Legal, Economic and Philosophical Perspectives*, Matthew D. Adler, and Eric A. Posner (eds.). Chicago: University of Chicago Press.

Sen, Amartya. 2001. "The Discipline of Cost-Benefit Analysis." In *Cost-Benefit Analysis: Legal, Economic and Philosophical Perspectives*, Matthew D. Adler, and Eric A. Posner (eds.). Chicago: University of Chicago Press.

Sheppard, S. 1999. "Hedonic Analysis of Housing Markets." *Handbook of Regional and Urban Economics 3*: 1595–1635.

Stiglitz, Joseph. 1998. "The Private Uses of Public Interests: Incentives and Institutions." *Journal of Economic Perspectives 12, 2*: 3–22.

Stokey, E., and R. Zeckhauser. 1978. *Primer for Policy Analysis*. New York: W. W. Norton.

Stone, Deborah. 2012. *Policy Paradox: The Art of Political Decision Making* (3rd Edition). New York: W. W. Norton.

Sunstein, Cass R. 2001. "Cognition and Cost-Benefit Analysis." In *Cost-Benefit Analysis: Legal, Economic and Philosophical Perspectives*, Matthew D. Adler, and Eric A. Posner (eds.). Chicago: University of Chicago Press.

Sunstein, Cass R. 2014. *Valuing Life: Humanizing the Regulatory State*. Chicago: University of Chicago Press.

Trumbell, William H. 1990. "Who has Standing in Cost-Benefit Analysis?" *Journal of Policy Analysis and Management 9*, *3*: 201–218.

Vining, Aidan R., and David L. Weimer. 2009. "Assessing the Costs and Benefits of Social Policies." In *Investing in the Disadvantaged: Assessing the Benefits and Costs of Social Policies*, Aidan R. Vining, and David L. Weimer (eds.). Washington, DC: Georgetown University Press.

Weimer, David L., and Aidan R. Vining. 2011. *Policy Analysis*. Boston, MA: Longman.

Whittington, D., and D. MacRae. 1986. "The Issue of Standing in Cost-benefit Analysis." *Journal of Policy Analysis and Management 5*, *4*: 665–682.

Zerbe, R.O. 1991. "Comment: Does Benefit Cost Analysis Stand Alone? Rights and Standing." *Journal of Policy Analysis and Management 10*, *1*: 96–105.

6
ANALYSIS AND MAKING RECOMMENDATIONS

A key step in policy analysis is the systematic comparison of the potential policy outcomes. Policy analysts must predict the most likely consequences of each alternative, were it selected, and weigh its strengths and weaknesses in light of the criteria specified for the analysis. They must recommend the policy alternative—or, in some cases, alternatives—that best address the values and concerns denoted by the criteria. Seldom will a single alternative show itself to be superior in all respects across all of the criteria. Almost always, each alternative will be stronger than others in some ways and weaker in others. It is the job of the policy analyst to evaluate these trade-offs and recommend the alternative that, on balance, is superior to the others.

In this chapter, we examine how analysts can estimate and compare the most likely consequences of each alternative. We first discuss prediction, or projecting the various outcomes of each alternative. We then turn to the comparison of these outcomes and how trade-offs should be addressed. In doing so, we illustrate the value of a matrix as a tool for analysis. The chapter concludes by returning to the child support case study, illustrating some of the key themes of this chapter through an analysis of options for reducing debt incurred by noncustodial parents.

Prediction and Estimation

Policy analysis is inherently uncertain as it is based on predictions of the future—whether near term or distant. Policy analysts must, to the best of their abilities, predict the most likely outcomes for each alternative in relation to the status quo, and across multiple dimensions. For each criterion, such as effectiveness, equity, cost, or feasibility, analysts must make appropriate estimations. To what extent will each address the problem (e.g., increase voter turnout, reduce child support debt)? How will the options affect the most vulnerable populations? What are the likely costs of each option? What are the key barriers to implementation?

In making these predictions, analysts must combine evidence and argumentation. Sometimes, analysts can draw from a rich body of empirical evidence to determine the likely outcomes of certain alternatives. Certain interventions may be thoroughly studied and documented, providing analysts with a solid evidentiary basis for predicting their effectiveness and understanding their costs. For example, in transportation there is a large literature on the impacts of highway expansion and public transportation investment on traffic congestion (e.g., Ossokina et al. 2023; Milam et al. 2017; Anderson 2013).

The Challenge With Prediction: Information Is Limited

More often, the available evidence is limited in scope or applies to only a portion of the issue. Some policies and programs may have been subject to little research and evaluation or may be completely untested, as would be the case if the policy is truly original. When policy alternatives lack a solid evidentiary record of their past performance, analysts must base their predictions mostly on logic and argumentation. But even when there are many well-documented examples of similar policies or programs, analysts must still explain why they expect previous outcomes to be repeated—or improved upon—in the current context.

For example, Mexico is known for a successful "conditional cash transfer" program (*Oportunidades*) that provides small financial incentives to impoverished families in rural areas to actively manage their health and keep their children in school. Would this approach work in the United States? New York City's mayor thought it might, and in 2007, the city adapted it to incentivize children and teens to attend school regularly, graduate from high school on time, and pass standardized tests. However, students showed no change in outcomes as a result of the incentive, and the city terminated the program ahead of schedule (Fawley and Juvenal 2010; Marsh et al. 2011). Notwithstanding the documented success of conditional cash transfers in Mexico, the approach failed to achieve its goals in New York City, perhaps because of differences in context and/or revisions to the model when applied in New York.

In estimating the effects of alternative policy options, it is important to consider them in relation to the status quo of letting current trends continue. For example, if a proposed change in election law would likely increase voter participation by 10 percentage points over five years, and voter participation is projected to increase by 5 percentage points in the absence of any intervention (i.e., the status quo), then the proposed change would increase voter turnout by 5 percentage points compared to the status quo. If voter participation is likely to *decline* by 5 percentage points under the status quo, then the proposed policy would increase participation by 15 percentage points.

The criteria selected to compare and assess the alternatives determine the specific kinds of predictions that must be undertaken. The number and types of predictions necessary to carry out the analysis depend on the criteria, as well as on the nature of the issue. The more criteria, the more predictions will be required. More predictions will be necessary, for example, if effectiveness is gauged in three discrete ways than if there is a single measure. Moreover, some criteria may require more predictions and estimations than others. Cost-benefit analysis, as discussed in Chapter 5, requires analysts to quantify the various effects of a potential program or policy and to assign monetary values to each one. Cost-effectiveness, on the other hand, usually focuses on a single potential impact.

Predictions and estimations for policy analysis do not always require the same degree of precision. As discussed in Chapter 4, some criteria may involve quantitative variables, while others may be categorical. Quantitative criteria require the analyst to arrive at an exact number for each alternative. For example, analysts might need to estimate the total increase in voter turnout for each alternative, or the total cost of implementing each alternative. Categorical criteria, on the other hand, require the analyst to assign the projected outcomes into two or more groups. A criterion might only require the analyst to determine if the alternative would satisfy a minimum threshold (e.g., increase turnout by at least 5 percentage points; cost less than $1 million)—or, it might require the analyst to estimate whether a particular outcome would qualify as "low," "medium," or "high" or some other set of categorical variables. As should be obvious, categorical criteria require less precision than quantitative ones. The analyst still needs to explain the reasoning behind an alternative's categorical rating, but the burden of explanation is less onerous compared to quantitative criteria. It is less difficult to explain why an alternative would increase voter turnout by between 20 percent and 50 percent as opposed to an increase of precisely 40 percent.

Next we discuss some of the key challenges associated with applying several of the most basic criteria, including effectiveness, equity, cost, and feasibility.

Effectiveness

Measures of effectiveness usually refer to the ability of the alternatives to address the central problem—or whether or not (or to what degree) the policy option will succeed. They require the analyst to estimate the most probable outcomes of each alternative with respect to specific aspects of effectiveness. For example, if the analyst is to recommend ways of reducing homelessness, the measures of effectiveness might include projected changes in homeless shelter populations, changes in the average duration of homelessness, or perhaps changes in size of specific homeless populations (e.g., veterans, elderly, children).

In making these estimates, the analyst might look at evidence from evaluations of other homeless programs instituted previously or elsewhere (see Chapter 7). However, in drawing from evidence on the outcomes of other programs, the analyst must take care to show that the current context would allow for similar results. Are there important differences in the political or legal environments surrounding the original program or policy and the place where a similar program or policy might be applied which could affect the outcome? Would these differences reduce or increase the effectiveness of the program or policy? Why?

Very often, it is impossible to marshal data from program evaluations or other sources to provide complete or credible estimations of all of the alternatives' potential effectiveness in addressing the problem. Such data may simply not exist, or may apply to some outcomes and not others—or the context surrounding the program or policy to be adopted may be so different from the current situation that any data regarding the performance of the original program or policy may not be very relevant. In such situations the analyst must employ various assumptions and develop arguments to apprise the effectiveness of the alternatives. Some of these assumptions may concern (i) the size of the population targeted by the policy or program, (ii) the likelihood that members of this population will participate in or comply with the program or policy, and (iii) the degree to which their participation or compliance will result in the desired change in behavior or otherwise address the problem. For example:

- What percentage of automobile buyers are likely to respond to tax incentives to purchase electric cars? What impact would the resulting increase in electric car use have on carbon emissions?
- Were the city to adopt congestion pricing, how many car owners would use public transportation or other alternative means of travel to commute to work if the fee were set at $10? What impact would this change have on traffic congestion?
- If the state were to institute a program to purchase firearms from residents, how many would participate if the price were set at $100? $500? What effect would the reduced number of firearms have on gun violence in the state?
- If a state were to restore voting rights to residents with felony convictions, what percentage of this population would register to vote? What percentage would vote in elections? What impact would this increase have on overall voter turnout?

To answer such questions, the analyst must decide on the appropriate assumptions and explain how they were determined. For example, if data are not available on the responsiveness of consumers to tax incentives for electric vehicles, perhaps one could adapt data on tax incentives or other financial incentives to purchase other kinds of durable goods. To estimate the impact of the incentive on carbon emissions, the analyst would also need to make assumptions about the amount of carbon emissions that would have been generated by gasoline-powered vehicles that consumers would have purchased (or retained) had they not acquired an electric vehicle as a result of the incentive.

Analysts may sometimes base their assumptions on economic, behavioral, or other kinds of concepts, models, and theories. For example, the concept of income elasticity of demand (which refers to the degree to which demand for different kinds of goods and services responds to changes in income) could help an analyst estimate the optimal size of a tax incentive to purchase electric vehicles, or how the incentive might vary with different income levels.[1] Behavioral economics may yield insights into the efficacy of different kinds of incentives (Thaler and Sunstein 2008). For example, one might apply the "EAST" framework (Easy, Attract, Social, Timely) developed by the United Kingdom's "Nudge Unit" (discussed in Chapter 3) to compare how well various policy proposals would increase voter turnout (Halpern 2015).

Analysts may not always be able to assign a specific number to each alternative (e.g., the estimated reduction in the homeless population). But they may be able to arrive at a likely range (e.g., 500 to 1,000). If it is impossible to come up with any credible quantitative estimates, analysts may still be able to categorically rank the alternatives in terms of their potential effectiveness. They may not be able to provide either exact figures or numeric ranges of the likely impact of the policy alternatives, but they may be able to provide convincing arguments as to why one alternative would be more effective than the others.

For example, it may not be possible to estimate the precise increase in voter turnout that would result from election day voter registration, from the use of social media to remind already-registered voters to vote or from expanded "early voting"—but it may be possible to rank these alternatives' most likely impact and provide credible arguments for this ranking. Reviews of the literature on electoral participation and interviews with experts in the field might indicate the relative efficacy of the alternatives in reducing various barriers to voting and in stimulating voter turnout. The information may not yield numeric estimates but can shed light on how the effectiveness of the alternatives compare.

If the original criteria require exact estimates of effectiveness, such as the percentage-point increase in voter turnout, and it turns out to be impossible to arrive at the required level of precision with any credibility, then the analyst may need to revise the criteria. Perhaps other quantitative variables might be substituted for the original, or, more likely, quantitative variables might be replaced with categorical ones. This once again illustrates the iterative nature of policy analysis: analysts must often revise assumptions and decisions made in previous stages in light of what is discovered in latter stages.

Taking uncertainty into account. Decision theory incorporates the probabilities of different possible outcomes to arrive at the overall effectiveness of each alternative (Hammond et al. 1999). Policy analysis texts (e.g., Wiemer and Vining 2005: 440) show how one can use decision trees to estimate the overall effectiveness of each alternative (see Figure 6.1 for an example). By specifying the most likely outcomes associated with each alternative, and the probability of achieving each of these outcomes, analysts can calculate the overall effectiveness of each alternative. For example, if one option for reducing homelessness has a 10 percent chance of decreasing the homeless population by 80 percent, and a 90 percent chance of reducing it by 20 percent—its overall effectiveness is estimated as the weighted average of these two outcomes, which is 26 percent (80 * .1 + 20 * .9 = 26). Another option might have a 20 percent chance of not impacting homelessness at all, a 40 percent chance of reducing it by 20 percent, and a 40 percent chance of reducing it by 60 percent. The weighted average effectiveness of this option would be 32 percent (.2 * 0 + .4 * 20 + .4 * 60 = 32).

All else being equal, analysts should take the weighted average of the various outcomes associated with each alternative as the overall outcome, as the expected value.

Most often, it is impossible to know with any precision the probability of each outcome. However, analysts can and should consider probabilities in a more general sense to estimate the most likely outcome of each option. For example, some options could be tremendously effective if several conditions are met—which is not very likely—but

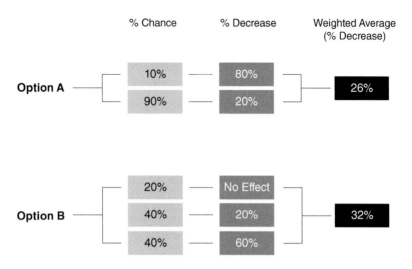

Figure 6.1 Using probability to estimate outcomes: options for reducing homelessness

may fail completely or be much less successful if only some preconditions are satisfied. Another option might be substantially less effective than the maximum potential effectiveness of the first alternative, but the outcome is much less sensitive to the satisfaction of preconditions. The analyst may not be able to determine the precise probability of each outcome, but he or she may feel comfortable in assuming that a probability is more than 50 percent, perhaps more than 75 percent, or less than 10 percent. For example, in assessing the effectiveness of a plan to make the streets safer for pedestrians an analyst might conclude that it had about an outside chance, perhaps one in five (20 percent) of reducing pedestrian deaths in the targeted area by as much as 40 percent, a 50–50 chance (50 percent) of reducing them by around 15 percent, and a very strong chance, certainly more than 75 percent, of reducing them by at least 5 percent.

In some cases, probabilities must be factored into estimates of outcomes in combination with other assumptions. For example, in estimating the most likely effect of a financial incentive to surrender one's firearms, the analyst would need to not only estimate the likelihood that gun owners would be willing to give up their weapons for a given price but also estimate the effect of the resulting decrease of guns in private ownership on overall levels of gun violence in comparison with other policy alternatives. In other instances, effectiveness may be measured by a single probability, such as the chances of different policy alternatives to convince utility companies to shift from coal-powered electrical generation to wind power or other "green" technologies.

Cost

Costs usually refer to the direct costs of administering a program or policy. In the context of cost-benefit analysis, however, they refer also to any negative impacts of the program or policy—impacts that must be quantified and monetized (see Chapter 5). In most cases, however, analysts focus on the direct costs associated with the initiative. In estimating costs, analysts must take into account the types of costs, the timing of the costs, and who bears the costs.

It is usually important to distinguish between capital and operating costs. Capital costs refer to the large, fixed expenses associated with major investments such as acquiring or constructing a building or purchasing new computer systems. Often, these costs are financed by debt (bank loans and bonds). These costs are usually "lumpy," occurring mostly at certain points in time, especially at the start of the program or policy. Operating costs, on the other hand, refer to the cost of labor, services, rent, supplies, and other ongoing costs. Operating costs are usually paid out of an organization's annual budget. They tend be ongoing and are usually in proportion to the scale of the program or policy.

In estimating the likely costs of each alternative analysts should take both capital and operating costs into account—although not all alternatives will require capital expenditures. The analysis will need to consider costs over some period of time. If some programs or policies will incur sizable start-up costs during the first year or so of its operation, it is particularly important to take a longer term perspective. As discussed in Chapter 5, the analyst must translate all costs estimated to be incurred in the future into their present-value equivalents, using an appropriate discount rate. Otherwise one runs the risk of favoring an option because its total *nominal* costs are lowest, even though the costs of another alternative has the lowest *present* value.

If a policy or program will incur costs over time, as most will, analysts may want to take inflation into account, or at least the probable increases in major expenses. For example, the analyst might apply forecasted increases in the Consumer Price Index to estimate operating costs in future years. If salary and wages are an expense item, the analyst might estimate future salary increases.

Sometimes, analysts must convert staff time into dollars. Some policies or programs may not require new staff positions. Instead, the work of existing personnel may be adjusted so that certain employees would staff the program or policy. The change might require all or a portion of an employee's time. In such instances, the policy analysts must estimate the number of full-time equivalent positions associated with the program/policy and the corresponding salaries. If a program would require the equivalent of one half-time position, that would be the staffing cost of the position. Just because the organization already employs the person doesn't mean that alternative has no labor costs. In estimating personnel costs, do not forget to include fringe benefits (health care, pension, etc.).

Finally, it is important to consider who will bear the costs. Often, the client's organization will be responsible for all of the costs of the alternatives under consideration. Sometimes, costs will be distributed across multiple organizations, or borne by private individuals and households. Cost-benefit analysis requires all costs to be accounted for. In other forms of policy analysis, the analyst must decide which ones to include. Nevertheless, the analysis is most credible when all of the major costs are taken into account and not just those that would be incurred by the client. If the client would be responsible for a minor portion of the costs, it can be misleading to claim that the costs of the alternative are low.

Equity

The equity criterion usually requires another set of predictions and estimations. As discussed in Chapter 4, equity can be defined in several ways. Most broadly, equity can concern outcomes or processes. In terms of outcomes, equity involves determining how alternatives may affect different groups of people, whether demarcated by income, gender, age, sexual orientation, disability, race, ethnicity, or other characteristics.

In assessing the differential effects of proposed policies or programs, one must consider the degree to which each option might favor or harm particular groups.[2] Will homeless programs serve certain populations to a much greater degree than others? Is this difference counterbalanced by other programs that give priority to these other groups? Are homeless housing sites located so that they are not overrepresented in certain neighborhoods and underrepresented in others? Are there systemic differences between these neighborhoods?

Process refers to opportunity, or access to the policy's benefits. This consideration does not take disparate outcomes into account but instead focuses on whether the process of participation, or towards achieving the desired outcomes, is fair. Are eligible populations equally likely to be informed about the availability of a program or service? Will certain groups have a stronger chance of participating than others?

As with effectiveness and cost, the analyst must provide evidence and/or argumentation to estimate how well the alternatives satisfy the selected indicator of equity. If, for example, equity is defined in terms of minimizing harm to low-income populations, the analyst will need to assess how the alternatives would affect different income groups.

Feasibility

Feasibility can refer to several distinctive (if related) concerns that can affect either the likelihood of a policy or program being approved and launched or, if it is established, its likelihood to succeed in reaching its goals. Political feasibility generally refers to the chances that policies or programs will receive sufficient support from key "stakeholders"—depending on the issue, elected officials, community leaders, program administrators, advocates, and the like. Which stakeholders are likely to oppose or support the policy program? How strongly are they likely to feel about the policy/program? What resources would they be able to mobilize in support or opposition? To what extent does the policy/program's adoption require the approval of other individuals or organizations? How many decision points are there? To what degree are the "gatekeepers" independent of the client—how likely will they comply with the client's wishes? Will they oppose it? Will they try to delay it?

In evaluating political feasibility, the analyst may draw from interviews with key stakeholders, as well as the past actions or decisions of government officials regarding similar issues. Has the governor supported similar policies in the past? Does the governor's previous decisions suggest he or she would support or oppose the rationale for the proposed policy? Has the governor's position held firm, or has it evolved over time? In addition to drawing on interviews, articles, and the like, the analyst might simply try to imagine how different stakeholders would respond to the policies under consideration, to put themselves in their proverbial shoes (see Bardach and Patashnik 2023).

Legal feasibility refers to the possibility that programs or policies might be challenged in court and whether there are sufficient legal grounds to counter such challenges successfully. What if any legal arguments might be used to contest the program or policy? How viable might these arguments be? Is the policy or program based on solid legal precedent? Would it require an untested legal argument? If one or more policy options do pose legal questions, the analyst will almost always need to consult with attorneys with appropriate expertise to assess legal feasibility.

Other aspects of feasibility concern ease of implementation. Whereas legal and political feasibility concerns the likelihood that a given policy or program can be launched at all, feasibility of implementation refers to various barriers that might prevent it from being executed as intended. In this sense, implementation relates directly to effectiveness. The more numerous and onerous the implementation challenges, the less likely the program or policy will achieve its goals (Pressman and Wildavksy 1984).

In assessing potential implementation challenges, policy analysts must keep several considerations in mind. These include the technical and organizational capacities of the entities that would carry out the program or policy; the complexity of the proposed policies or programs and the degree to which each element is essential to its success; the degree to which the success of the program or policy depends on the continued leadership of a single individual; and the degree to which the policy or program's operation is under the client organization's direct control or is contingent on the participation and/or support of external partners. Closely related to ease of implementation is what Bardach and Patashnik (2023) call "robustness." By this, they refer to the ability of a policy to achieve its aims when one or more of its core elements go awry. For example, some policies may still function, at least in part, if certain agencies charged with their administration drop out, or if a court issues a ruling that invalidates certain eligibility requirements. Other policies may collapse entirely if one or more components fails to operate as planned.

Additional Considerations When Projecting Outcomes

Sensitivity Analysis

Policy analysis, since it requires prediction of future outcomes, almost always involves some degree of uncertainty. Nearly all estimates and predictions are subject to error. The behavior of people and organizations may not unfold as predicted, and even when a policy does effect the desired change in behavior, this change—if it is not an end in itself—may not address the problem as thoroughly as expected. Given this inherent uncertainty, policy analysts should almost always conduct sensitivity analysis. In other words, they should examine the potential outcomes of the alternatives when key assumptions are changed. In some cases, the outcomes will show relatively little variation; in others the outcomes may vary a lot. At a minimum, analysts should discuss the results of the sensitivity analysis with the client; in some cases they may want to reconsider the recommendation, especially if slight variations in the assumptions would change the ranking of the alternatives.

Unintended Consequences

In addition to using criteria to predict the most likely outcomes of each alternative, it is also important to consider the possibility of unintended consequences, even if they fall outside the realm of the criteria. If the analyst identifies potentially negative outcomes that could result if an alternative is implemented, they might revise the criteria to take these outcomes into account, modify the alternative so as to prevent this outcome from occurring, or eliminate the alternative altogether. At a minimum these outcomes should be discussed.

For example, if policy analysts and their clients had given greater consideration to the ramifications of jailing and otherwise penalizing indigent parents, they might have adopted more nuanced policies that differentiated between parents with financial resources and parents who can afford to pay very little in child support. Perhaps if the impact of child support enforcement on low-income parents were included as a criterion, then some of the adverse consequences of child support policy could have been averted.

Several economic and other concepts can point to possible unintended consequences.

- *Free riders*: will the policy or program bring into its sweep people who are not intended to benefit? For example, would a debt forgiveness program include parents who can afford to pay their child support debt?
- *Moral hazard*: will a policy or program induce risky behavior by providing some level of protection against these risks. For example, would the availability of debt relief for noncustodial parents tempt some to stop paying child support?
- *Rent seeking*: will individuals or organizations find ways of exploiting the program for financial gain or otherwise serve their private interests? For example, policies intended to address the "disruptive" effects of technology on the taxicab and hotel industries might run the risk of suppressing competition in these industries and allow them to increase prices above what would otherwise be possible.

Comparison of Outcomes

After the analyst has estimated the likely impacts of the alternatives in light of the criteria, the next step is to compare them and decide which to recommend. A key tool for this comparison is a matrix that links the criteria and the alternatives. Reading down the columns, the matrix shows how the alternatives (or their projected outcomes) compare across each criterion. Reading across shows how each alternative rates with respect to all of the criteria. We present a sample matrix in Table 6.1, which has been completed for purposes of analyzing options for increasing voter turnout.

ANALYSIS AND MAKING RECOMMENDATIONS 207

Table 6.1 Analysis of Options for Increasing Voter Participation in Elections

		Criteria			
		Effectiveness: Change in Voter Turnout	Cost	Political Feasibility	Time to See Results
Alternatives	Mandatory Voting	**High** Would require all eligible adults to both register and vote	**Low** Would depend on intensity of enforcement and degree of compliance	**Low** No precedent in the United States; would be vociferously opposed by Republicans on the basis of infringement of liberty, among other claims	**2 years**
	Universal Vote-by-mail	**Medium** Modest turnout increases in general/presidential elections; more meaningful turnout increases for primary and local elections; may increase new registrants at the margin	**Medium to High** Depends on processing of mail-in ballots (e.g., entirely via mail or using drop boxes); potential for administrative savings for day-of voting	**Low to Medium** Would be popular if risk, or perception of fraud, were abated; would need to overcome belief that it disproportionately benefits Democratic candidates	**2 years**
	Voting Incentive (lottery)	**Low** Could increase turnout and perhaps increase registration among low-income adults (evidence in the United Kingdom shows no effect for higher-income voters)	**Low** Would depend on the lottery rewards and on its administration	**Low to Medium** Possible confidentiality concerns and ethical concerns about creating selective financial incentives for meeting basic civic duties like voting	**2 years**
	Automatic Registration	**Medium to High** Would reduce registration as a barrier to voting; could indirectly lead to increased turnout	**Medium** Start-up costs would be substantial, but ongoing costs would be low due to automation	**Medium** Significant support, except from factions opposed to any increase in the electorate	**2 years**

The matrix provides a birds-eye view of the analysis, a visual summary of the results. It indicates the strengths and weaknesses of each alternative and enables the reader to identify which options are most promising. The matrix can also be useful in ensuring that the analysis is consistent and thorough, that there are no gaps, and that all of the alternatives have been examined in light of all of the criteria.

Using the Matrix

In filling out the matrix, the analyst inserts a measure or rating for the alternatives according to the relevant criteria. Sometimes, the content of a cell may be very specific (e.g., a dollar figure for cost). Sometimes, it will be a more general rating such as good, poor, excellent. If the criteria refer to evaluative ratings such as "good," "high," or a number on a numeric scale, it is often wise to include a few explanatory words that justify the ratings. These notes will remind the analyst—and the client—about the underlying rationale for the rating.

Each cell in the matrix should be filled. Analysts should not leave cells blank or put "NA" (not applicable/not available) when they have difficulty arriving at a rating. Otherwise, it isn't possible to compare the alternatives across all of the criteria. If analysts find that it is not possible to apply a criterion to one or more alternatives, then they may need to rethink that criterion. This situation can occur when analysts consider very different kinds of interventions to address a problem. For example, if the analyst is assessing such varied ways of addressing the opioid epidemic as public education about the dangers of opioid use, increased funding for drug treatment, increased availability of naloxone to treat overdoses, stricter regulation of prescriptions for opioid-based pain medications, and a crackdown on street sales of heroin and other opiates, the criterion for effectiveness must be sufficiently broad so that it can apply to all of these alternatives. While projected change in the number of opioid overdose fatalities might encompass all of the alternatives, projected increases in the number of arrests for illegal distribution, sale or possession of opioids would not.

As discussed in Chapter 4, criteria can take different forms and involve varying degrees of precision. Some criteria can be binary—pass/

fail—while others are quantitative. In the case of binary criteria, the important thing is to *satisfice*. The analyst is interested in whether the alternatives satisfy a minimum requirement, not in the extent to which they exceed this requirement.

Some criteria may be more important than others, and therefore weighted more heavily. In some instances, certain criteria may determine if an alternative is acceptable at all, regardless of how it rates under the other criteria. In other words, if alternatives are to be considered further they must satisfy this criterion. If they fail to do so they are eliminated from further consideration. If some criteria are weighted more heavily than others, it often helps to highlight these criteria in the matrix by positioning them first—for example, to the left of the other criteria so they are read first. This can provide a visual cue to help the client and other readers interpret the matrix.

Box 6.1 Should Costs Always Be Included in the Analysis?

If the alternatives cost about the same, should cost be omitted as a criterion? In general, criteria that show no variation across the alternatives do not contribute directly to the comparison of trade-offs, and their removal from the matrix would not influence the final recommendation. However, clients and other audiences are almost always concerned about costs, and failure to refer to costs may raise doubts about the credibility of the analysis. Therefore, the analyst might either retain costs in the matrix to show that they were indeed estimated. Alternatively, the analyst could discuss costs separately, explaining how they were estimated and why they do not figure in the comparison of the policy options.

Rarely will one alternative be clearly superior to the others in all respects. When that is the case, the desired course of action may be so obvious that there is little if any need for policy analysis. Almost always the alternatives will present trade-offs. They will have strengths and weaknesses. Some alternatives may be superior to the others under some criteria but not others; other alternatives may be superior vis-à-vis other criteria. One of the most difficult aspects of policy analysis is in sorting through and weighing these trade-offs.

Eliminate "Dominated" Alternatives

A first step in the process of comparison is to winnow out any options that offer no meaningful strengths relative to the other alternatives. Such alternatives are said to be "dominated" by others. That is, they perform as well as or worse than the other alternatives across all the criteria. Given that they offer no distinct advantage over the others, such alternatives may be safely discarded.

Sometimes an alternative will be only slightly superior to other alternatives under one or more criteria, but are otherwise weaker. For example, its feasibility may be slightly better than that of the other options, but it rates much lower with regard to cost and effectiveness. The modest advantage is clearly outweighed by more substantial weaknesses. In such instances the alternative is "practically dominated" by other options (Hammond et al. 1999).

Table 6.1 illustrates both types of dominance. Four distinct alternatives for increasing voter turnout are assessed on the basis of four criteria: effectiveness in increasing the percentage of potentially eligible voters (adult citizens) who vote in elections, cost, political feasibility, and time to see results. The four options under consideration are mandatory voting (requiring all citizens to vote), universal vote-by-mail (allowing citizens to vote by mail without requiring excuses), voting incentives (a lottery that randomly awards cash prizes to voters), and automatic registration (voter registration is activated automatically once citizens become of age to vote).

Of the four options, the lottery is dominated by the others. It is the least effective in increasing voter turnout and fares no better than the other three alternatives with regard to the other criteria. The universal vote-by-mail option is practically dominated by the automatic registration alternative. It would cost somewhat less than automatic registration—at least initially—but would be less effective in increasing turnout, and would be no more politically feasible or take less time to be implemented.

Omit Invariant Criteria

Another way to simplify the analysis is to omit criteria that show little or no variation across the alternatives. If the alternatives rate similarly with respect to a particular criterion, that criterion will not factor into the analysis; it will not illuminate any differences across the alternatives. For this reason, that criterion may be removed from the matrix so that the analyst and client can focus on the trade-offs. Such criteria may still be important. They may serve as prerequisites for inclusion in the analysis, but they do not play a role in determining the final recommendation. For example, analysts must always consider the cost of the alternatives. However, if the options cost about the same, the analyst may note this fact in their report, but omit cost from the final comparison of the alternatives. Similarly, the analyst may need to show that there are no major obstacles to implementation facing the recommended alternatives, but if implementation is feasible for all of the alternatives, then it doesn't need to be included in the matrix.

Box 6.2 Is it Useful to Create a Total "Score" or "Grade" Across Criteria?

Sometimes, analysts calculate an average or total "score" or "grade" for each alternative, for example, by summing the individual ratings across the criteria. They then recommend the alternative with the best score. This procedure should be avoided. It can cause analysts to overlook "fatal flaws"—key deficiencies of alternatives that otherwise seem very compelling. It can also obscure important trade-offs across alternatives. A key purpose of the matrix is to compare and assess the relative strengths and weaknesses of the alternatives. Aggregate ratings can elide over these distinctions.

In the voter turnout example discussed earlier, time required for implementation was constant across all four options at two years. It therefore played no role in evaluating the strengths and weaknesses of the alternatives and might therefore have been discarded as a criterion.

This is not to say that time is unimportant. It may serve as a prerequisite for selecting potential alternatives. It could also be an initial criterion in the analysis, but one that can be omitted once the analyst realizes that it does not vary across the alternatives.

Weighing Trade-Offs

Once dominated and practically dominated options are eliminated and invariant criteria are taken out of consideration, the analyst can now focus on the most compelling alternatives. It is here that trade-offs come into play. Choosing between alternatives with varying strengths and weaknesses is a matter of judgment. The analyst is quite literally trading the strengths of one option for those of another; the weaknesses of one for those of another. How the analyst makes these choices depends in part on the priorities and values of the analyst and her or his client.

A good starting point is effectiveness. All else equal, the analyst would choose the alternatives that are most effective in addressing the problem. However, all else is seldom equal. Alternatives that would seem most effective may also be extremely costly, may favor certain populations far more than others, may be politically infeasible. In addition, if more than one measure of effectiveness is involved, the same alternative may not always come out on top; alternatives may be ranked differently in light of different forms of effectiveness. For example, an alternative that is most effective in reducing the number of homeless people sleeping on the streets on a given night of the year might be less effective than another option in reducing the total number of people who are homeless during the course of a year.

One way of weighing trade-offs is to consider what is gained or lost when shifting from the alternative that seems most effective to one that appears less effective. Is there a small or large difference in effectiveness? How does this difference compare with changes in the other criteria, such as cost, equity, or feasibility? If one alternative is only slightly less effective than the top-rated option, but is far more equitable, the analyst might prefer the gain in equity over the loss in effectiveness. Similarly, if the effectiveness of the top-rated option is greater than that of the runner-up, and its cost is substantially higher too, the analyst must decide if the increment in cost between the two options is worth the increase in effectiveness.

Returning again to the example of voter turnout, with the elimination of incentives and universal vote-by-mail, the choice is between mandatory voting and automatic registration. The trade-off here would seem to be between the potentially greater effectiveness of the former against the relatively greater political feasibility of the latter. Mandatory voting, by requiring all eligible citizens to vote (perhaps with certain exemptions), would clearly result in a major increase in voter participation. The option would not only require citizens above a minimum age to register to vote, it would also require them to show up at the polls and vote. In the nations that have enacted compulsory voting, including Australia and Brazil, turnout increased from 7 to 16 percentage points (Matthews 2015). The automatic registration alternative, on the other hand, would remove registration as a barrier to voting, but it does not guarantee that registered voters will actually vote. States with easier registration laws have a higher representation of lower-income voters compared to states with more stringent laws. However, in Oregon, one of the first states to mandate automatic registration, the easier requirements elevated turnout among people already inclined to vote while doing little to lift voting among the most disenfranchised citizens (Beitch 2016).

On the other hand, there is no precedent for compulsory voting in the United States, and proposals to enact it would likely face stiff political resistance—perhaps because of the potential for increased voter fraud, or because some may see it as an infringement on personal liberty, or because it may force people to vote who are completely unfamiliar with the candidates or the issues.

In the current climate, all efforts to increase voter participation face formidable political obstacles, but compulsory voting would confront particularly strenuous opposition. The political viability of automatic registration is certainly not assured either, but this option most likely would receive more support than compulsory voting. In addition, the proposal would be an incremental change from measures that states have already taken, as 32 states have introduced or expanded some form of automatic registration in recent years (Brennan Center for Justice 2018).

Perhaps most analysts would favor automatic registration over mandatory voting because of its greater political feasibility. But others may recommend mandatory voting because of its superior effectiveness in increasing turnout. These analysts may argue that since both alternatives face formidable political obstacles it makes sense to choose the one that would, if adopted, stimulate the most turnout.

Of course, analysts need not always give priority to effectiveness. Another approach might be to establish a minimum level of effectiveness, and among the options that meet this minimum standard choose the alternative that rates highest on other criteria.

If some criteria are weighted more heavily than others, trade-offs may be less of an issue. If, for example, effectiveness is weighted twice as heavily as the other criteria, then alternatives that rate highest in effectiveness would almost always be selected over those with other strengths. When an alternative performs far better than the others under the most heavily weighted criterion, its deficiencies in the other criteria would need to be quite severe to select a different option.

Trade-Offs Involving Cost-Benefit Analysis and Cost-Effectiveness

One might think that the need to address trade-offs is reduced, if not eliminated, if the analysis involves cost-benefit analysis (CBA) or cost-effectiveness analysis (CEA). As discussed in Chapter 5, these criteria combine costs and effectiveness into a single criterion. With CBA, the analyst quantifies and monetizes as many effects of the proposed alternatives as possible, and subtracts total costs from total benefits. Cost-effectiveness is more limited in scope than CBA. It usually takes the ratio of a single measure of effectiveness to total cost. While CBA and CEA may in some situations eliminate the need to deliberately weigh effectiveness against costs, they do not obviate other kinds of trade-offs.

In Chapter 5 we discussed how it is often impossible to quantify and monetize all of the major costs and benefits of policy alternatives. If the analyst decides that certain impacts of a proposed policy (e.g., environmental, psychological) should not be subject to CBA, then these outcomes must be considered *in addition* to net benefit (i.e., the difference between the total benefits and total costs of the elements included in the CBA). In other words, net benefit may be one of several criteria that the analyst must consider. In such situations analysts often need to trade off net benefit against other considerations that cannot or should not be assigned monetary values. Cost-effectiveness is less comprehensive than CBA, usually encompassing a single aspect of effectiveness, and limiting costs to the direct costs of implementing the policy or program. As a result, analysts often need to weigh a number of other factors that are not captured by CEA.

Making Recommendations

The final outcome of policy analysis is a recommendation, or advice on how to address the issue at hand. Recommendations can be conveyed in a variety of ways. The analyst may present a single recommendation for the client, and explain why, on balance, it is preferable to the other options. However, alternatives are not always mutually exclusive. Sometimes analysts may recommend a combination of alternatives, especially if they complement each other, by addressing different aspects of the problem or offsetting each other's weaknesses. However, the client may not be able to adopt and implement multiple policies or programs simultaneously. It may not have the time, the staff, or other resources. If more than one alternative is recommended, the analyst should consider the relative priority of each option and the sequencing of their implementation. Analysts should avoid recommending all of the alternatives—"all of the above." Doing so obviates the very need for analysis, which is fundamentally the consideration of the alternatives' strengths and weaknesses.

Recommendations should flow directly from the analysis. The recommended course of action must be one of the options that was assessed in light of the criteria; otherwise, it is impossible to know if the recommendation is more desirable than other possible options. Indeed, recommending a wholly new alternative undermines the very purpose of policy analysis. Similarly, analysts must not refer to new criteria when justifying a recommendation. The recommendation should flow from the preceding analysis.

Sometimes, analysts recommend a hybrid of two or more alternatives in a new option that combines different aspects of some of the alternatives that were part of the analysis. Such options may indeed be superior to the other options, but they should be subject to the same analysis as the others. Once the analyst realizes the potential value of a hybrid option, he or she should treat it as a discrete alternative and subject it to the same analysis as the other options. The analyst may add it to the alternatives already under consideration or substitute it for one or more of these options.

There can be instances when analysts do not present formal recommendations to the client. Instead, they may list the most promising alternatives along with their key strengths and weaknesses. Here, the role of the analyst is to present several choices to the client on how to address a particular issue and to present a framework for comparing options in a transparent and systematic way. The client may ultimately ask the analyst for a recommendation, but that is by no means inevitable.

Preliminary Versus Final Analysis

Throughout this book we have emphasized that policy analysis is an iterative process and that the analyst often cycles back and forth between the steps, revising previous portions in light of what is learned in later ones. Indeed, the analysis of alternatives presented in a memo, Microsoft PowerPoint presentation, or report may bear little resemblance to earlier versions of the analysis. In predicting and comparing the likely outcomes of the alternatives, analysts may realize that alternatives would be improved by various modifications. Perhaps aspects of two separate alternatives might be combined into a single option. Perhaps a single alternative might be split into two separate alternatives. Perhaps the analyst may decide to consider a combination of two alternatives as a discrete option while also including each component as separate alternatives to themselves.

Early versions of the analysis may also cause analysts to reconsider some of the criteria. The analyst may decide to modify how criteria are defined or calibrated. If the analyst or the client is uncomfortable with the recommendation that emerges from the analysis, even if it clearly rates best on all of the most important criteria, this could suggest that the analyst has omitted one or more criteria that should have been included.

In other words, the analyst may have neglected important values that should have been taken into account. By introducing new criteria in a subsequent iteration these values may now be incorporated into the analysis, yielding a more compelling recommendation.

One way of ensuring that the analysis does not omit key values and other important considerations is to present preliminary versions of the analysis to the client or perhaps to other knowledgeable audiences (with the client's permission). In "workshopping" the analysis, and fielding questions about the nature of the problem, the alternatives, criteria, and the trade-offs, the analyst can find important ways of improving the work.

Summary

In this chapter we have examined the two key facets of analysis: how to **estimate** and how to **compare** the most likely **outcomes of the policy alternatives** under consideration. We have discussed how the criteria indicate the outcomes of interest, and that the outcomes must be assessed relative to the status quo, of letting current trends continue.

We have emphasized that analysis involves a high degree of **uncertainty**, as it requires the analyst to predict the future. Moreover, the data available to analysts to help them estimate future outcomes are seldom comprehensive or directly relevant to the case at hand. Analysts must therefore draw on the **evidence** that is available and make defensible assumptions, to estimate the most likely outcomes of the alternatives vis-á-vis the criteria. They must be able to explain the reasoning behind these projections, and to articulate a coherent argument.

In comparing the most likely outcomes of each alternative, we employed a **matrix** to ensure that the analysis is thorough and consistent. We have shown how analysis ultimately involves the **weighing of trade-offs**, or choosing which combination of strengths and weaknesses is most preferable. In doing so, it often helps to see if any alternatives can be eliminated from consideration because they are "**dominated**" by one or more other alternatives. Sometimes, an alternative may be slightly superior with respect to one criterion (usually one of lesser importance), but is otherwise dominated by another alternative. In such situations the alternative is said to be "**practically dominated**," and is also removed from further consideration. In addition to showing if any alternative can be dropped for reasons of dominance, the matrix also makes clear whether or not the criteria actually reveal differences in the alternatives' projected outcomes. If there is no variation in outcomes under a criterion, that criterion will not influence the ultimate recommendation and can therefore be omitted from further consideration.

The search for dominated alternatives and invariant criteria enables the analyst to then focus her or his attention on trade-offs between the remaining alternatives. We have discussed how it is often helpful to look first at the alternatives that appear most effective in addressing the issue and to consider its degree of superiority relative to other leading alternatives. That is, are deficits in one or more measures of effectiveness outweighed by the advantages of another alternative vis-à-vis other criteria such as equity or cost? Ultimately, the resolution of trade-offs reflects the values and priorities of the analyst and her client.

Throughout the chapter we have discussed the **iterative** nature of policy analysis. As the analyst goes through the process of projecting and comparing outcomes, he or she may discover that the criteria need to be revised, or decide to revamp one or more alternatives. After making these changes the analyst must return again to the task of estimating and comparing the alternatives' outcomes. Even if the analyst does not definitively put forth a single alternative, the matrix provides the client with a method for **ranking** the possible options in light of the evaluative criteria.

Child Support Debt Case: A Recap

In Chapter 3 we presented four policy options to reduce child support debt incurred by low-income noncustodial parents. These alternatives were as follows:

- Participation Incentive Program (PIP): forgive debt owed to the state after the noncustodial parent pays child support for 12 and 24 months.
- Match Plus Outreach (MPO): for every dollar of child support paid, 50 cents of debt is forgiven. The program applies to state debt and, if the custodial parent agrees, debt owed to custodial parents. It includes outreach to custodial parents.
- Workforce Development (WD): the state forgives debt for noncustodial parents who enroll in workforce development program and obtain and retain employment.

- Automatic Forgiveness of Arrears due to Incarceration (AFAI): the state automatically forgives arrears that noncustodial parents accrued while incarcerated in the state's prison system.

In Chapter 4 we presented six criteria to evaluate these alternatives:

1. *Effectiveness: Maximize the number of noncustodial parents eligible for debt reduction.*
2. *Effectiveness: Maximize the amount of state debt reduction.*
3. *Effectiveness: The possibility of custodial parent debt reduction*
4. *Equity: Maximize ease of compliance by noncustodial parent.*
5. *Minimize cost of implementation.*
6. *Maximize political acceptability.*

Child Support Debt Case: Analysis of Policy Options and Recommendation[3]

Having developed several potential policy options to reduce child support debt and formulated criteria to evaluate these options, we now proceed to the analysis of these options in light of the criteria. We first estimate each alternative's most likely outcomes with respect to the criteria. We then compare these outcomes and weigh key trade-offs between them.

Alternative 1: Participation Incentive Program

Effectiveness: Maximize the Number of Noncustodial Parents Eligible for Debt Reduction

All noncustodial parents with child support arrears are eligible for the Participation Incentive Program: **100 percent**

Effectiveness: Maximize the Amount of State Debt Reduction

The PIP program would forgive **100 percent** of the NPCs' arrears if they make the required child support payments over a 24-month period (i.e., every month for 24 months). After 12 months of payment **50 percent** of the arrears would be forgiven.

Effectiveness: Possibility of Custodial Parent Debt Reduction
No. PIP would apply to state debt only.

Equity: Maximize Ease of Compliance by Noncustodial Parent
Low. Noncustodial parents must pay child support for a minimum of 12 months for partial debt forgiveness and 24 months for total debt forgiveness. Participants are disqualified from the program and receive no debt reduction if they miss three payments over the 24-month period.

Cost: Minimize Cost of Implementation
We assume that participant recruitment and program oversight and administration can be carried out by existing child support staff, augmented by ten additional full-time-equivalent staff positions, amounting to **$900,000** annually, including benefits.

Maximize Political Acceptability: Likelihood and Intensity of Opposition to Proposed Options From Key Stakeholders
High. There seems to be strong political support for debt forgiveness programs such as PIP. Political support for the Maryland program on which this option is based is strong.

Table 6.2 Analysis Summary for Participation Incentive Program

Alternative	Maximize Number of Noncustodial Parents Eligible for Debt Reduction	Maximize Amount of State Debt Reduction	Possibility of Custodial Parent Debt Reduction	Maximize Ease of Compliance by Noncustodial Parent	Minimize Cost of Implementation	Maximize Political Acceptability
Participation Incentive Program	Approx. 80%	50 to 100% of outstanding arrears (50% after 12 months; 100% after 24)	No	Low	$900,000	High

Alternative 2: Match Plus Outreach

Effectiveness: Maximize the Number of Noncustodial Parents Eligible for Debt Reduction

All noncustodial parents with child support arrears are eligible for Match Plus Outreach: **100 percent**

Effectiveness: Maximize the Amount of State Debt Reduction

Unlike PIP and WD, which forgive a set percentage of debt after the attainment of particular milestones (e.g., regular payment of child support over a set number of months), MPO would reduce a noncustodial parent's debt by 50 cents for every dollar he pays in child support or for back debt. If the noncustodial parent pays $3,000 in child support over a 12-month period, he or she would be forgiven $1,500 in child support debt. Nationally, the average amount of state child support arrears is $10,800. In order to eliminate that amount of debt in one year under this alternative, a noncustodial parent would need to pay nearly $22,000 in child support ($1,833 per month) or $11,000 over 24 months ($916 per month). These sums would be very difficult for most low-income noncustodial parents to afford—for example, someone working full-time at $15/hour would earn $31,200 before taxes. If the participant earns less, or works part-time, his or her income and ability to pay child support would be reduced further. **Overall, we estimate that MPO would reduce state child support arrears by about 10–25 percent annually for participating noncustodial parents**.

Effectiveness: Possibility of Custodial Parent Debt Reduction

Yes. As discussed in Chapter 2, state child support debt has declined rapidly in recent years both in absolute terms and as a percentage of total child support debt.[4] As of 2022, only 27 percent of all noncustodial parents with child support debt were in arrears to the state, and state debt accounted for only 17 percent of all child support arrears (Office of Child Support Enforcement 2023). However, states do not have authority to modify in any way the amount of child support debt owed to custodial parents. They may forgive debt owed to the state, but not debt owed to custodial parents. Custodial parents almost always have the option of forgiving some or all of the debt owed to them, but that decision is entirely up to them.

MPO is the only policy option that has the potential of reducing debt owed to custodial parents. It includes various ways of informing custodial parents about the potential benefits of debt forgiveness, including its positive effect on child support payments and parental involvement. Child support agency staff would tell custodial parents about the option of forgiving child support debt through the Match program. They would also provide pamphlets explaining the operation of the program and the benefits it provides. The state would also advertise the Match program to custodial parents through its websites and social media (including testimonials from custodial parents who have forgiven child support debt). There is insufficient evidence to support a prediction of how many custodial parents would agree to forgive child support debt through the Match program. However, a study of five debt-forgiveness programs found that when custodial parent debt is addressed, "the reaction is more likely to be positive than negative" (Pearson et al. 2012: 54).

Equity: Maximize Ease of Compliance by Noncustodial Parent

High. Although MPO forgives less debt, on average, than the other policy options, it is easier for participants to qualify for debt reduction. Unlike the other options, participants can begin reducing their debt immediately and this debt reduction is permanent regardless of the consistency of payments in the future.

Cost: Minimize Cost of Implementation

MPO would require ten full-time-equivalent staff positions for participant recruitment and program oversight and administration, amounting to $900,000 annually, including benefits. The program would also require ten additional staff to inform custodial parents about debt forgiveness and to train existing child support workers on how to approach custodial parents to discuss this option. Assuming each outreach worker is paid $75,000 (including benefits), this component would cost about $750,000 annually, bringing the total annual cost of MPO to **$1,650,000**.

Table 6.3 Analysis Summary for Match Plus Outreach

Alternative	Maximize Number of Noncustodial Parents Eligible For Debt Reduction	Maximize Amount of State Debt Reduction	Possibility of Custodial Parent Debt Reduction	Maximize Ease of Compliance by Noncustodial Parent	Minimize Cost of Implementation	Maximize Political Acceptability
Match Plus Outreach	Approx. 80%	Varies, probably 10% to 25% of debt forgiven annually	Yes	High	$1.65 million	Moderate

Maximize Political Acceptability: Likelihood and Intensity of Opposition to Proposed Options from Key Stakeholders

Moderate. MPO might elicit more political opposition than the other alternatives. The governor and legislature will need to be convinced about the merits of public outreach to encourage custodial parent debt forgiveness. As discussed earlier, nearly all debt forgiveness programs focus on state-owed debt and few attempt to address debt owed to custodial parents. Some states are wary of trying to influence custodial parents to accept a debt reduction, and some are concerned about the possibility of litigation if they are perceived to be pressuring parents to forgive debt (Pearson et al. 2012). Yet it does not appear that efforts to educate custodial parents about the pros and cons of debt forgiveness should be exceptionally controversial. If presented in a sympathetic way, the governor and legislature should be persuadable.

Alternative 3: Workforce Development

Effectiveness: Maximize the Number of Noncustodial Parents Eligible for Debt Reduction

Workforce Development would benefit a much smaller share of all eligible noncustodial parents compared to the other options, as it would require participants to complete a ten-week educational program and then obtain

Table 6.4 Analysis Summary for Workforce Development

Alternative	Maximize Number of Noncustodial Parents Eligible For Debt Reduction	Maximize Amount of State Debt Reduction	Possibility of Custodial Parent Debt Reduction	Maximize Ease of Compliance by Noncustodial Parent	Minimize Cost of Implementation	Maximize Political Acceptability
Workforce Development	5%	25% to 100%	No	High	$2.72 million	High

paid employment. The capacity of these educational programs would be limited, at least initially, to around 200 slots per ten-week period, serving about 1,000 noncustodial parents annually. This is **about 5 percent of all noncustodial parents who are in arrears to the state**.

Effectiveness: Maximize the Amount of State Debt Reduction
WD would also forgive 25 percent of all noncustodial parents' debt upon the completion of the ten-week educational program, and the remaining 75 percent would be forgiven after the noncustodial parent completes six months of employment. **Therefore, 100 percent in total**.

Effectiveness: Possibility of Custodial Parent Debt Reduction
None. WD would forgive state debt only.

Cost: Payroll and Other Costs to State Government and Partner Organizations
WD would be the most expensive of the four options as it involves an educational component as well as case management. The state will need to cover the costs of developing and operating a ten-week workforce development program. As a rough approximation, this program would cost $2,000 per participant. If the state serves 1,000 noncustodial parents per year (200 people per cohort, with five cohorts per year), the educational component would cost about $2 million annually. In addition, participant recruitment, employer recruitment, and program administration would require a full-time-equivalent staff of perhaps eight people,

which would cost about $720,000 (assuming an average staff salary, including benefits, of $90,000). In total, the alternative would cost about **$2.72 million** annually.

Equity: Likelihood of Compliance (Months of Child Support Payment Required for State Debt Reduction)
High. As noted earlier, WD would forgive 25 percent of total state debt after ten weeks (completion of the educational program) and the remaining 75 percent after six continuous months of employment. In other words, 100 percent of state debt could be forgiven after **8 1/2 months**. Moreover, debt reduction is not contingent on payment of child support.

Maximize Political Acceptability: Likelihood and Intensity of Opposition to Proposed Options from Key Stakeholders
High. There seem to be few if any objections to this approach. For example, the former county executive of Westchester County, New York, a conservative Republican, was a staunch advocate for that county's debt forgiveness program (Wogan 2017).

Alternative 4: Automatic Forgiveness of Arrears Due to Incarceration

Effectiveness: Maximize the Number of Noncustodial Parents Eligible for Debt Reduction
AFAI applies to a subset of all noncustodial parents with child support debt owed to the state: only noncustodial parents who fell into arrears as a result of incarceration, specifically in the state's prison's system. Arrears accumulated while in the federal prison system, in the prisons of other states, or in local jails would not be reduced. Nationally, about 40 percent of all noncustodial parents with child support orders are currently or were formerly incarcerated (Haney and Mercier 2021: 14) Five years ago the state initiated a policy of automatically suspending the child support orders of all parents entering state prison. These individuals have not incurred arrears during their incarceration, but this policy change did not affect noncustodial parents who were previously

Table 6.5 Analysis Summary for Automatic Forgiveness of Arrears Due to Incarceration

Alternative	Maximize Number of Noncustodial Parents Eligible For Debt Reduction	Maximize Amount of State Debt Reduction	Possibility of Custodial Parent Debt Reduction	Maximize Ease of Compliance by Noncustodial Parent	Minimize Cost of Implementation	Maximize Political Acceptability
AFAI	22%	About 50%	No	High	$50,000 in year 1 only	Medium

incarcerated. We will assume that 25 percent of the NCPs in the state accumulated child support debt during incarceration in the state's prisons and are therefore eligible for automatic arrears reduction (Haney and Mercier 2021), and that the state will be able to successfully match the child-support and prison records of 85 percent of these NCPS (21 percent of all NCPs)

Effectiveness: Maximize the Amount of State Debt Reduction
The amount of debt that is forgiven under AFAI would depend on the extent to which the outstanding debt was accrued while the noncustodial parent was incarcerated (the state did not charge interest on child support debt). These circumstances may account for all of the debt incurred by some noncustodial parents but a smaller percentage for others. Some parents were in arrears prior to prison, and many continued to accrue debt after their release, in part because of difficulty finding and retaining employment (Haney 2022). We will therefore assume that on average AFAI will eliminate about **half** of an eligible parent's outstanding child support debt.

Effectiveness: The Possibility of Custodial Parent Debt Reduction
None. AFAI applies only to debt owed to the state.

Equity: Maximize Ease of Compliance by Noncustodial Parent (Duration and Stringency of Child Support Payments Required for State Debt Reduction)

High. Debt reduction under AFAI is automatic and unconditional, requiring no action on the part of the noncustodial parent. The debt is erased in recognition of the fact that it was impossible to provide child support while incarcerated, and that the resulting debt was not incurred fairly. Therefore, the debt relief is not contingent on any behavioral change or expectations on the part of the noncustodial parent.

Cost: Minimize Cost of Implementation
We assume that the matching of child support and state prison records can be executed by current staff. A total of $50,000 may be required for start-up costs (computer programming, training)

Maximize Political Acceptability: Likelihood and Intensity of Opposition to Proposed Options from Key Stakeholders
Medium. Debt forgiveness for low-income noncustodial parents currently enjoys a significant amount of political support, as evidenced by the increasing number of programs in place to forgive child support debt owed to the state. Moreover, support of debt forgiveness is bipartisan. Political opposition to AFAI is particularly unlikely since it focuses on debt that was accumulated when the noncustodial parent had virtually no ability to pay child support—when incarcerated. However, some law makers may balk at the automatic, unconditional aspect of this option—that debt reduction would not require beneficiaries to pay down the rest of their debt or meet their current child support obligations, or otherwise demonstrate "personal responsibility." Moreover, the state would be setting a new precedent, becoming the first to automatically reduce child-support arrears incurred during incarceration. As discussed in Chapter 3, several states automatically suspend current child support orders when parents become incarcerated, but none have applied the same procedure to reduce arrears accumulated during incarceration.

Comparison of Alternatives and Their Trade-Offs
Having estimated the outcomes of the four policy options in light of the criteria, we can now turn to their comparison. Table 6.6 summarizes the results so far.

Table 6.6 Comparison of Debt Forgiveness Alternatives Criteria

	Maximize Number of Noncustodial Parents Eligible For Debt Reduction	Maximize Amount of State Debt Reduction	Possibility of Custodial Parent Debt Reduction	Maximize Ease of Compliance by Noncustodial Parent	Minimize Cost of Implementation	Maximize Political Acceptability
PIP	Approx. 80%	50 to 100% of outstanding arrears (50% after 12 months; 100% after 24)	No	Low	$900,000	High
MPO	Approx. 80%	Varies, probably 10% to 25% of debt forgiven annually	Yes	High	$1.65 million	Moderate
WD	5%	25% to 100%	No	High	$2.72 million	High
AFAI	25%	About 50%	No	High	$50,000 (year 1 only)	Moderate

The first step in comparing the alternatives is to see if any can be eliminated from further consideration because they are "dominated" by the others; that is, they rate no better than the other alternatives across all of the criteria. None of the alternatives are dominated. Each alternative has at least one area of strength compared to the others.

However, one could argue that WD is "practically dominated" by AFAI. AFAI's outcomes are equal or superior to WD across all but one criterion: political feasibility. Whereas WD is highly feasible, AFAI's feasibility is moderate because of possible objections to its unconditional design. For this reason we will focus our attention on the other three alternatives: PIP, MPO, and AFAI.

In comparing the three remaining options, it is useful to see if differences in certain measures of effectiveness are outweighed by others. Two options, PIP and MPO, would be available to most, if not all, noncustodial parents with child support debt owed to the state. AFAI would be available to fewer noncustodial parents. The options also vary with regard to the amount of debt that could be forgiven, the likelihood that noncustodial parents will satisfy the requirements for debt forgiveness, and whether there is opportunity for reduction of debt owed to custodial parents.

While the PIP program can forgive 100 percent of all arrears, the amount reduced by AFAI will depend on the extent to which debt was incurred as a result of incarceration but is likely to average around 25 percent. With MPO, less debt is likely to be forgiven over one or two years as compared to the other two programs.

However, participants in MPO and AFAI are more likely to succeed in seeing their debt forgiven because these options would not claw back any debt reduction of participants who fail to satisfy programmatic requirements such as failing to make child support payments. With PIP, 50 percent of child support debt is forgiven after 12 months of consistent payments, and 100 percent after 24 months. Participants who fail to make three complete child support payments during the 24-month period would be dropped from the program and receive no debt reduction at all. In other words, although the program is open to a large number of noncustodial parents, it is likely to see more attrition than the others due to its requirements.

MPO is the only alternative that attempts to help noncustodial parents obtain debt forgiveness from **custodial parents**. Child support debt to custodial parents is now far more pervasive than child support debt owed to the states. If this option achieved even a modicum of success in reducing debt owed to custodial parents, it would greatly increase both the number of noncustodial parents who could see their child support debt reduced and the total amount of debt that is reduced. Moreover, the option would enable the state to learn from its outreach experience about the most effective ways of obtaining permission from custodial parents to forgive child support debt.

The cost of the alternatives vary widely. AFAI is least expensive because it would not require any additional staff, only up to $50,000 in start-up expenses for computer programming and training. PIP would cost about $900,000 annually and MPO about $1.65 million. Nevertheless, none of the programs would be prohibitively expensive for a large state government agency. As a result, differences in costs are unlikely to be determinative considerations.

Although MPO would result in less debt forgiveness for the average noncustodial parent compared to the other two options, the program, as with AFAI, rates highly in ease of compliance. The program would be more expensive than AFAI but costs less than $1 million annually. MPO and AFAI both rate moderate for political feasibility. MPO would require some political persuasion to be adopted given the sensitivities surrounding the fact that government cannot require custodial parents to forgive debt. But if the option is presented so that clear safeguards would be in place to prevent custodial parents from feeling pressured or otherwise coerced into debt forgiveness, it is likely that the governor and the legislature would support the program. AFAI, as noted, may encounter opposition to the fact that it does not require any behavioral change among noncustodial parents in exchange for debt forgiveness (e.g., sustained child support payments; employment), and some lawmakers may be hesitant to launch an untested policy that has not been adopted elsewhere.

In sum, MPO is on balance the most compelling alternative. It would be available to about 80 percent of all NCPS, the same as PIP. Although it would not forgive as much debt in the same amount of time as the other options, it offers the key advantage of being the only option with the potential for forgiveness of custodial parent debt. Like AFAI it also rates high for ease of compliance as debt reductions would be irrevocable. Also like AFAI it is moderately politically feasible.

The WD option is far more expensive than the other alternatives and would operate at a much smaller scale. For this reason, it is not recommended. However, if experience shows that many noncustodial parents are unable to participate in MPO because they lack the workforce skills necessary for steady employment, then the state should also consider adopting programs that combine debt reduction with workforce development, case management, and job placement.

The preceding analysis has assumed that the alternatives are mutually exclusive. Is this always the case? Would it be possible to automatically forgive all child-support arrears incurred during incarceration AND give noncustodial parents the opportunity for additional debt reduction, perhaps through PIP or MPO?

Similarly, a major advantage of MPO is the potential for gaining permission from custodial parents to forgive debt owed to them. The outreach component of this alternative refers to outreach to custodial parents. While the state does not have legal authority to automatically reduce arrears owed to custodial parents, there is no reason why the outreach component of MPO could not be part of PIP and WD.

The possibility of revising the alternatives and criteria and repeating the process of estimating and comparing the outcomes of the modified alternatives once again underscores the provisional and iterative character of policy analysis.

Notes

1 See Stokey and Zeckhauser (1978) for a discussion of the application of several types of models in policy analysis. See also Patton et al. (2013).
2 See Chapter 4 and Stone (2012) for a discussion of multiple ways of defining equity.
3 Child support debt is a complex issue, and to facilitate its use as a case study to illustrate the process of policy analysis, we have simplified it in certain respects. For example, the case does not deal with individuals who have child-support debt but no longer have active child-support cases (e.g., their children are now adults). Also, the technical term for child-support debt forgiveness is debt compromise (Office of Inspector General 2007). Finally, note that all of the options under consideration are restricted to low-income noncustodial parents.

4 As discussed in Chapter 2, the amount and proportion of child support debt owed to the states has declined sharply since the early 2000s. A key reason for this decrease is that participation in the nation's welfare program—Temporary Assistance for Needy Families (TANF)—has diminished steadily since the program was created in 1996, replacing Assistance for Families with Dependent Children (AFDC) (Sorensen 2014).

References

Anderson, Michael L. 2013. "Subways, Strikes, and Slowdowns: The Impacts of Public Transit on Traffic Congestion." *National Bureau of Economic Research, Working Paper No. 18757*. www.nber.org/papers/w18757.pdf

Bardach, Eugene, and Eric M. Patashnik. 2023. *A Practical Guide for Policy Analysis: The Eightfold Path to More Effective Problem Solving* (7th Edition). Los Angeles, CA: CQ Press.

Beitch, Rebecca. 2016. "Oregon's First Test of Automatic Voter Registration has Mixed Results." *Pew Charitable Trusts: Stateline* (November 16). www.pewtrusts.org/en/research-and-analysis/blogs/stateline/2016/11/16/oregons-first-test-of-automatic-voter-registration-has-mixed-results

Brennan Center for Justice (New York University School of Law). 2018. *Automatic Voter Registration*. www.brennancenter.org/analysis/automatic-voter-registration

Fawley, Brett, and Luciana Juvenal. 2010. "Mexico's Oportunidades Program Fails to Make the Grade in NYC." *Federal Reserve Bank of St. Louis* (July). www.stlouisfed.org/~/media/Files/PDFs/publications/pub_assets/pdf/re/2010/c/opportunity_program.pdf

Halpern, David. 2015. *Inside the Nudge Unit*. London: WH Allen.

Hammond, John S., Ralph L. Keeney, and Howard Raifa. 1999. *Smart Choices: A Practical Guide to Decision Making*. Boston, MA: Harvard Business School Press.

Haney, Lynn. 2022. *Prisons of Debt: The Afterlives of Incarcerated Fathers*. Berkeley, CA: University of California Press.

Haney, Lynne, and Marie-Dumesie Mercier. 2021. *Child Support and Reentry*. Washington, DC: National Institute of Justice. www.ojp.gov/pdffiles1/nij/300780.pdf

Marsh, Julie A., Matthew G. Springer, Daniel F. McCaffrey, Kun Yuan, Scott Epstein, Julia Koppich, Nidhi Kalra, Catherine DiMartino, and Art Xiao Peng. 2011. *A Big Apple for Educators New York City's Experiment with Schoolwide Performance Bonuses. Final Evaluation Report*. Santa Monica, CA: Author. www.rand.org/pubs/monographs/MG1114.html

Matthews, Dylan. 2015. "Obama Suggested Making it Illegal not to Vote. Here's How that's Worked in Australia." *Vox* (March 18). www.vox.com/2014/11/11/7155285/australia-compulsory-voting-turnout-midterm

Milam, Ronald T., Marc Birnbaum, Chris Ganson, Susan Handy, and Jerry Walters. 2017. "Closing the Induced Vehicle Travel Gap Between Research and Practice." *Transportation Research Record 2653*: 10–16.

Office of Child Support Enforcement. 2023. *Preliminary Report FY2022*. Washington, DC: Author. www.acf.hhs.gov/sites/default/files/documents/ocse/fy_2022_preliminary_report.pdf

Office of Inspector General. 2007. *State Use of Debt Compromise to Reduce Child Support Arrearages*. Washington, DC: US Department of Health and Human Services. OEI-06–06–00070 (October). https://oig.hhs.gov/oei/reports/oei-06-06-00070.pdf

Ossokina, Ioulia V., Jos van Ommeren, and Henk van Mourik. 2023. "Do Highway Widenings Reduce Congestion?" *Journal of Economic Geography 23, 4*: 871–900.

Patton, Carl V., David S. Sawicki, and Jennifer J. Clark. 2013. *Basic Methods of Policy Analysis and Planning* (5th Edition). Boston, MA: Pearson.

Pearson, Jessica, Nancy Thoennes, and Rasa Kaulnelis. 2012. *Debt Compromise Programs: Program Design and Child Support Outcomes in Five Locations*. Report submitted by Center for Policy Research to US Office of Child Support Enforcement. www.ywcss.com/sites/default/files/pdf-resource/debt_compromise_improving_child_support_outcomes_final_report_nov_14_2012.pdf

Pressman, Jeffrey, and Aaron Wildavksy. 1984. *Implementation* (3rd Edition). Berkeley, CA: University of California Press.

Sorensen, Elaine. 2014. "Major Change in Who is Owed Child Support Arrears." *US Office of Child Support Enforcement, Child Support Fact Sheet Series, Number 4*. www.acf.hhs.gov/sites/default/files/programs/css/changes_in_who_is_owed_arrears.pdf

Stokey, Edith, and Richard Zeckhauser. 1978. *A Primer for Policy Analysis*. New York: W. W. Norton.

Stone, Deborah. 2012. *Policy Paradox: The Art of Political Decision Making* (3rd Edition). New York: W. W. Norton.

Thaler, Richard H., and Cass R. Sunstein. 2008. *Nudge: Improving Decisions About Health, Wealth, and Happiness*. New Haven: Yale University Press.

Wiemer David. L., and Aidan R. Vining. 2005. *Policy Analysis: Concepts and Practice* (4th Edition). Upper Saddle River, NJ: Prentice-Hall.

Wogan, J.B. 2017. "A New Strategy for Collecting Child Support: Debt Forgiveness." *Governing* (June 27). www.governing.com/topics/health-human-services/gov-child-support-westchester-new-york-debt-foregiveness.html

7
RESEARCH AND POLICY ANALYSIS

Research is essential for policy analysis. From problem definition through analysis of alternative options, nearly all elements of policy analysis require evidence and knowledge. The purpose of this chapter is to discuss the role of research in policy analysis and examine the most important methods and data sources.

The Role and Purpose of Research in Policy Analysis

A distinction is often made in the social, natural, and physical sciences between basic and applied research. Basic research serves to advance our understanding of a phenomenon or problem, perhaps by uncovering new knowledge or developing or improving a theoretical explanation. The research is valued as an end in itself. Applied research, in contrast, is more instrumental, a means to achieve certain goals. In biology, for example, basic research may help understand the functioning of human cells, while applied research may focus on the development of new medications. Basic research in biochemistry may generate vital insights that are integral to the development of new medications, but these pharmaceutical innovations are not the primary objectives of basic research.

Policy analysis is a form of applied research. Its purpose is to understand the nature of the issue to be addressed, to identify potential solutions, and to compare these alternatives in light of specific criteria. It is shaped by the context of the issue and the time and other resources available to the analyst. Research for policy analysis tends to be synthetic, to cover a range of questions, draw from a variety of sources, and involve a mix of methods. The questions and methods are shaped in large part by the nature of the issue to be addressed and the types of policies to be considered. In the social sciences, on the other hand, the focus is usually much narrower. The "agenda of inquiry is largely established by the internal logic of existing disciplines" (Moore 1980: 273), and research often serves to uncover new knowledge or support or refute theoretical propositions.

Another key difference between research in policy analysis compared to other fields is the amount of time and resources that are available. Whereas the time frame for basic research and some forms of applied research is usually measured in years or months, for policy analysis it is compressed into weeks or even days. In addition, policy analysts, from necessity, are more receptive than their peers in the social sciences to imperfect information and uncertainty (Moore 1980; Behn 1985).

Similarly, whereas research in the physical, biological, and, to a lesser degree, social sciences is funded through grants from government agencies and foundations, policy analysts seldom if ever have access to external funding for research. This means that policy analysts are usually unable to purchase proprietary databases or specialized computer software (unless their employer has the resources and inclination to do so), contract for opinion polls, or hire research assistants. Articles in peer-reviewed academic journals may also be prohibitively expensive unless the analyst's employer subscribes to a bibliographic database. Given these constraints, research for policy analysis typically revolves around activities that require little more than the analyst's time: interviews, focus groups, reviewing documents available at no or nominal cost, and analysis of publicly available data sets. Fortunately, thanks to the Internet, policy analysts enjoy instant access to millions of policy-relevant documents and many data sets.

The Research Plan

Given the multitude of questions to be addressed and the variety of data sources and research methods that can be required, it is often useful to prepare a research plan. Otherwise, analysts risk becoming bogged down researching topics that are tangential or irrelevant, or plunging into more detail than is necessary, and perhaps neglecting the most essential questions. Policy analysts have only a limited amount of time to arrive at their recommendations. It is therefore essential to be as efficient and strategic as possible in researching the issue.

A research plan can serve as a guide for the project, linking the questions to the pertinent data sources and research methods, and specifying how the research will contribute to policy analysis (e.g., helping to illuminate the nature of the problem, identifying possible alternatives, evaluating the alternatives). It also forces the analyst to decide on the relative importance of each question and the amount of time and resources that should be dedicated to it. If a team of analysts is collaborating on a project, the research plan can also designate which team member(s) is responsible for each task (see Table 7.1 for an example of how a research plan might be structured for the child support debt case.).[1]

Almost all policy analyses involve a combination of research methods. They almost invariably include literature reviews, interviews (individual or group), and often analyses of quantitative data. Sometimes, research can involve observation of public meetings or hearings and attendance at conferences and other events.

The research that policy analysts carry out, and the questions they seek to address, is to a large degree shaped by the kinds of policy alternatives the analysts consider and the criteria they choose to evaluate them. Analysts always need to research the nature of the problem, including its evolution over time, its causes, and its consequences. Analysts will want to explore how the issue—and perhaps similar or analogous ones—is addressed elsewhere or has been addressed previously. Depending on the criteria they adopt to assess the alternatives, analysts need to obtain information necessary to apply these criteria. For example, analysts may need to research the principal costs of each alternative and seek out evidence of their effectiveness. If equity is a concern, the analysts may need to look at the distributional impacts of programs and policies similar to those being proposed. In order to assess political feasibility, the analysts may need to gauge the degree to which key

Table 7.1 Research Design for Child Support Case, Selected Questions

Question	Hypothesis	Information Source	Priority	Plug In	Responsibility
What do you need to know?	What is your best guess?	Where might you go for the information? What will you do when you find the source? Interview? Get a report? Examine the files?	How critical is the information to your analysis? (Which question[s] must be answered first?)	How will this information help your analysis? (Where will it fit in?)	Which team member(s) is assigned to get this question answered?
What is the total child support debt, and how has it changed over time?	Tens of billions of dollars; little change	Office of Child Support Enforcement annual reports, academic studies, other reports	Very important	Nature of the problem	
What is the distribution of child support debt among noncustodial parents? What is the average debt amount?	Highly skewed towards a relatively small portion of parents with high amounts of debt	Office of Child Support Enforcement annual reports, academic and other studies	Very important	Nature of the problem, analysis of alternatives	
What are the key reasons for accumulation of debt?	Failure to pay, retroactive obligations, interest and fees	Literature review, interviews with experts	Very important	Nature of the problem, analysis of alternatives	
What are the consequences of child support debt—for custodial and noncustodial parents, and for children?	Varied	Literature review, interviews	Important	Nature of the problem	

Question	Findings	Sources	Importance	Section
How have federal, state, and local governments and other organizations attempted to reduce outstanding child support debt? What are their costs? How effective have they been?	In a variety of ways, some of which involve various requirements on the part of the noncustodial parent (continuous payment of child support, participation in classes). Few evaluations	Literature review, interviews	Very important	Identification and analysis of alternatives
Could programs currently or previously in place to reduce other kinds of debt be adopted for child support debt? Which ones?	Perhaps, it depends on context	Literature review, interviews	Important, but not essential	Identification of alternatives
To what degree is there political support for debt reduction?	Mixed, but increasing	Literature review, interviews	Important	Nature of the problem, analysis of alternatives

stakeholders (e.g., elected officials, advocates) would oppose or support the alternatives under consideration.

Documents

Policy analysts draw heavily on many kinds of documents. The list that follows illustrates the variety of documents that can provide valuable information and insights. We define "document" broadly. In addition to texts—whether hard copy or electronic—we also include audiovisual materials. In an era of YouTube and podcasts, more and more videos and audio productions are available on issues relevant to policy analysis. For example, it is now common practice to "live stream" speeches, panel discussions, symposia, and entire conferences, and these videos are often archived and available to the public.

- Books
- Peer-reviewed journal articles
- Newspaper and magazine articles
- Internet blogs
- Government reports
- Academic reports/studies
- Program evaluations
- Reports produced by advocacy organizations
- Reports produced by membership organizations and trade associations
- Doctoral dissertations
- Legislation and associated rules and regulations
- Judicial decisions and related documents
- Public hearing testimony and supportive documents
- Minutes and videos of town halls and public meetings of regulatory boards and commissions
- Budget documents
- Annual reports
- Meeting minutes
- Radio/television programs, including transcripts
- Transcripts, audio, or video of speeches, panel discussions

- Webinars
- Microsoft PowerPoint presentations
- Podcasts
- Documentaries

Documents, of course, can vary in their accuracy and balance. In an era of "fake news," it is not difficult to find diatribes and patently false information in blogs and newsletters that, from the standpoint of their professional-seeming format and editing, appear reputable and credible. It is therefore crucial at all times to be cognizant if not skeptical of the source for all documents.

One way of reducing the risk of basing policy analysis on misleading or false information is to "triangulate." In other words, like journalists, policy analysts should try to confirm important or potentially controversial statements or observations with other sources such as documents or people. This is especially important when the statement in question comes from sources that are not well known or that are known for being partisan or one-sided.

Voting Case: Dueling Views on Voting Policy

As a politically contentious issue, information on voting policies, and how it is presented, can vary widely depending on the positions taken. The most prominent organization working on voting rights in the United States is the Brennan Center, based at the New York University Law School. While the Brennan Center is nonpartisan and provides thorough, peer-reviewed research on voting policy, the Center openly advocates for voter rights and increased access to the polls. In contrast, the Heritage Foundation, a conservative think tank, has picked up the mantle of documenting voter fraud. At first glance, the two organizations may seem to provide counter-balancing evidence; however, a closer look shows a considerable degree of difference in the depth of research and evidence on voting policy, and a distinctly partisan agenda by the Heritage Foundation. A truly bipartisan approach to voting policy can be found at the National Conference of State Legislatures, which provides research on election law in states across the country.

Peer-reviewed journals, university presses, and newspapers "of record" are among the most reliable sources of information and analysis. Other important sources include governmental agencies that provide research and policy analysis to the executive and/or legislative branches. For example, the federal Government Accountability Office publishes rigorous reports on a wide array of topics in response to Congressional requests. Many federal agencies also publish high-quality studies, including program evaluations. State and local government oversight bodies, auditors, and related entities publish research on many topics germane to public policy. For example, New York City's Independent Budget Office issues reports on municipal finance, education, environment, housing, social services, and other subjects (Independent Budget Office of the City of New York 2024).

Policy analysis can seldom if ever rely exclusively on peer-reviewed sources for their work. Depending on the topic, these sources can be extremely important and useful. However, they may not be particularly current—in part because of the amount of time required for book and journal manuscripts to be reviewed and revised, and the time it takes for publication. In addition, some topics are covered more thoroughly than others, and some issues may be very idiosyncratic or local, and require information and insight from other sources.

It may be inevitable that policy analysts must draw on articles and other documents that were not peer reviewed, but this does not mean that non-peer-reviewed documents are of equal credibility. Some are far more authoritative than others. Policy analyses based primarily on the likes of the Huffington Post or Wikipedia will carry far less weight than analyses that draw from reports published by, say, nonpartisan think tanks and research organizations such as the American Enterprise Institute, the Brookings Institution, or the Center on Budget and Policy Priorities. While the Huffington Post and Wikipedia publish many excellent articles, these websites do little to fact check or otherwise vet their submissions. For example, Wikipedia entries are monitored, edited, and updated by volunteers, who often correct or flag for deletion erroneous or misleading language—but there is no guarantee that particular statements will be noticed and corrected, and false statements may linger for a long time before being corrected or deleted (Wikipedia

2024). In contrast, commentary and analysis published by the American Enterprise Institute, Brookings, or the Center on Budget and Policy Priorities may reflect these organizations' political and ideological proclivities (respectively, conservative, centrist, liberal), but are generally respected as thoughtful, thorough, and evidence-based.

Advocacy organizations can also be an important source of information and analysis. True, they may publish reports and articles to advance their agenda, or their position on a particular issue, but this does not mean that their work should be dismissed. Many advocacy groups are highly respected for the quality and rigor of their research and data analysis and for the cogency of their arguments. Moreover, the credibility and effectiveness of many advocacy organizations rests on the quality of their work. Blatantly misleading data analysis or analysis that is otherwise flawed can undermine a group's ability to persuade decision makers to adopt their position and can, in the longer run, cause them to lose influence and access.

When reviewing documents published by advocacy organizations, policy analysts should always be mindful of the organization's reputation for the quality of its research and analysis. Is the organization's work often cited? Are the authors recognized as experts on the topic? If the analyst is not familiar with the advocacy organization, it is essential to do some due diligence before using the group's publications. If possible, it's always advisable to draw from multiple sources so that it doesn't appear that the analysis is based entirely on the work of an advocacy (or other) organization.

How to Find Relevant Documents

With just a few keystrokes, Google or other Internet search engines can produce links to hundreds or even thousands of documents germane to the topic of interest. However, these documents can vary widely in their relevance, quality, and credibility. As a result, analysts must spend a substantial amount of time scanning and assessing the value of the documents revealed through an Internet search.

Moreover, not all documents are accessible through standard search engines. Google Scholar allows users to identify journal articles and other specialized publications on numerous topics, but these publications may not be available for free, unless the analyst's employer subscribes to a full-text bibliographic database (e.g., jstor, ProQuest) or can access these databases through a library. Some peer-reviewed journals are "open access," available free of charge. Some academic journals designate a small number of articles to be "open access" as well. However, the vast majority of peer-reviewed journals are behind a paywall. If analysts do not have access to a library database and need to access a limited number of journal articles, they may still be able to acquire the articles without having to pay the publisher. Sometimes, PDFs of individual articles are available online (often in draft form). If not, analysts can ask colleagues, friends, and relatives with access to university libraries to download the article. Another option is to contact the author directly and request the article. It is usually not difficult to obtain email addresses for academics by searching for their CVs or scanning the website of their university departments. ResearchGate also enables people to request publications from the author.

In addition to Internet searches, another productive way of identifying and accessing documents is to search for reports published or sponsored by government agencies. As noted earlier, the federal Government Accountability Office issues scores of reports every year on a wide array of topics, such as criminal justice, housing finance, child welfare, and national defense. Almost every federal agency has a research or statistical unit that is a depository of reports and data sets (see Table 7.2). The websites of many state agencies and of large cities may also provide important documents and data. Congressional committees also produce reports, and hold hearings, on numerous topics that can be extremely valuable.

An excellent source for federal documents of many kinds is FDsys (Federal Digital System). Sponsored by the US Government Printing Office, FDsys is a searchable database of a host of government documents, including regulations, hearing transcripts, Congressional bills, Congressional reports, and much more. Another useful resource is the Library of Congress website, http://Congress.gov, which provides comprehensive information of current and previous legislation.

Table 7.2 Statistical and Research Agencies of the Federal Government

Government Department	Agency
Administration for Children and Families	Office of Planning, Research, and Evaluation
Board of Governors of the Federal Reserve System (FRB)	NA
Centers for Disease Control and Prevention	NA
National Academies of Science, Engineering and Medicine	NA
National Science Foundation	National Center for Science and Engineering Statistics
US Congress	Congressional Budget Office Congressional Research Service Government Accountability Office Library of Congress (http://Congress.gov)
US Department of Agriculture	Economic Research Service National Agricultural Statistics Service
US Department of Commerce	Bureau of Economic Analysis Census Bureau
US Department of Education	National Center for Education Statistics
US Department of Energy	Energy Information Administration
US Department of Health and Human Services	National Center for Health Statistics
US Department of Housing and Urban Development	Office of Policy Development and Research
US Department of Justice	Bureau of Justice Statistics
US Department of Transportation	Bureau of Transportation Statistics
US Environmental Protection Agency	Office of Research and Development Laboratories Office of Research and Development Research Programs
US Social Security Administration	Office of Research, Evaluation, and Statistics

Nonpartisan think tanks and research organizations also publish reports on numerous topics of concern to policy analysis. At the national level, almost every policy domain (e.g., health care, national defense, education, technology) is covered by one or more such organizations. Some research groups also focus on particular states and cities. Table 7.3 lists a sampling of the most prominent think tanks.

Table 7.3 Selected Policy-Related Research Organizations With a National or Global Focus

Organization	Website
Abt Associates	www.abtassociates.com
American Enterprise Institute	www.aei.org
Aspen Institute	www.aspeninstitute.org
BiPartisan Policy Center	https://bipartisanpolicy.org
The Brookings Institution	www.brookings.edu
Center on Budget and Policy Priorities	www.cbpp.org
The Century Foundation	https://tcf.org
Economic Policy Institute	www.epi.org
Inter-University Consortium for Political and Social Research	www.icpsr.umich.edu/icpsrweb
Lincoln Institute of Land Policy	www.lincolninst.edu
Mathematica Policy Research	www.mathematica-mpr.com
MDRC	www.MDRC.org
National Bureau of Economic Research	www.nber.org
Pew Research Center	www.pewresearch.org
Policy Link	www.policylink.org
RAND Corporation	www.rand.org
Resources for the Future	www.rff.org
Urban Institute	www.urban.org

Internet searches—including, if possible, searches of library databases—are not the only way of identifying and obtaining useful documents. As Bardach and Patashnik (2015) put it, "documents lead to documents," and "people lead to documents."

Documents Lead to Documents

Once the analyst obtains one useful document, that document can lead to many more. Its bibliography and/or footnotes may refer the analyst to other important documents, and the references provided in these other documents can lead the analyst to still others.

People Lead to Documents

When interviewing subject experts, program administrators, journalists, or anyone else, you should always ask about any books, articles, reports, or other documents that may be pertinent to the issue. Sometimes, interviewees may be able to identify, and perhaps provide, documents that are not accessible on the Web or that are still in draft form (always bring a flash drive to any meeting so that you can readily obtain documents that are offered). It's also smart to obtain annual reports, newsletters, and other materials about or published by the interviewee's organization, especially if the organization currently is involved in the issue or could play a role in implementing one of the potential alternative options. This information may provide, among other things, important information about the capacity of the organization. In addition to printed materials, the interviewee's website may also contain or provide links to valuable documents.

Interviews and Focus Groups

Rare is the policy analysis that does not entail interviews.[2] Interviews can be essential for all aspects of policy analysis. They can shed light on the nature of the problem, educate analysts about potential policy options, and shed light on their strengths and weakness, including their political and technical feasibility. Interviews can vary in their length and formality and in the number of people involved. They can be conducted in-person or remotely by phone, Zoom and other videoconferencing platforms, or email. In this section we discuss the role of interviews in policy analysis and provide guidance on selecting interview subjects, in conducting interviews, and in summarizing the interview results. Afterwards, we will discuss focus groups, a form of group interview.

Whom to Interview?

Depending on the kind of information and perspectives to be obtained, policy analysts may interview a wide range of people. They may include the client and other staff and colleagues at his or her organization. They may include experts on the topic, including academics, journalists, advocates, and researchers at think tanks and other organizations. They may include individuals directly affected by the issue at hand. They may include elected officials. They may include officials and other staff at public agencies, nonprofit organizations, and private companies, including those who operate programs that might serve as alternative options for solving the problem. Interviewees may be local or may be based in other states or countries. In selecting interview subjects, it is crucial to keep in mind the purpose of the interview—how the interview will contribute to the policy analysis—and to focus the questions on these topics.

It is seldom difficult to identify people to interview. Let's say you are the analyst. Most often, you will be able to speak with only a fraction of the potential interviewees you have identified. Once started on the project, the number of potential interviewees will snowball quickly, as each document and each interview can point to new people to interview.

Some interviews will always be easier to arrange than others. While some people respond quickly and affirmatively to requests for interviews, others are more elusive. It is rare for people to refuse requests for interviews. They are far more likely to ignore or put off these requests.

As a rule, people most readily agree to interviews when they already know the person requesting the interview—provided, of course, they do not dislike him or her. However, in most cases, policy analysts will not be personally acquainted with many—or any—of the people they wish to interview. The next best thing to knowing the person you wish to interview is to establish a connection through someone the person does know. For example, several key interviewees may be colleagues or acquaintances of the client. If that is the case, it is ideal to ask the client to contact these people directly and inform them that you will be reaching out to them for an interview. Other interviewees may also be willing to communicate directly with colleagues to encourage them to speak with you. If the client—or anyone else—isn't willing or able to contact prospective interviewees directly, you should ask permission to use their name when requesting interviews.

Most often, analysts will send interview requests by email. In composing the email, it's always advantageous to refer in the subject line to someone the prospective interviewee knows. For example, the subject line in an email requesting an email might say "Interview request: _____ suggested I speak with you." In the body of the text, you should again state that you are contacting the interviewee at the suggestion of the person they know—whether it is the client or someone else.

You should also explain the purpose of the interview. You should ask the person to contact you by email or phone to schedule the interview. Be as succinct as possible. Few people want to read more than a paragraph or two from a stranger. If you do not hear from the interviewee within a few days—and no more than a week—you should send a quick note to the person stating that you are following up on your previous email to set up a time to talk, or you might call the person's office and say that you are following up on your email to schedule an interview.

Interviews should be scheduled as quickly as possible to ensure that the subjects are able to fit the interviews on their schedules. However, some interviews should be scheduled earlier than others. It usually makes sense to first speak with people who can provide important background information and refer you to other informants. These may include scholars and other researchers who have written extensively on the topic as well as journalists who frequently cover the topic. It may also be useful to interview advocates at this stage as well. A second wave of interviews might focus on people associated with organizations, policies, or initiatives that could influence some of the policy options.

A third group of interviews might include individuals who can speak about the feasibility and other implementation challenges of the potential alternatives. If you need to speak with top officials and others with extremely busy schedules, it is usually best to hold these interviews towards the end of the project. This increases the chances that the official will be able to find the time for the interview and allows time for you to formulate the most important questions. Given the short amount of time that many people may have available, most analysts should focus on the questions that only the interviewee can answer or those for which it is essential to know the subject's views. Also, asking questions that reflect a substantial knowledge of the issue, and of the interviewee's background, may impress the interviewee and elicit more candid and thorough responses.

Finally, if the issue is especially contentious or controversial, the last people to interview are likely opponents of the recommended course of action who, once aware of the project, might seek to squelch the analyst's research by discouraging people in his or her network from cooperating. This is not to say, however, that you should always put off interviewing opponents of the proposed alternative. We are only referring to individuals who, once informed of the project, are likely to try to impede or derail it.

Preparing for the Interview

Analysts can expect interviews to last no more than 30 to 60 minutes, and when the interviewee is a government official or a top executive of a nonprofit organization or private corporation, the time allotted for the interview can be especially tight. It is therefore essential to focus on the topics for which the interviewee's perspectives are particularly valuable. These may include information that only the interviewee can provide or topics on which it is vital to know the interviewee's perspective.

Most interviews are open-ended. The interview is a conversation guided by a set of questions. While the analysts may ask some yes/no or other fixed response questions (e.g., "on a scale of 1 to 10, how would you rate the importance of X"), the purpose of most interviews is to learn from the subject's knowledge and opinions. This information is best conveyed in responses to open-ended questions.

In preparing for an interview, the analyst should compose a set of guiding questions. These questions should ask about the key topics to be explored. They may include, for example, questions about the origins of the problem, clarifications about a program, interpretations of the political viability of different potential programs to address the problem, or the capacity of different organizations to implement a program. Sometimes an interview guide will include a list of several main questions to be explored, plus some subsidiary questions related to the principal questions. The latter may serve as prompts in case the interviewee's initial response to the main question does not fully address the analyst's needs. It is crucial that the number of questions be in line with the amount of time available for the interview. If there are only 45 minutes allotted to the interview, it will probably be impossible to get through 20 open-ended questions. Of course, some people are very succinct and can respond fully to more questions than those who are more loquacious and like to illustrate their points with anecdotes and perhaps go off on tangents. Given that it may not be possible to cover all of the questions in the interview, put the most important questions towards the beginning of the interview and leave the less essential ones toward the end.

In preparing for the interview, the analyst must make the most of information already available from published sources as well as from previous interviews. Asking people about basic information about their organization or the issue to be addressed not only wastes valuable time, but it also conveys the impression that the interviewer is ill-prepared and/or uninformed. Moreover, if it is evident that the interviewer has done his or her "homework" and is familiar with the issue and the respondent's background, the interviewee will probably be all the more likely to take the interview seriously and be more generous with his or her time and perhaps his or her connections as well.

Interviewing in Person, by Video Conference, Phone, and Through Other Means

Policy analysts will usually conduct interviews in person or remotely by phone or video conferencing (e.g., Zoom). Interviews can also be conducted via email, with the subject responding in writing to a series of questions. In-person interviews tend to take the most time, as they usually require the analyst to travel to the subject's office or to another agreed-upon location (e.g., coffee shop).

The advantages of in-person interviews are substantial. Perhaps most important, they enable the analyst and interviewee to develop some rapport and trust—especially if they have not met previously. In-person interviews also enable the interviewer to read the "body language" of the subject—to see facial expressions and gestures that may convey excitement, frustration, impatience, distraction, and other positive and negative emotions. Such body language can provide clues about the subject's level of interest in the issue and signal when to probe deeper into a topic or move on to a new one. That the analyst is willing to travel to meet with the subject can also signal that the analyst is serious about the topic and is genuinely interested in learning about his or her views. Also, people may be willing to allocate more time to an in-person meeting than to a phone call or Zoom session and also may be more willing to extend the interview beyond its scheduled end time. Finally, being present at the subject's office may allow the interviewer to be introduced on the spur of the moment to colleagues who might also be useful sources and to obtain relevant reports and other hardcopy documents (although in a time when almost everything is online, this is less important than previously).

The principal disadvantage of in-person interviews is that they take more time, including travel, than other formats. Of course, in-person interviews are usually only possible when the interviewee is located nearby—say within a 30-minute drive or subway ride. When the subject is based in another city or country, the only feasible option is phone, videoconferencing, or email.

Conducting the Interview

Regardless of the mode of interview and the topics on the agenda, it is always important to do the following:

1. Briefly summarize the purpose of the interview and overarching project.
2. If you would like to record the interview, be sure to ask permission. Also, be sure to say that you're happy to turn off the recorder at any time for off-the-record comments.
3. Confirm the amount of time available for the interview.
4. Avoid asking leading questions. Do not pose questions in ways that encourage or discourage particular responses.
5. Always ask for recommendations on who else to interview (people lead to people). You should also ask if it's OK to tell these individuals that the respondent suggested you speak with them.
6. Always ask about any reports or other documents that might be useful (people lead to documents). The interviewee might be able to download them for you on a flash drive that you provide—or email them or links to them.
7. Always ask if you can contact the interviewee again for any follow-up questions.

8   When nearing the end of the allotted time of the interview, it is sometimes good to ask if the respondent is able to continue longer, especially if the discussion is illuminating and if he or she seems highly engaged.
9   Always follow up by sending emails to the interviewees thanking them for their time and confirming what items they owe the analyst and what the analyst will follow up on.

To Record or Not

Analysts may wish to record their interviews. Journalists almost always record their interviews, and individuals who are frequently interviewed by the media are often accustomed to being recorded and may even expect it. Other people may not be comfortable being taped and even those who are OK having some interviews recorded may not want others to be recorded.

There are advantages and disadvantages to recording interviews. Perhaps the most important advantage is that recording (if the technology works) provides a verbatim record of the interview and can be used to settle any misunderstandings or disputes that may arise about quotations or summaries of the interviewee's comments. Recordings also enable the analysts to clarify any gaps or ambiguities in the interviewer's notes and to extract exact quotes from the interview. On occasion, the analyst may want to transcribe some or all of the interview recordings as appendices to the report or perhaps as grist for computer-aided content analysis (e.g., summarizing the number of times that certain themes were aired.).

A key disadvantage of recording interviews is that it can be intimidating and make people more restrained and cautious in their remarks than would be the case if they were not recorded. This may be especially true of people who are not used to being interviewed. Sometimes, these concerns may be eased by telling the interviewee that you are happy to stop the recording at any time in the interview and that you will not record any comments that the interviewee wishes to be "off the record."

Another disadvantage of taping is that it takes time and effort to replay recordings and search for specific quotes or other sections of the interview. It also takes time and effort to produce transcripts of taped interviews. Voice recognition software may make it easier to produce transcripts, but it remains essential to double-check any quotations from the original recording.

Taping can also make it easier for the interviewer to lose focus. Because the interviewer knows the conversation is being recorded, analysts may feel less need to listen closely to the subject's comments or may at times allow their concentration to wane. As a result, the interviewer may fail to ask the subject to elaborate on certain points or ask important follow-up questions. Taping may also tempt interviewers to take less extensive notes than they would in the absence of a recording.

Finally, while recording is often essential for conveying verbatim quotes, such quotes are not often so important. What is more important is that the analyst capture key information from the interview (e.g., factual matters as well as impressions and opinions). Most often, the exact wording used in these discussions is not essential. Of course, the analyst may sometimes want to quote from an interview—especially if the statement is especially eloquent, insightful, or surprising. In such cases, the analyst may be able to write the quote down in its entirety.

After the Interview

As soon as possible after each interview it is essential to write up a summary—whether or not the interview is recorded. One way of doing so is to draw from the interviewer's memory and notes and summarize the interviewee's responses to each question in the interview guide. The longer one waits to summarize the interview, the less he or she will remember. If done right away, the analyst may be able to elaborate on incomplete or confusing notes; otherwise, he or she may not be at all able to interpret the notes or recollect what the interviewee was referring to.

One Interviewer or More?

If a team of analysts is collaborating on a policy analysis, it can be advantageous for two or more team members to participate in interviews. With two interviewers involved, one can take the lead in guiding the conversation and the other can focus mostly on note taking. With two sets of ears, the interviewers may be more alert to comments that are ambiguous or contradict what the analysts have gleaned from other research and thus be able to ask appropriate follow-up questions. There is less chance of important questions being overlooked. Moreover, if the interview was not recorded, having two analysts present can generate a more complete summary of the interview. If the interviewee is particularly knowledgeable about the issue, or is otherwise central to its resolution, it can be beneficial for the entire team to participate in the interview.

Focus Groups and Group Interviews

Sometimes, analysts will conduct group interviews, speaking with two or more people at once. For example, an analyst may interview the executive director of a nonprofit organization along with a program director who operates one of the organization's initiatives. Another form of group interview is the focus group, whereby around 6 to 15 or so people discuss their experiences and/or views relating to a certain issue.

When the analyst is interviewing only a few people at once, the procedures are not very different from when there is a single interviewee—although the interview may need to last longer if it is to cover the same number of topics. However, note taking may be more difficult—and if the interview is recorded, it may be difficult to identify each speaker, and the sound quality of the recording may be uneven, depending on the position of the microphone and the volume of the speaker's voice. If possible, it is almost always beneficial to have more than one analyst participate in group interviews. Of course, group interviews need not only be conducted in person; they are also easy to carry out with conference calls and videoconferencing such as Zoom.

Focus groups can provide valuable insight regarding the way problems and programs are perceived. They generally involve people who may be affected by an issue and are less likely to include subject experts (government or official) or the leadership of nonprofit organizations or private companies. One benefit of focus groups is that they can enable participants to build off each other's comments and perhaps generate insights that would not be possible in a one-on-one interview. Focus groups, in other words, make it possible for participants to react to others' experiences and opinions and engage in a robust discussion. Focus groups require considerable skills on the part of the facilitator. Among other things, the facilitator needs to ensure that all participants have ample opportunity to speak freely and to prevent individual participants from dominating the discussion. The facilitator also needs to keep the discussion on track but also ask questions in ways that are open-ended enough so that they do not foster particular kinds of responses.

Focus groups require more planning than other interviews. Participants need to be recruited. An appropriate space must be found. Funds must be available to cover the cost of refreshments. Sometimes, especially when focus groups involve private citizens who are not participating in the discussion as an employee of an organization or as a government official, it is desirable to provide a small honorarium as compensation for their time. Focus groups almost always require the support of several people to run successfully. They are generally easier to carry out than surveys, but they require more time and resources than other types of interviews.[3]

Public Events and Site Visits

Policy analysts can also gain valuable information and insights by attending public events and, in some cases, visiting places of interest. In many instances, policy analysts can conduct research by listening and observing. If the timing is right, there may be opportunities to attend speeches, town halls, public meetings, workshops, seminars, conferences, or hearings on the topic at stake. For example, an analyst looking at strategies to preserve affordable housing might learn that the city council is holding a hearing on just that topic, in which case it would behoove her or him to attend. The hearing might feature a range of perspectives on the subject, reveal information or arguments new to the analyst, and enable the analyst to meet key experts and other stakeholders.

Site visits may also be very informative. They enable the analyst to observe first-hand the physical context surrounding the issue and to speak with some of the people most directly affected by it. For example, if an issue concerns changes in land use, such as the redevelopment of a particular neighborhood, visiting the site targeted to change may give the analyst a more tangible sense of its possibilities and limitations, and of the positive and negative consequences for local residents, employees, businesses, and other organizations. Site visits also enable analysts to speak at least informally with some of the people who would be most directly affected by proposed policies and perhaps by some of the people who would be responsible for their implementation. Some client projects carried out by students for the New School's Urban Policy Lab illustrate the value of site visits:

- For a study of possible redevelopment of an area in Brooklyn, students visited the site several times, photographing it and interviewing pedestrians, business owners, and other local stakeholders about their reactions to different redevelopment scenarios.
- For an analysis of possible ways to reform the bail system in New York City's criminal justice system, students observed court proceedings and visited several jails and other locations where people pay bail for relatives and friends, and interviewed more than 20 of them.
- For an analysis of ways to increase employer engagement in the design and delivery of vocational education at a community college, students visited the college, observed classrooms, and spoke with students and instructors.

Data Sets

In addition to written documents and interviews, policy analysts often need to draw on quantitative data. These data can be essential for framing the context of an issue, describing the nature of the problem, identifying policy alternatives, and analyzing these alternatives. Relevant data, depending on the topic, might include demographic and socioeconomic characteristics, employment trends, crime rates, budgetary trends, greenhouse gas emissions, public transit usage, housing costs, reading and math test scores, health indicators, voting patterns, public opinion polls, and much more.

Often, policy analysts can draw on data analysis conducted by others, such as statistical tables in journal articles or in reports. The analyst can then create new tables or graphs from these sources, with appropriate attribution. However, there will be times when the analyst is unable to locate published data summaries that address the issue at hand. Then, the analyst must work with larger data sets, and create his or her own tables, graphs, and maps.

Many data sets are readily available in the public domain, accessible for downloading from the Internet. The US Census Bureau, for example, publishes the decennial census and the American Community Survey, which provides a very wide range of demographic and socioeconomic data from the census tract level to the nation as a whole. http://Data.gov is a searchable clearinghouse of nearly 200,000 governmental databases. It focuses on data from federal agencies but also provides information on data sets developed by state and local governments (http://data.gov 2024). Fedstats is another online database that provides access to official statistical information produced by federal governmental agencies. The Inter-University Consortium for Political and Social Research at the University of Michigan provides access to more than 65,000 data sets that cover many topics relevant to policy analysis. The Pew Research Center provides to the public polling and other data on several topic areas, including science and technology, religion, demographic and social change, and politics (Pew Research Center 2024).

Box 7.1 A database on child support

An essential database for studies of child support is the Future of Families and Child Wellbeing Study. Originally known as the Fragile Families and Child Wellbeing Study (FFRC), this collaborative project overseen by researchers at Columbia and Princeton Universities, follows a cohort of nearly 5,000 people born in large US cities between 1998 and 2000. The study is based on wide-ranging interviews conducted with mothers, fathers, and/or primary caregivers of the children. The interviews took place at birth and when the children were ages 1, 3, 5, 9, and 15. Supplementing the interviews are in-home assessments of children at ages 1, 3, 5, 9, and 15 (Bendheim-Thoman Center for Research on Child and Family Wellbeing 2024). More than 1,400 articles, books, and other reports have been published that draw on FFRC data, covering a wide range of issues (Future of Families and Child Wellbeing Study 2024). Several of these studies assess the effects of the

> child support system in general and child support debt in particular on families. Emory et al. (2020) employed FFRC data to study the impact of incarceration on nonresident fathers' cash and in-kind contributions to their children's "household economy." Nepomnyaschy et al. (2021) used the FFRC to examine the effects of child support arrears on the socioemotional health of 9- and 15-year old children of nonresident fathers. Um (2019) drew on the FFRC to study the extent to which child support debt affects depression and alcohol abuse among nonresident fathers. Cozzolino (2018) utilized the FFRC to estimate the likelihood that nonresident fathers will acquire a formal child support order, accrue child support debt, and be jailed for this debt.

In addition, analysts can access the websites of individual government agencies for data. In some cases, especially if the analyst knows what data set to use, it can be most efficient to go to the website of the government agency that hosts it. Table 7.2 lists various statistical and research agencies of the federal government. Each provides numerous data sets.

A large and growing number of city, state, and federal agencies have created "open data" platforms, which are websites that make it easy to access a wide array of data on government services and related topics. Some of these open data platforms can be accessed through the previously mentioned http://data.gov website.

Budgets are another important form of quantitative data that can be very important for policy analysis. Government budgets, including information on expenditures, revenue, assets, and liabilities are almost always in the public domain and are often accessible on relevant websites. The budgets—or financial statements—for nonprofit organizations are also available to the public. Many nonprofits post their annual reports on their websites. Tax returns (IRS Form 990) of more than 1.8 million tax-exempt nonprofit organizations can be downloaded free of charge from Guidestar, a clearinghouse of information about nonprofit organizations. Public for-profit corporations are also required to make their annual financial statements available to the public.

The ready availability of large databases enables policy analysts to quickly construct tables, graphs, and maps to illustrate key patterns and

Table 7.4 Monthly Housing Costs in the United States in 2022

(One-Year Estimates)

Monthly Housing Costs	Total Households
Less than $100	371,839
$100 to $199	1,489,755
$200 to $299	3,959,968
$300 to $399	5,174,198
$400 to $499	5,674,680
$500 to $599	5,852,084
$600 to $699	6,021,159
$700 to $799	6,248,684
$800 to $899	6,392,490
$900 to $999	6,419,027
$1,000 to $1,499	28,745,380
$1,500 to $1,999	20,911,572
$2,000 to $2,499	12,312,316
$2,500 to $2,999	6,877,701
$3,000 or more	11,169,292
No cash rent	2,250,783
Total Households	129,870,928

Source: American Community Survey

trends. This requires some facility with spreadsheets, statistical software, and mapping (geographic information systems, or GIS) programs. Sometimes, the analyst will need to simplify statistical tables published by governmental agencies to make them more digestible to the client, to make patterns and trends easier to discern. This can involve combining categories and/or variables. For example, a table from the American Community Survey (ACS) shows monthly housing costs in $100 and $500 increments in 16 separate categories, from less than $100 to $3,000 or more, as shown in Table 7.4. To provide greater clarity, an analyst could consolidate some of the categories and include percentages so that the client can see the relative share of each category. In addition, the analyst might also include the median value, which can be obtained from a separate table in the ACS. Table 7.5 shows how the data might be presented in order to provide a clearer overview of housing costs in the United States.

Table 7.5 Monthly Housing Costs in the United States in 2022

(One-Year Estimates)		
Monthly Housing Costs	Total Households	Percent Share
Less than $600	22,522,524	25.2%
$600–$999	25,081,360	25.2%
$1000–$1,499	28,745,380	22.7%
$1,500–$2,499	33,223,888	18.7%
$2,500 or more	18,046,993	8.2%
No Cash Rent	2,250,783	
Median	1,268	

Source: American Community Survey

Sometimes, the only data available are highly disaggregated (e.g., with the unit of analysis at the individual level). In such cases, the analyst may need to aggregate the cases to a larger category, such as neighborhoods, cities, or states. For example, a database that shows the reading and math scores of individual students may need to be aggregated to show the average scores per school or school district.

In addition to census and other federal data that provide current and historical information on the population, economy, environment, and other important domains, policy analysts often make use of *administrative data*. Administrative data documents key aspects of an agency or department's activity and performance. They may include, among other things, service requests, response times to these requests, the nature of the requests, and the outcome of the requests. Data from a school system might include test scores, graduation rates, teacher turnover, and many other indicators.

Governments at all geographic levels have become increasingly involved in collecting and analyzing administrative data since the 1990s, partly reflecting the salience of performance-based management, which requires government to track service delivery and other functions in light of various metrics. Many agencies now publish data on these indicators of service provision and overall efficiency. For example, New York City's Mayor's Management Report provides longitudinal data on key performance indicators for every municipal agency.[4]

Not all administrative data are in the public domain. Some information may be collected but not published. Policy analysts should always ask program managers or other officials in a government agency or nonprofit organization for administrative data if such information may be helpful. Sometimes, such information is readily available, or sometimes a staff person at the agency may need to extract it from a database. Administrative data, especially when in raw form, varies in its reliability and can require a substantial amount of time to "clean up" or eliminate incomplete or faulty records. Data may not be aggregated and, depending on the number of records, may require the analyst to sample a subset of cases for further analysis.

In addition, administrative data may cover only a subset of all cases. It is always important to ask if an administrative data set is comprehensive in scope or if it is based on a sample. If it is a sample, who or what is included, and how were they selected? Who or what may be excluded?

These questions about the methods and assumptions used to generate administrative data also apply to other data sets as well, including large surveys conducted by the US Census Bureau and other agencies. In particular, as Ruth Hanf discusses in an essay on "the use of social science data for policy analysis," analysts should be mindful of (i) the methodology used to collect the data and (ii) adjustment of the data. Regarding the methodology, analysts should consider, among other things, the reliability of the sample and response rates. Data adjustments may include the treatment of missing values and duplication of counts (Hanft 1980: 258).

In addition, Hanft also cautions that analysts should be alert to key differences in the sampling frames and purposes of data sets that pertain to similar issues. For example, the federal government publishes two annual estimates of homelessness in the United States. One study, based on "street surveys" and counts of people in various kinds of homeless shelters, estimates the total number of homeless people at a single point in time (usually a night in January). The second study excludes the unsheltered homeless population and estimates the number of people who have stayed at least one night in a homeless shelter during the previous 12 months. Even though the latter study excludes homeless people who have not stayed in shelters, it shows a much higher prevalence of homelessness than the point-in-time study (1.2 million versus 653,000). That is because homelessness is usually an episodic experience, and the people who are sheltered on a single night represent only a portion of those who have stayed in a shelter at some point during the preceding year (US Department of Housing and Urban Development 2023a, 2023b).

> **Voting Case: Selected Databases on Elections and Voting**
>
> The National Conference on State Legislatures maintains several databases on state legislation involving election administration, campaign finance, and related topics. The State Elections Legislative Database covers all state-level legislation on elections from 2011 to the present, and is updated weekly. Topics include, among many others, absentee voting, election day holidays, internet voting, mail voting, automatic registration, and voter identification. For more information, go to www.ncsl.org/elections-and-campaigns/state-elections-legislation-database.
>
> The US Election Assistance Commission provides data on voter registration, absentee voting, state election laws and procedures, and other topics. The Commission also publishes studies on voter registration and related topics. For more information go to www.eac.gov/research-and-data.
>
> The International Institute for Democracy and Electoral Assistance provides an international database on voter turnout for presidential and Parliamentary/legislative elections from 1948 to the present. For more information, go to **www.idea.int/data-tools/data/voter-turnout**.
>
> The US Elections Project provides up-to-date information on election laws, statistics and research reports on the US electoral system. It hosted by a faculty member and elections expert in the Political Science department at the University of Florida. www.electproject.org/home.
>
> The US Census collects data on the characteristics of American voters. Since 1964, the Census has reported on the number of registered voting-age citizens; the number of voters; and a host of characteristics, such as their race, ethnicity, age and sex. www.census.gov/topics/public-sector/voting.html.

Surveys

An advantage of publicly available data sets is that they can usually be analyzed quickly and can be readily converted to tables, graphs, and maps. However, in some cases existing data sets may not cover the issue at hand adequately. They may not address the particular questions at stake, and/or the geographic scale of the data set may not be appropriate (Hanft 1980). For example, data sets based on a nationally representative sample of public housing residents may not be an accurate representation of public housing residents in a particular city or in a particular public housing development. A nationally representative survey of relatives of prison inmates may not be representative of the relatives of the inmates in a particular area or in a particular correctional facility. If the policy issue relates to a topic or population not covered in available data sets, it may be necessary to carry out a survey.

The Internet has made it much easier to design and administer surveys and analyze their results, yet analysts should be extremely wary about surveys. Surveys can take a lot of time to design, and it can take weeks to obtain a numerically adequate response, and it may be difficult to control for biases in the survey results.

Prior to the development of online survey platforms (e.g., Survey Monkey, Qualtrics, FormSite, Google Forms), surveys usually needed to be conducted in person, by phone, or by mail. In most cases (especially with mail surveys), survey results needed to be manually entered into a computer database. With online surveys, the researcher needs to prepare a questionnaire and distribute Internet links to the questionnaire to prospective respondents (e.g., public housing residents, police officers, child support case workers). The survey software automatically records and aggregates the survey results. While online systems eliminate the need to manually enter questionnaire forms and can produce instant summaries of the results, they do not eliminate all of the risks of using surveys for policy analysis.

First, it is not easy to craft a well-designed questionnaire. Questions that may seem obvious to the researcher may be ambiguous or confusing to the respondent. Surveys also often rely on categorical responses—the categories put into the survey may not be sensitive to the variation in the respondents' responses. Some categories may be too broad, encompassing nearly all respondents, while others are too narrow or only cover extreme cases.

Second, there is no guarantee that an adequate number of people will respond to the survey. To be statistically meaningful, surveys usually need at least 30 responses, and ideally many more. If the analysis will focus on a subset of respondents (e.g., women, people in their 20s) or conduct multivariate analysis, larger samples are essential. It can also take too much time for an adequate number of responses to accumulate.

Third, even if an adequate number of people respond to the survey, it can be difficult to know if the respondents are representative of the population of interest. For example, the fact that the survey is based on Internet technology and in English only may mean that the respondents have higher levels of education, are younger, and are more likely to speak English than the overall population. People who take the time to complete the survey may differ in systemic ways from other members of the target population. In technical terms, this is the risk of selection bias.

Even though online surveys take less time to execute than phone or mail surveys, they can still require substantial amounts of time to complete and analyze. First, as noted earlier, it can take weeks to accumulate an adequate number of responses. Second, if the survey includes open-ended questions where respondents can answer questions in sentences or paragraphs, these responses can take considerable time and effort to analyze. Sometimes, these responses can be coded into discrete categories that can then be subject to quantitative analysis. In addition, analysts will need to read these open-ended responses and use them to illustrate key findings from the survey.

Yet, notwithstanding these concerns, surveys can be indispensable for some policy issues. If the analyst must carry out a survey, it is always helpful if he or she can get the client or other organizations to spread the word about the survey—including its Web address—to the targeted population. It is also very helpful if the analyst can obtain feedback on the quality of the survey instrument (questionnaire), including its design, length, and the wording of the questions. If at all possible it is highly desirable to test out the survey with a small number of subjects and refine it afterwards before launching it formally.

Given the inherent risks of survey research, and the possibility of delays in each step in the process of designing and executing the survey, it is always wise to have a Plan B for gathering the information and insights expected of the survey. For example, instead of surveying noncustodial parents about the possible changes in child support enforcement policies, one might interview lawyers and social workers with extensive experience working with these parents. Alternatively, the analyst might convene a focus group of ten or so noncustodial parents to discuss the options. The results won't be statistically representative but could generate valuable insights, and there is no guarantee that a survey's results would be bias-free and statistically significant.[5]

Box 7.2 Informal In-Person Surveys

Policy analysis can often benefit from informal surveys, especially when they involve contact with people most directly affected by the issue at hand. For example, analysts may speak with residents and workers in a neighborhood targeted for redevelopment to gain some understanding of their concerns and priorities even if the informants do not constitute a random sample and the discussion is informal and is entirely qualitative. Moreover, informal surveys may generate important topics and questions to ask in a larger-scale survey with closed-end questions.

However, analysts must exercise caution about interviewing children or particularly vulnerable populations. Interviewing children may require the permission of parents or teachers. When interviewing people in an institutional setting, such as a correctional facility, the analyst must be cognizant of any risks the interview may pose to the interviewee, especially if other people are aware of the interview.

Case Studies and "Best Practices"

As discussed in Chapter 3, policy analysts often look to other programs, policies, and initiatives as models for possible solutions to the issue they are addressing. Analysts may develop alternative options from current or past efforts carried out elsewhere. For example, if an analyst is tasked to find ways to increase the composting of degradable household waste so as to reduce the growth of landfills, he or she might look at how other jurisdictions have promoted composting, or how they have dealt with similar or analogous issues such as the recycling of paper, glass, and plastic. Initiatives that are believed to be particularly effective are often considered to be "best practices."

In tackling almost any issue, the policy analyst will want to look for possible models to adopt or build on. Therefore, an initial research priority is to scan through literature reviews and interviews for promising precedents that could become the basis of one or more policy options. Once precedents are identified, the analyst will need to explore these policies or programs in greater depth. If they are to be foundational to the policy alternatives, the analyst will need to collect information on the background of these programs or policies, the details of their operations, and, if possible, their effectiveness. In other words, policy analysts must often produce case studies of efforts conducted in various places and at various times to address issues similar to the one at hand.

These case studies may draw from reports written about the policy or program, news articles, conference proceedings, and other documents. They may also involve interviews with key participants and observers. Information about the context surrounding the policy; the motivation; the characteristics of the key actors involved; and details about the structure, size, and growth of the program can generate ideas for establishing a similar policy or program. They can also provide clues for assessing the feasibility of adopting such a program now and for modifying it so that the program better aligns with the current political, institutional, and economic environment.

It is highly desirable to obtain information on the performance and effectiveness of the model policies or programs. Data on the outcomes of the policy or program can be crucial for the comparative analysis of the policy options. Ideal is a rigorous program evaluation, but most policies and programs are not evaluated at all, much less subject to state-of-the-art evaluations. Nevertheless, it is not difficult to find evaluations and related reports on all sorts of initiatives, large-scale and small.

Case studies of programs or policies should include the following elements:

1 Program/policy overview. Describe key features of the program. Discuss why the program or policy is germane to the issue at hand and why it might be considered a "best practice." What makes it innovative or interesting? What aspects of the program are particularly important?

2   Contextual information. Who established the program or policy? When? Why? Discuss the factors that led to the development of the program or policy. If appropriate, provide background information on the geographic setting and the organizations most directly involved in launching it.
3   Evidence. Provide evidence of the program or policy's accomplishments. Refer to any evaluations of the program or policy. In addition, or if it has not been evaluated, refer to data on program outcomes and costs from other sources.
4   If the case study refers to programs or policies from the past, those of a different jurisdiction (city, state, country), or those of a different kind of organization, discuss how these differences might impinge on the adaptation of the policy or program for the current context—for example, the client's jurisdiction. If the policy or program was created in Los Angeles, what changes might be needed for it to be adapted in Boston?

Summary

In this chapter we have discussed the role of research in policy analysis. Policy analysis is a form of **applied research**, usually drawing from a variety of data sources and involving multiple research methods. Research serves multiple functions in policy analysis, from documenting the nature of the problem to providing evidence on the effectiveness, cost, and other aspects of the policy alternatives. We have discussed the value of a **research plan** as a guide to a policy analysis project, linking key questions to pertinent data sources and research methods. We have also emphasized the interconnections between information sources: documents not only lead to additional documents but also to people to interview; people lead to additional people to interview, and also to documents.

We have discussed several key forms of research for policy analysis and examined some of their strengths and weaknesses. They include the following:

- **Literature reviews**: how to identify relevant documents and how to assess their credibility.

- **Interviews and focus groups**: identifying interview subjects; selecting an appropriate interview format; preparing for the interview; conducting the interview; summarizing the interview.
- **Public events and site visits**: the value of attending hearings, workshops, town halls, and other public events as well as visits to places directly affected by the policy issue.
- **Data sets**: identifying potential quantitative data sets and the challenges of the interpretation and analysis of data sets.
- **Surveys**: advantages and disadvantages of surveys for policy analysis; alternative means of conducting surveys; informal in-person interviews.
- **Case studies and "best practices"**: guidelines for developing case studies of programs or policies that could serve as models for policy options.

Child Support Debt Case: Research Methods and Data Sources

The variety of research methods involved in policy analysis is well illustrated by the child support case. A literature review, involving Internet search engines and bibliographic databases, revealed numerous articles and other documents that shed light on the evolving nature of the problem and ways by which it has been and might be addressed. These publications described the structure of the child support system and how it varies from state to state; the ways by which child support payments are determined and enforced; the effect of the system on families, including noncustodial parents; and evaluations and related studies of state and local efforts to reform child support enforcement, including debt reduction.

In addition to various texts, we also drew from data on child support caseloads, payments, arrears, and other related topics. The federal Office of Child Support Enforcement (renamed in 2023 as the Office of Child Support Services) publishes these and other statistics in its annual reports to Congress, which is available on the office's website.

We were also fortunate to interview Vicki Turetsky, commissioner of the federal Office of Child Support Enforcement from 2009 to 2017, who responded to numerous questions we had about recent changes in the child support system and situated these changes within a broader historic context. She sent us numerous documents, including PowerPoint presentations, strategic plans, fact sheets, and regulations (people lead to documents). One of the co-authors met her at a conference in New York City on child support debt and asked if we could interview her by phone.

Although we have not done so, we could easily interview many others, including researchers, attorneys, and advocates, federal and state officials in the child support system. One can imagine convening focus groups of noncustodial parents to discuss, among other topics, their assessment of potential ways of reducing child-support arrears. One could also imagine a focus group of custodial parents to discuss their concerns about the current child support system and the circumstances under which they might forgive some of the child support debt owed them.

Table 7.6 lists some of the most useful publications and other documents that we identified. They include a peer-reviewed journal article that documents the inequities of the current child support system, an international comparison of child support policies published by a research center based at a British University, summaries of recently enacted federal guidelines, and evaluations and related studies of various initiatives aimed at reducing child support debt.

Table 7.6 Selected Sources for Child Support Policy Analysis

Source	Relevance
Robles, Frances, and Shaila Dewan. "Skip Child Support. Go to Jail. Lose Job. Repeat." *The New York Times* (April 19)	Op-ed on the police killing of Walter Scott and its connection to child support debt.
Brito, Tonya L. 2012. "Fathers Behind Bars: Rethinking Child Support Policy toward Low-Income Fathers and Their Families." *The Journal of Gender, Race & Justice 15*: 617–673	Historical account and critique of the child support system, focusing on its impact on low-income noncustodial parents and suggestions for reform.
Skinner, Christine. Jonathan Bradshaw and Jacqueline Davidson. 2007. "Child support policy: An international perspective." London, UK. *Department for Work and Pensions Research Report* No. 405	International comparison of child support polices.
Haney, Lynn. 2022. *Prisons of Debt: The Afterlives of Incarcerated Fathers*. Berkeley, CA: University of California Press.	Ethnographic study of the impact of the child support system on formerly incarcerated fathers.

(*Continued*)

Table 7.6 (Continued)

Source	Relevance
Heinrich, Carolyn J., Brett C. Burkhardt, and Hilary M. Shager. 2010. *Reducing Child Support Debt and Its Consequences: Can Forgiveness Benefit All?* Report Prepared for Wisconsin Department of Workforce Development	Evaluation of a demonstration program developed to help noncustodial parents with large child support debts reduce their debt while simultaneously increasing child support paid to families. Also includes literature review of debt reduction programs.
U. S. Department of Health and Human Services, Office of the Inspector General. 2007. *State Use of Debt Compromise to Reduce Child Support Arrearages.* OEI-06–06–00070.	Survey of state programs to reduce child support debt.
Office of Child Support Enforcement, Preliminary Report, FY 2022	State and federal data on a wide array of child support topics, including total caseloads, total collections, and total arrears.
Office of Child Support Enforcement, National Child Support Strategic Plan for 2015–2019	Summarizes the key elements of the Obama Administration's reforms of Child Support enforcement.
Flexibility, Efficiency and Modernization rule: 81 Fed. Reg. 244:93492, 93516, OCSE-AT-16–06, on Dec. 20, 2016	Text of federal Child Support rule of 2016 specifying major changes in determination and enforcement of child support payments.
Ascend at the Aspen Institute & Good+Foundation. 2020a. "Implementing Sensible Debt Reduction Strategies." *Child Support Policy Fact Sheet.* https://ascend-resources.aspeninstitute.org/wp-content/uploads/2020/08/2_ChildSupport_Reducing_Arrears.pdf	Profiles of state and local debt forgiveness programs.

Notes

1 Table 7.1 provides a small sample of the possible questions and the related research tasks. A complete research design would take up several pages.
2 Numerous textbooks on qualitative research methods, as well as policy analysis, provide detailed instruction on interviewing. See Rubin and Rubin 2011; Seidman 2012; Bardach and Patashnik 2015; Patton et al. 2013.
3 For extensive guidance on the use of focus groups, see Krueger and Casey 2014.
4 Mandated by the New York City charter, the Mayor's Management Report "serves as a public account of the performance of City agencies, measuring whether they are delivering services efficiently, effectively and expeditiously" (New York City Mayor's Office of Operations 2017).
5 For further guidance on survey research methods, see Fowler 2013; Ruel et al. 2015.

References

Ascend at the Aspen Institute & Good+Foundation. 2020a. "Implementing Sensible Debt Reduction Strategies." *Child Support Policy Fact Sheet*. https://ascend-resources.aspeninstitute.org/wp-content/uploads/2020/08/2_ChildSupport_Reducing_Arrears.pdf

Bardach, Eugene, and Eric M. Patashnik. 2015. *A Practical Guide for Policy Analysis* (5th Edition). Los Angeles, CA: Sage Publications.

Behn, Robert D. 1985. Policy Analysts, Clients, and Social Scientists. *Journal of Policy Analysis and Management 4*, *3*: 428–432.

Bendheim-Thoman Center for Research on Child and Family Wellbeing. 2024. *Future of Families and Child Wellbeing Study*. https://crcw.princeton.edu/fragile-families-and-child-wellbeing-study

Cozzolino, Elizabeth. 2018. "Public Assistance, Relationship Context, and Jail for Child Support Debt." *Socius: Sociological Research for a Dynamic World 4*: 1–25. https://doi.org/10.1177/2378023118757

Data.Gov. 2024. www.data.gov.

Emory, Allison Dwyer, Lenna Nepomnyaschy, Maureen R. Waller, Daniel P. Miller, and Alexandra Haralampoudis. 2020. "Providing After Prison: Nonresident Fathers' Formal and Informal Contributions to Children." *Russell Sage Foundation Journal of the Social Sciences 6*, *1*: 84–112. www.rsfjournal.org/content/6/1/84

Fowler, Floyd J. 2013. *Survey Research Methods* (5th Edition). Los Angeles, CA: Sage Publications.

Future of Families and Child Wellbeing Study. 2024. *Publications Archive*. https://ffcws.princeton.edu/publications

Hanft, Ruth S. 1980. "Chapter 10: Use of Social Science Data for Policy Analysis and Policymaking." In *Ethics, the Social Sciences, and Policy Analysis* (pp. 249–270), D. Callahan, and B. Jennings (eds.). New York: Plenum Press.

Independent Budget Office of the City of New York. 2024. *Publications*. www.ibo.nyc.ny.us/publications.html

Krueger, Richard, and Mary Anne Casey. 2014. *Focus Groups: A Practical Guide for Applied Research* (5th Edition). Los Angeles, CA: Sage Publications.

Moore, Mark. 1980. "Chapter 11: Social Science and Policy Analysis." In *Ethics, the Social Sciences, and Policy Analysis* (pp. 271–291), D. Callahan, and B. Jennings (eds.). New York: Plenum Press.

Nepomnyaschy, Lenna, Allison Dwyer Emory, Kasey J. Eickmeyer, Maureen R. Waller, and Daniel P. Miller. 2021. "Parental Debt and Child Well-Being: What Type of Debt Matters for Child Outcomes?" *The Russell Sage Foundation Journal of the Social Sciences 7*, *3*: 122–151. www.rsfjournal.org/content/7/3/122

New York City Mayor's Office of Operations. 2017. *Mayor's Management Report (MMR)*. http://www1.nyc.gov/site/operations/performance/mmr.page

Patton, Carl V., David S. Sawicki, and Jennifer J. Clark. 2013. *Basic Methods of Policy Analysis and Planning* (3rd Edition). Boston, MA: Pearson.

Pew Research Center. 2024. www.pewresearch.org/download-datasets/

Rubin, Herbert J., and Irene S. Rubin. 2011. *Qualitative Interviewing: The Art of Hearing Data* (3rd Edition). Los Angeles, CA: Sage Publications.

Ruel, Erin, William E. Wagner, and Brian J. Gillespie. 2015. *The Practice of Survey Research: Theory and Applications*. Los Angeles, CA: Sage Publications.

Seidman, Irving. 2012. *Interviewing as Qualitative Research: A Guide for Education and Social Sciences* (4th Edition). New York: Teachers College Press.

Um, Hyunjoon. 2019. *The Role of Child Support Debt on the Development of Mental Health Problems among Nonresident Fathers*. Princeton, NJ: Princeton University.

US Department of Housing and Urban Development. 2023a. *The 2023 Annual Homeless Assessment Report (AHAR) to Congress. PART 1: Point in Time Estimates of Homelessness*. www.huduser.gov/portal/sites/default/files/pdf/2023-AHAR-Part-1.pdf

US Department of Housing and Urban Development. 2023b. *The 2021 Annual Homeless Assessment Report (AHAR) to Congress. PART 2: Estimates of Homelessness in the United States*. www.huduser.gov/portal/sites/default/files/pdf/2021-AHAR-Part-2.pdf

Wikipedia. 2024. *Wikipedia: Researching with Wikipedia*. https://en.wikipedia.org/wiki/Wikipedia:Researching_with_Wikipedia#Notable_weaknesses_of_Wikipedia

8
Policy Analysis in Practice

In this chapter, we discuss in more detail the professional context of policy analysis. We touch on three aspects of being a professional policy analyst: the nature and diversity of policy analyst positions, the role of communication in policy analysis, and the ethical challenges of conducting policy analysis. We make the case that policy analysts, and more specifically the skills and tools they employ, are assets in a range of settings. While their public service orientation often sets them apart from other analytical practitioners, their strategies for decision making and argumentation more generally are broadly relevant and transferrable to a range of positions and sectors. Like other professionals, analysts also confront ethical challenges in their work, what Tong (1986) aptly refers to as the "ethics of expertise." We address these here and discuss how ethics are treated when the public's interest is at stake, as it often is in policy analysis. We identify several concerns about policy analysis and ethics and offer an approach for incorporating ethical practices into policy analysis while still maintaining the integrity of the technical work.

Where Do Policy Analysts Work?

Individuals trained in policy analysis can employ their skills in many settings (Radin 2003). The analyst's role depends as much on the environment of where he or she works (e.g., a government agency versus a private firm) as the kind of role he or she assumes (i.e., rationalistic technician versus policy advocate) (Jenkins-Smith 1982). As we have demonstrated in the chapters that precede this one, policy analysis is fundamentally an approach for evidence-based decision making and a framework for weighing trade-offs across potential policy options. Analysts need to know how to communicate clearly and succinctly and to negotiate towards a particular position. These skills are valuable in any sector and for jobs that entail "number-crunching" analytics, advocacy, and many forms of advice giving. Paul Light (2001) uses the term "new public service" to describe how graduates of public affairs programs are increasingly dispersing across the sectors, often interfacing with all of them through the span of their careers.[1]

There are two common themes throughout the kinds of jobs described in this chapter. First, policy analysts tend to work on issues that pertain to the public good or interest in some way. While the prioritization of other, often private, interests can also be central to the analyst's work, the problem and subsequent options under consideration usually intersect with the public domain.

Second, policy analysts are doing their job in the context of some set of constraints, whether they are time-, resource-, or information-based. The work usually entails culling and combining massive amounts of disparate information into a streamlined problem-solving approach. The analyst needs to be nimble, responsive, and persuasive.

Policy Analysts Work in All Sectors

Policy analysts can employ their skills in different ways, and in a wide range of settings. Jenkins-Smith (1982) identifies three types of roles that policy analysts assume:

- *The objective technician*: in this kind of role, the analyst relies on metrics of efficiency (like cost-benefit analysis) to identify the "best" option and uses a framework that very closely follows the rational model. It is most feasible to carry out this style of analytics in settings where the analyst is not committed to the organization or client (so those preferences or objectives do not cloud the "objectivity" of the work).

- *The issue advocate*: in this kind of role, the analyst "acts to serve specific values and goals" (p. 93) and to be an active participant in the political process (rather than removed from it, like the *objective technician*). The analyst might still work towards maximizing social welfare or economically efficient programs but in a less detached way: the interests of the beneficiaries supersede those of the client. It is most feasible to carry out this style of analytics when the client or decision maker is either uncommitted to the issue or aligned with this prioritization. The analyst needs a good degree of autonomy to act as an issue advocate.
- *The client's advocate*: in this kind of role, the analyst is also very active in the political process, but in pursuit of the goals set forth by their client (versus more abstract values, as with the *issue advocate*). It is most feasible to carry out this style of analytics where the analyst has strong allegiance to the organization and is working with a committed client.

Moreover, the analyst will assume these roles in the context of different organizational environments. The settings create different incentives and norms for the analyst, establishing a range of expectations with respect to process and outcomes. Not only will roles and environments determine the nature of the work, but they will also present different ethical considerations (we elaborate on this later).

Here, we consider variations in settings as they relate to the sector of the organization. Policy analysts are found in public, nonprofit, and private-sector organizations, and we provide some examples of the roles they play in each.

It is no surprise that policy analysis is used in the *public sector*. Many government agencies have policy research and strategic planning arms where analysts work to assess existing policy programs and project the potential impacts of policies that are new or in development. Government administrators, such as mayors or governors, and legislators always have people on their teams who help in developing policy priorities and strategies. While many of these actors are involved in the process due to their topical expertise (for example, on health care or transportation), there are also those trained in analysis. Policy analysts often serve as advisors or aides to government officials and agency heads. Policy expertise is important, especially for crafting options and connecting to the relevant stakeholders. However, getting policies from idea to reality involves strategy and negotiation. Policy makers, broadly conceived, are constantly presented with an array of problems and potential solutions. Similarly, they are confronted with limited resources and other constraints that prevent them from addressing all of them. How can they go about prioritizing the issues? This is where policy-analytical skills are essential: a policy is only as good as its ability to ascend the agenda and get adopted.

Box 8.1 Featured Job in the Public Sector

Position title: Housing Policy Analyst
Company: California Department of Housing and Community Development

Description
The Housing and Community Development Representative is seeking an analyst to provide technical assistance, policy analysis, research, reviews of documents, program development, and implementation and other policy development functions. Responsibilities include but are not limited to data analysis and research, report preparation, stakeholder outreach, and technical assistance activities. The analyst also provides policy and legislative analyses, technical assistance, advice, and recommendations on housing and community development policies and coordinates with public and private sector representatives on housing policy and statutory interpretation related to housing policy development and implementation.

Activities also include developing and maintaining a project charter and timeline, conducting team meetings, presenting to the deputy director and other division leadership, and utilizing other project management tools and resources as necessary. The analyst is also expected to work in a team environment on continuous improvement projects, such as strategic planning initiatives, priority work areas, and policy development review as appropriate.

Responsibilities and Qualifications

- Experience in land use, community development, and housing planning and policy development.

- Experience communicating with (written, verbal, and interpersonal) and presenting to a variety of stakeholders.
- Experience with the areas of California state government or other policy making practices such as the legislative process.
- Ability to work independently and as part of a team.
- Experience preparing, writing, editing, and/or presenting policy reports, memoranda, or analyses on complex, sensitive, and/or controversial topics to internal or external stakeholders.

Source: http://Publicservicecareers.org (some content is adapted)

The *nonprofit sector* is composed of mission-driven organizations that either substitute for or partner with the public sector to fulfill social and economic services. Therefore, it is also not surprising that policy analysis takes place in nonprofit organizations. Since many nonprofits are small and often financially unable to sustain in-house analysts, individuals engaging in analytical work are either brought in from the outside or are also involved in a host of other activities and responsibilities at the nonprofit organization. Policy analytical skills are also useful when the organization has to interact with government actors, which is inevitable. The majority of nonprofit organizations either rely on public funding or partner with government agencies in the provision of services (Salamon and Abramson 1981; Salamon 1987, 1995; Gidron et al. 1992). Usually, only the very large operations can support policy analysis expertise in-house.

Box 8.2 Featured Job in the Nonprofit Sector

Position title: Policy Director
Company: Open Communities Alliance (Connecticut)

Description
Open Communities Alliance (OCA) seeks a policy director to join our growing team. This position is ideal for a mission-driven advocate ready to assist with the development of research and policy recommendations to counter the legacy of housing segregation. The policy director will

also be deeply engaged in outreach and education in urban and suburban areas about the benefits of such policies as OCA continues to develop an urban-suburban interracial coalition to support its work.

Responsibilities and Qualifications

- Work as part of a collaborative team to guide the research and policy work of OCA.
- Manage multiple fair housing policy areas, including conducting appropriate analysis, providing commentary, and generating creative and workable policy solutions.
- Conduct qualitative and quantitative research on existing or potential policies and their fair housing implications.
- Analyze and/or map data for various affordable housing programs, zoning, and other metrics as needed.
- Produce a variety of written products (such as reports, articles, or fact sheets) to reach a range of stakeholders.
- Cultivate strong relationships with select branches of government and key constituencies including the non-profit community, funders, and coalition members.
- Prepare comments or testimony on proposed legislation and/or rule-making, in collaboration with other staff, on behalf of OCA.
- Present OCA research findings to colleagues, partners, and decision makers at educational events and community meetings.
- Strong research, mapping, and data analysis skills.
- Exceptional analytic, presentation, research, and written and oral communication skills.
- Strong interpersonal and relationship building skills.
- Excellent time management skills and ability to prioritize under pressure and meet tight deadlines.
- Strong organizational skills, ability to troubleshoot, multitask, and manage several projects at once.
- Attention to detail is critical for this position.

Source: Adapted from posting on http://furmancenter.org

Less obvious is the role that policy analysts play in the *private sector*. Large private for-profit organizations have "policy" arms or "intergovernmental" departments that strategize and oversee the company's involvement in public policy and governmental affairs more generally.

In addition, private organizations still operate within a broader regulatory and policy environment, and they need to plan internal courses of action in the context of (and sometimes alongside) these more public circumstances. Lobbying firms or trade associations also hire policy analysts to strategize in favor of particular policies or respond to proposals put out by other entities or interests. There has also been an uptick in socially minded private entities that operate with "triple bottom lines" accounting for financial, social, and environmental outcomes (Schultz 2015; Salamon 2014). Therefore, the workforce needed to achieve the organization's financial, social, and environmental goals is one that is technically capable but also publicly and politically savvy. Finally, there are private organizations whose main purpose is to consult or provide analytical expertise to other (private and public) entities. Positions in these kinds of firms offer individuals the opportunity to apply their analytical skills to a range of issues on projects that usually have set time frames.

Box 8.3 Featured Job in the Private Sector

Position title: Policy Analyst
Company: Booz Allen Hamilton (Virginia)

Description
We are seeking an analyst to work with Navy and Marine Corps clients' operations and help them meet mission requirements by developing innovative solutions to their most pressing challenges in the areas of infrastructure, energy, resiliency, and the environment. As a general management consultant, you will apply critical thinking, policy writing, and analytical skills to help our team's efforts supporting the Navy and Marine Corps mission every day.

On our team, you'll learn to use discussions with stakeholders and support staff to help identify client challenges and collaborate with our team on solutions. Once you have a thorough understanding of organizational challenges and mission requirements, you'll review the path forward—and the expected results—with your team lead and clients. This is your chance to gain experience in DoD policy, analytics, and decision-making while establishing your consulting skills.

Responsibilities and Qualifications

- Experience with using Microsoft Office software, including Word, Excel, and PowerPoint
- Experience with using data analytics software, including R or Python
- Experience with technical writing
- Ability to perform data analysis, policy implementation, and client support
- Knowledge of federal or DoD programs related to infrastructure, energy, resiliency, or the environment is preferred by not required
- Ability to work well in a fast-paced team environment

Source: http://Indeed.com (some content is adapted)

The tools presented in this book can also be applied to private matters, like problems internal to a particular organization or particular to a specific individual. For example, one organization may have goals of expanding their services and need to figure out which ones to invest in first. Another may have newly vacated space that it needs to purpose in some way—it would need a method for prioritizing potential uses since the space can house only one. Organizations may be faced with a crisis and need to consider options for managing it internally and externally. Individuals are faced with decisions every day, and the model presented in this book can also be a guide for those moments. For example, when faced with choices on where to live, what to do for an occupation, or how to travel from Point A to Point B, individuals regularly use criteria to prioritize options. Whether done more formally or impromptu, a framework for weighing trade-offs in order to achieve a set of objectives can be applied widely (Hammond et al. 2015).

Can Policy Analysts Be Policy Advocates?

Policy analysis and policy advocacy have traditionally been seen as incompatible. It is not uncommon to find analysts and advocates operating in isolation of one another. We have already made the case that policy analysis is best applied in a multi-dimensional and multi-modal way, incorporating aspects of both ground-up processes and technical facility. The same can be said about advocacy: individuals engaged in these activities, which often employ different strategies than policy analysis, can still benefit from the tools necessary for shaping and assessing policy options. Schick (1976) asserts, "[t]he fact that advocacy and analysis are different crafts does not mean that they cannot be united in a common cause" (pp. 200–221). Indeed, advocates and organizers must interact with policy makers and government officials in order to lobby or negotiate their positions on issues. Majone (1989: 34) agrees that it is "artificial and difficult" to maintain the division between policy analysis and advocacy. The tools of persuasion, research, and communication that are core to policy analysis are effective complements to the strategizing and mobilizing skills inherent to organizing. They are often even more important for policies that are new and untested; it may take time for evidence to emerge about their effectiveness and therefore advocacy and organizing can be critical to sustaining attention around the issue. Dunn (1983) describes analysts as "coalition builders as well as information accumulators" (p. 49). Advocates also use an analytical framework to put forth policies, even if their selection of and motivation for criteria may differ from those of a more neutral technician (Stone 2012). The combination is also a good mechanism for ensuring that analysts leave their desks to confront up close the realities that public policies set out to address.

While analysts can work side by side with policy advocates, they are still responsible for doing their work in an inclusive way. That is,

Table 8.1 Online Resources for Job Searches

Online Resources for Policy Analyst Job Postings
http://Publicservicecareers.org
www.Indeed.com
http://Idealist.org
Hiring sites for federal, state, and local government agencies
Job advertisements via field-specific professional and policy organizations, for example: • Association for Public Policy Analysis and Management (http://appam.org) • Urban Land Institute (http://uli.org) • American Society for Public Administration (http://aspanet.org)

while the analyst may be aligned with a particular interest or party, the integrity of the analysis is still secured by studying all sides of the issue and employing evidence towards the arguments behind one strategy or another. The analyst has to avoid undermining the trustworthiness of the work by using a one-sided approach or by assuming that they have all of the answers. Majone suggests "multiple advocacy" (p. 40), or the process of collecting competing ideas and viewpoints, as a way to maintain a range of perspectives. Therefore, the analyst avoids relying solely on the input from advisers who share similar views with the clients. Indeed, policy analysts can also be policy advocates as long as they argue for the soundness of their position (and the deficiencies of others) using well-rounded criteria and evidence-based projections.

Policy Analysts Need Good Communication Skills

As the sample job postings demonstrate, communication skills are desirable assets of a policy analyst. Conducting a robust analysis is only part of the job; the analyst often needs to be able to communicate their work to multiple audiences. The analyst needs to communicate their methods, findings, and recommendations in a clear and accessible way, and should be comfortable doing so in a range of modalities. Analysts often have to communicate their work in written, oral, and visual forms. Here we briefly discuss some general pointers for communicating effectively in all three forms to a range of audiences.

Know the Audience

Every version of communication should be tailored to the targeted audience. Before even embarking on drafting a memo or presentation, the analyst needs to understand the background, interests, and attention span of the particular audience. How informed are they on the issue at hand? What is their stance on the issue (do they have a preference for more or less intervention)? What do they have at stake with respect to the issue?

Unless the audience is comfortable with technical terminology and concepts, the presentation of information should be jargon-free and comprehensible without a deep expertise in the topic. If the presentation requires some technical components or issue-specific terminology, it is useful to make sure everyone is on the same page by introducing those concepts at the beginning or in an appendix or handout. This way, audience members who are not knowledgeable about the topic have something to reference as they receive the presentation or report. The analyst will need to do some research on the audience to figure out how nuanced the presentation or report should be. There are two goals for the analyst. First, the analyst should provide enough information so that the audience can follow the argument and fill in gaps by fielding questions when necessary. Second, the analyst should provide enough information to convey to the audience that any simplification of terms or concepts is intentional for presentation purposes, and not an omission due to lack of mastery of the topic. The audience needs to be able to digest the information and, at the same time, trust that the analyst has done a comprehensive job in their research.

Box 8.4 The Value of Outlines

Outlines, or sketches of the content and organization of a document or presentation, are not for very long products only. Outlines can be very useful even for one-page memos. For example, Microsoft PowerPoint can be used for outlining ideas. PowerPoint slides are convenient devices for organizing points, testing visualizations, and mapping out the logic of an argument far ahead of any actual presentation. Here is why:

- Outlines ensure that the communication stays within set page limits or time limits.
- Outlines ensure that the communication is complete and coherent—the logic of the argument is thought out from beginning to end.
- Outlines are a useful touchstone to make sure all team members (and clients) are on board with the communication content and structure before putting time into writing up the final product.

Organization and Brevity Matter

Clients often have very busy schedules and might have a short window of time available to attend a presentation or read a memo. Therefore, the information needs to be presented in a way that can be digested easily. For oral presentations, Microsoft PowerPoint presentations are very useful for helping audience members to follow the logic of an argument and visuals help with processing complex ideas or processes. For written communication, memos should be brief (no more than a few pages), and longer reports should always be accompanied by a shorter executive summary that captures the key take-aways. Written documents can also include graphics and visual cues to draw attention to particular concepts and take-aways. For example, the formatting of bolded, italicized, or underlined words or phrases signals that they are important; bullets and tables make lists or sequenced terms easier to process; descriptive headers of paragraphs tell the reader right away about the content of that section. Even something as simple as using an active voice, like "I propose" or "the organization implements" (rather than passive voice, like "it is proposed that" or "it is implemented by the organization") in written communication can make a difference—the information is conveyed more directly and assertively, and it saves space, to boot.

Box 8.5 Less Is More

Visual presentations are "busy" when they have a lot of content in a single viewing. For example, a single slide of a PowerPoint presentation can have too many lines of text or too many competing images. With very few exceptions, most audiences will better tolerate cleaner and simpler visual presentations.

- There is no need to put everything on the slide or image, as some of the information can be provided by the presenter's talking points.
- Keep background designs to a minimum: avoid visual distractions that will make it harder for the audience to process the central take-aways.
- Each slide should have one or two take-aways: these main points should be reflected in the talking points and the title of the slide (avoid boilerplate titles—use titles to highlight the main content of that particular slide).
- Be wary of dynamic presentations: there are presentation tools available, like Prezi, that create interactive and dynamic presentations. Even PowerPoint has an animation functionality. Depending on the audience, too many bells and whistles can disorient more than engage.

Make a Good Impression

In any form of communication, details matter. Every written piece of communication should be proofread for typos and grammatical errors—this is true even of more informal methods, like email. Even one error can send a signal to the client that the analyst is not careful; indeed, where there is one error, more usually follow. It is always a good idea to have a fresh set of eyes on any document before it gets distributed to a new audience—it is not uncommon for those very familiar with the topic to gloss over, or automatically fill in, errors due to their deep knowledge of the topic.

With oral communications, the presenter should be without notes. If the presenter is reading from notes, it makes it more difficult to respond in the moment to comments and to make eye contact and engage with members of the audience. This means the analyst will have to practice the presentation in order to feel comfortable without notes—this, along with the deep knowledge of the topic that is naturally developed while working on the analysis, is the best kind of preparation. In addition, the PowerPoint, or any kind of visual presentation, can be a useful point of reference for the presenter. The main points and order of items should be captured in the visual presentation and the analyst can use these as guideposts. However, the analyst must avoid using the slides as a script, reading the text aloud to the client.

Box 8.6 Good Resources for Help With Written and Oral Presentations

- Publicases has a series of guides on writing effective memos available at www.publicases.org/case/writing-effective-memos/
- The Center for an Urban Future. 2002. *The Big Idea: A Step-by-Step Guide to Creating Effective Policy Reports*. City Limits Community Information Service, Inc.
- RAND's Guidelines for Preparing Briefings (1999; a bit dated, but still useful).
- Pennock, Andrew S. 2023. *The CQ Press Writing Guide for Public Policy* (2nd Edition). Thousand Oaks, CA: Sage Publications. Some useful pointers are available at http://presentationzen.blogs.com/presentationzen/2005/09/whats_good_powe.html

An Ethical Code for Policy Analysts?

Policy analysts, like any other professionals, face ethical challenges in carrying out their work. As Fischer and Forester observe, "policy analysis lies squarely (if uncomfortably) between science and ethics" (Patton et al. 2013: 33). Ethics pertain to the moral imperatives of a profession or field, or a general understanding of what is the "right" thing to do. Ethics are often synonymous with values. These standards tend to vary by field, since the nature of the work, and therefore the expectations of conduct, varies considerably. For example, the legal profession operates by a different ethical code than the medical profession or the mental health profession. These fields all have codes of ethics to which their professionals are held. The American Bar Association puts out its *Model Rules of Professional Conduct*, which provides guidelines on practices, such as client–lawyer relationships, advocacy, and pro bono work.[2] This serves as the model for ethics and professional responsibility for most states in the United States. Similarly, the American Medical Association publishes its *Code of Medical Ethics*, which guides patient–doctor relationships, professional relationships, and the use of technology and treatments.[3] Neither of these published codes is binding. However, they are issued by the fields' leading professional associations, and they have governed professional practices for decades. Therefore, their sway is pervasive.

Common across these professions is the presence of a client or patient and the privileged position of the professional. The lawyer or doctor has access to and information from the client or patient that is not publicly available. In addition, the professional imparts knowledge and advice that is backed by a certified credential—therefore, their input holds weight and influence over the client or patient.

The professional positioning of policy analysts is both similar to and distinct from that of lawyers, doctors, or therapists. It is similar in that policy analysts work with clients and receive and impart privileged information. Depending on the nature of the project, clients may share closely held information with the analyst. Policy analysts are brought in to provide advice and guidance on how to address a particular problem, which is conveyed through both technical and topical expertise. Trust is a core component of all these relationships, and policy analysts usually have to instill it quickly and in the crosshairs of a partisan environment (Hill 2003; Nelson 2002; Orr 2002). While policy analysts may not regularly confront the literal "life or death" scenarios as doctors or lawyers, they do deal with topics that could have significant welfare implications for large swaths of people. If the public perceives the analytical process to be politicized or captured, then their advice is delegitimized (Benveniste 1984). The analyst's responsibility to the public interest is a unique feature that needs to be considered when thinking about their ethical conduct (Tong 1986).

There are also distinct circumstances and expectations for policy analysts. Policy analysts do not have a common code of ethics to reference (Benveniste 1984). Policy analysis is a multidisciplinary field, making it hard to unify around a single set of values. The field, and social science more broadly, is given a lot of latitude in terms of research methods and scientific standards of significance and replication (Warwick and Pettigrew 1983). Analysts rely on both quantitative and qualitative methods to gather information, and the definition of "significant effects" from interventions varies depending on where the study is published or the field from which the author comes. In addition, it is difficult to assess the methodological rigor of some evaluation studies, making causal inferences tenuous. There is also great variation in the kinds of roles that analysts hold, from advisors to advocates to technicians, and the environments within which they operate; therefore, ethical expectations are similarly diverse (Jenkins-Smith 1982). Finally, policy analysts are usually doing their work within very short time frames, which is in contrast to the long-term processes that lawyers or medical professionals often oversee. It can be challenging to be methodical about ethics in such pressure-ridden circumstances.

Ethical Analyses Versus Ethical Practices

In the context of policy analysis, it is important to distinguish between ethical analyses and ethical practices. Much of what we've covered in the book addresses the challenges of and strategies for achieving ethical analyses. As Amy (1984) asserts, ethics are incorporated into the analysis when there is a "systematic investigation of the normative dimensions of policy issues" (p. 573). We talked at length about making sure that all interests, especially those without a seat at the table, are reflected in the analysis and that metrics of fairness and distributive burden (and benefit) are included. We stressed the importance of reconsidering the problem statement from various perspectives and situating it in the appropriate context. We also explained how to be transparent about the limitations of certain metrics, especially those that come out of cost-benefit analysis. All of these strategies will ensure that the analysis itself is balanced and inclusive, both highly ethical aspirations.

Ethical practices for the policy analyst should go hand-in-hand with the standards set earlier for analyses. However, practices pertain more to how analysts conduct themselves and how they reconcile their own values with getting the job done (Dunn 1983). One of the greatest ethical challenges for analysts is to come to terms with the philosophical and moral differences they may have with the various parties involved. Patton et al. (1993: 45) point out four perspectives from which ethics should be considered:

1 that of the analyst;
2 in relation to employers and clients;
3 in relation to colleagues and the profession; and
4 in relation to third parties and the general public.

What we propose here is not a universal ethics code but rather a call to be reflective on the ethical conflicts and to be aware of where they are resolved and where they remain at odds. For example, consider a scenario where an analyst is employed by or contracted by a state child support agency to explore options for increasing child support collections. The state has a responsibility to maintain its fiscal integrity, and increasing the collection of child support can help it achieve that. Fiscal mandates, however, may come at the expense of social welfare outcomes (for the noncustodial parent and, possibly, the children). Depending on where the analyst's own alliances lie (for example, if they identify with the plight of noncustodial parents), this tension could be an ethical challenge to completing an analysis that prioritizes the fiscal responsibilities of the state over the social justice repercussions.

Ultimately, the analyst is not expected to make a policy decision—usually that is in the hands of the client or policy maker. The analyst is tasked with providing a set of recommendations, or a framework for assessing the trade-offs across potential policy strategies. However, there is no consensus on whether or not the analyst is responsible for the decision that the client ultimately makes. One could argue that the analyst is offering up information and the client is solely responsible for how the information is put to use. Like in the case of policy research, it is often out of the hands of the author to control all of the ways in which the findings could be promulgated. On the one hand, this is consistent with the "fiduciary model" of analyst–client relationships (Tong 1986). On the other hand, the analyst has a duty of transparency in his or her methods and content and should be held accountable to how recommendations are positioned. Patton et al. (1993), for example, assert that the analyst should be held responsible for the consequences of their advice. Tong (1986) discusses the "personal model of responsibility," which imposes moral responsibility for an outcome if the analyst knowingly omits something to induce it.

Majone (1989) also makes a case for accountability. He views analysts as having a key role in creating and sustaining policy discourse more broadly. They play important roles in shaping ideas around an issue and, when necessary, breaking down systems that perpetuate stereotypes. They are the arbiters of information, especially in circumstances where it is being suppressed (Tong 1986). This is done through argument, debate, persuasion, and rhetoric. Majone asserts that the process of policy analysis is just as important (if not more) than the technical aspect of it. Therefore, the analyst carries a responsibility that extends beyond the specific project at hand. There is a moral imperative to be cognizant of their broader, and more permanent, effects on the narrative around issues.

Challenges to Incorporating Ethics Into Policy Analysis

Incorporating ethics into the practice of policy analysis is often met with skepticism. As we mentioned earlier, the field is diverse in terms of ideological perspectives, methodological tendencies, and analytical sophistication. Therefore, it is difficult for the field to coalesce around a common set of norms (Benveniste 1984). In addition, many contend that ethics-based approaches to policy analysis are inconsistent at best and impossible at worst. Amy (1984) summarizes the four main reasons why it is challenging to combine policy analysis and ethics.

It is impossible. The most prevalent critique is that ethics is theoretical, subjective, and incompatible with the rational and pragmatic intent behind policy analysis (Kenny and Giacomini 2005; Dunn 1983). How can the analyst objectively weigh the evidence while also incorporating value-based judgments? Amy states that "preferences do not usually require justifications, but moral stands do" (1984: 575). Analysts should not get into the business of evaluating moral positions as "true" or "false."

It is unnecessary. Another response claims that ethics and values will be addressed through the political process (Amy 1984). The analyst is responsible for presenting the policy options (and the trade-offs among them) and then political negotiations reconcile ethical discrepancies and priorities.

It is impractical. The study of ethics is considered to be too abstract and philosophical to incorporate into a technical process like policy analysis. Indeed, how could the analyst operationalize or measure items pertaining to ethical standards? The argument could become one of moral positions rather than facts and evidence. It also could undermine the analyst-client relationship if moral clashes cannot be resolved.

There is a fear of introducing bias. Since ethics are perceived as subjective and normative, the acknowledgement of the analyst's personal views could muddle the objective nature of the analysis. The irony is that by putting ethics out front the analyst could in fact avoid introducing unintended biases into the analysis.

Amy concludes that these arguments are weak and are more of a reflection of political, professional, and institutional resistance to ethical considerations. He advocates for a move away from the technocratic nature of policy analysis and towards a more ideological frame to effectively merge ethics and policy analysis. Next, we go through the details of a strategy for maintaining the methodological and ethical integrity of policy analysis.

> **Voting Case: Voter Mobilization, Information Mining, and Deception**
>
> Policy problem: how to increase voter turnout?
> Dilemma: Social pressure has proven to be an effective tactic for voter mobilization (see Gerber et al. 2008 for a summary). However, a number of these tactics rely on massive data mining (of individuals' very personal information) and sometimes excessively persuasive communication. Consider, for example, "neighbor mailer" initiatives, which, via paper mailers, provide information on the voting behavior of individuals' neighbors or divulge plans to share that individual's voting behavior with their neighbors. These initiatives have come under scrutiny for how aggressively they apply social pressures and what kind of personal data they use. An analyst could be confronted with the following questions:
> - How severe are the repercussions from excessive social pressure?
> - What are the political, legal, and social implications for using deceptive communication?
> - Can social pressure tactics be implemented effectively with minimal mining of personal information?
>
> Resolution: A decent body of research and evidence can be tapped to answer these questions and weigh the benefits of social pressure tactics over the costs. For example, evidence shows that aggressive social pressure mailings work no better than milder forms of persuasion (for example, Mann 2010) and that the messenger might matter more than the message itself (Sinclair 2012). The analyst should also self-reflect and consult the client on personal comfort levels related to information mining and communication policies.

How to Conduct Ethical Policy Analysis

Skeptics of ethics-oriented policy analysis may assume that pushing values aside will keep the analysis sound. However, we advocate for tackling questions related to ethics and values from the start of the analytical process. Without doing so, the risk is that values, or ethical assumptions, will seep into the analytical process without proper disclosure or acknowledgment. Furthermore, since policy analysis is usually a short-term, fast-paced exercise, there is little time to correct for this "conceptualization bias," or the tendency to use mental shortcuts or biases to frame issues (Warwick and Pettigrew 1983). As we discussed in earlier chapters, if the analyst leaves these predispositions unchecked, the analysis (and the recommendations that come out of it) could unintentionally perpetuate structures and perceptions that disadvantage certain groups and prop up others. The analyst has an ethical responsibility to do as much as possible to prevent this from happening. Here we propose four principles for lifting up the ethical issues in analysis.

1 *Do some self-reflection*: the analyst should take stock of their own assumptions and predispositions with respect to the issue at hand. This includes reflecting on one's values, documenting them, and assessing how they might align or conflict with those of the client, the other stakeholders involved and the public at large.
2 *Talk to others*: the analyst needs to do some due diligence and talk to other stakeholders, especially those who hold divergent views or opinions than the analyst on the issue (Breedlove 2002). Schick (1976) observed, in his consideration of policy analysis on Capitol Hill, that "a prime objective of analysis is to improve the outcomes of political bargaining by introducing a new set of participants" (p. 221). This approach is consistent with elements of design thinking, a practice that relies heavily on "empathizing" with the user or consumer of the good or service (Allio 2014). Expanding the point of reference serves as a good check to make sure that the analyst is not approaching the project in isolation but rather with a spectrum of moral issues in mind.
3 *Maintain the integrity and transparency of the analysis*: the analyst can work to influence the client's perspective on the issue by providing well-rounded knowledge. However, the analyst cannot control the views or actions of the client. The analyst can, on the other hand, control the integrity and rigor of the analysis. The analyst should stay true to the goals of the analysis and problem, as defined at the outset. The analyst can control how information is conveyed. In both advocacy and analysis, evidence is always used towards persuasive arguments; however, inconvenient facts should not be

omitted for purposes of furthering a particular position. Dunn (1983) calls this "communicative ethics," or the practice of instilling trust in the public and in clients. It is reasonable, and often strategic, to present proposals differently to different audiences. However, these different presentations cannot contradict one another—the various forms of communication have to hang together.

4   *Do no harm*: doctors follow this oath, and it seems equally appropriate in the context of policy analysts. As we've stated earlier, much of what policy analysts do will ultimately impact the public, with potentially significant welfare effects. Be respectful of others' rights and opinions; disagreement is not synonymous with virulence. The analyst has an obligation, at the very least, to protect basic rights and to minimize the infringement on any one individual's well-being.

It may be the case that the analyst comes up against a client whose values clash with their own and whose commitment to those values is unwavering even in the face of facts and evidence that suggest other views on the issue. Perhaps the client is already committed to a particular outcome and expects the analyst to create a rationale to support it regardless of how questionable the assumptions or standards might be. Should the analyst stay on the project? This is a very personal choice, and one that depends not only on personal ethical views but also on financial and professional circumstances. The magnitude of the disagreement might be determinative. The professional stage or status of the analyst might matter—individuals at earlier stages of their career may feel less confident about making such a move. Patton et al. (1993) offer up an important reminder: it is often harder to make change from the outside. This is particularly true if the analyst does not have the autonomy to put forward advice or analyses that may not align with the interests or goals of a particular organization (Jenkins-Smith 1982). For this reason, they recommend exiting the client relationship only in very extreme situations. An analyst's job often entails both the interrogation of the problem at hand and the brokering of knowledge and evidence to those less informed on the topic (which could, at times, include the client).

> **Box 8.7 When to "Trust Your Gut"?**
>
> Analysts, like any human beings, experience gut reactions. They have instincts, which are honed by personal experiences and, over time, professional experiences. This intuition is hard to suppress. As with personal biases or expectations, we encourage the analyst to respond to their gut reactions, rather than ignore them. This includes the following:
>
> - Reflection: recognize and articulate what the gut reaction is and what motivated it.
> - Expression: share it with colleagues and possibly the client to see if the same impression is sensed by others.
> - Confirmation: conduct research and collect evidence to either confirm or question the gut reaction.
>
> This intuition can spark additional research and lines of argument. The key is to back it up by evidence from a range of sources. As Fischer and Forester (1993) assert in their seminal book, *The Argumentative Turn in Policy Analysis and Planning*: "We should be more suspicious than ever of policy arguments that cannot meet public tests of evidence. If we cannot distinguish policy argument from sales talk, we should consider it propaganda undeserving of the name 'analysis'" (p. 3).

Summary

In this chapter, we addressed the kinds of jobs that policy analysts typically assume and the ethical challenges with carrying out both morally and technically robust analyses. The skills that policy analysts develop, both in their training and on the job, are transferrable across settings and sectors. However, the way in which the skills are applied, and to what end, vary depending on the institutional environment. While some analysts may engage solely in technical exercises, relying heavily on quantitative data and methods (like cost-benefit analysis), other analysts work in the context of more mission-driven organizations that use these technical analyses to further policy goals and shift the discourse more broadly. More and more, policy analysts are employing their commitment to public service in **all three sectors**.

Communication skills are an integral part of being an effective policy analyst. Analysts need to be equipped to present their work in written, oral, and visual forms and to a wide range of audiences. This means understanding the knowledge base and interests of the audience and turning, often complex, issues and analyses into clear, concise, and accessible presentations. There is no room for careless mistakes: whether big or small, any form of communication with the client or another audience is an opportunity to make an impression and convey the integrity of the analytical and research work.

Due to the diversity of methods, application, and training among analysts, it is difficult for them to unify around a single code of ethics. However, "public policy is an inescapably moral enterprise" (Kenny and Giacomini 2005: 247), and analysts need to figure out ways to simultaneously confront the ethical challenges of their work and maintain the methodological integrity of the process and product. We recommend that analysts be both **self-reflective** and proactive in reaching out to and involving **as many stakeholders as possible**. It is critical that the analyst be honest about their ideological and personal commitments, with themselves and with the client. The analyst also needs to seek out a wide range of inputs, especially those that diverge from the inclinations of the client.

Unlike other professionals relating with clients on a regular basis, policy analysts are beholden to a third party: **the public**. This bestows a moral obligation that goes beyond a single technical exercise, and one that is typically demanded under great time, resource, and political constraints. Depending on where analysts are in their career trajectory, they may or may not have control over the projects they take on. Therefore, it is important that analysts consider their personal ethical framework as they enter and navigate the field. Inevitably, it is a question that will arise sooner or later.

Child Support Debt Case: Ethical Dilemmas

Here we present two hypothetical scenarios related to addressing debt reduction among noncustodial parents. Each one presents an ethical dilemma facing a state's Department of Social Services and an example of how that dilemma may be overcome. These scenarios are based on actual considerations in the context of debt reduction policy (Turetsky 2018).[4]

Eligibility for Debt Reduction

Policy Problem: Should those incarcerated for domestic violence be eligible for debt reduction programs?

Dilemma: The reason for the incarceration of the noncustodial parent (e.g., domestic violence) is inconsistent with the intent of helping those parents overcome prohibitive child support debt. Should this kind of opportunity be awarded to those with a track record of dangerous behavior that threatens the safety of the custodial parent and children?

Resolution: The state's Department of Social Services was presented with a new rule that would make ineligible for debt reduction those who had been incarcerated for domestic violence. The ethical support for this rule was clear and accepting it would have been politically feasible. The state, however, opted to reject the rule. This decision was based on the following:

- A clear understanding of OCSE's policy goals: the office was charged with reducing the unbearable burden of child support debt. It was not an extension of the criminal justice system, and making decisions based on the criminal history of a noncustodial parent blurred this distinction.
- A reliance on facts: the evidence definitively demonstrated that time in prison increased child support debt, and therefore any exemption due to the nature of incarceration would exacerbate the debt accumulation—the exact problem OCSE was tasked with solving. The Department's mandate was to incorporate ability to pay into child support orders, and the proposed exemption would undercut that goal. This is an example of where evidence-based analysis superseded any issue-based advocacy interests.

Adjusting Child Support Orders Due to Incarceration

Policy problem: How long should a person be incarcerated before child support orders are adjusted down?

Dilemma: Longer thresholds (i.e., more time in jail or prison) increase the debt burden and risks of other negative outcomes related to incarceration. However, there are administrative limits to how quickly child support orders can be thoroughly reviewed.

Resolution: The Department was presented with a proposal to decrease from 180 to 90 days the maximum length of incarceration before which child support orders are subject to adjustment. At the time, individuals needed to be incarcerated for 180 days before their child support orders were adjusted; the proposed rule would decrease the period to 90 days in order to diminish the growth of unpayable child support debt. The Department decided not to accept the shortened time frame. This decision was based on the following:

- A clear understanding of the Department/s policy goals: the proposed extension was due to administrative constraints; it was not possible to thoroughly review child support cases in 90 days. This problem was outside the scope of the Department's mandate (of basing child support obligations on ability to pay), and, unlike the first scenario, they could not draw on an analytical principle to reject the proposed rule.
- Addressing multiple interests: the Department came to understand the nature of the problem (i.e., the state's administrative constraints) by talking with and accounting for multiple interests. Rather than simply focusing on the needs and interests of the parents and families, the office also incorporated the circumstances of state administrators.

Notes

1 Henderson and Chetkovich (2014) empirically document this trend in their study of MPP graduates in 2004–2005.
2 Available at www.americanbar.org/groups/professional_responsibility/publications/model_rules_of_professional_conduct/.
3 Available at https://code-medical-ethics.ama-assn.org/.
4 These scenarios reference comments recorded in the final rule, Flexibility, Efficiency and Modernization in Child Support Enforcement Programs, 81 Fed. Reg. 93492 (December 20, 2016); available at www.federalregister.gov/documents/2016/12/20/2016-29598/flexibility-efficiency-and-modernization-in-child-support-enforcement-programs.

References

Allio, Lorenzo. 2014. *Design Thinking for Public Service Excellence.* Singapore: UNDP Global Centre for Public Service Excellence.

Amy, D.J. 1984. Why Policy Analysis and Ethics are Incompatible. *Journal of Policy Analysis and Management 3,* 4: 573–591.

Benveniste, G. 1984. "On a Code of Ethics for Policy Experts." *Journal of Policy Analysis and Management 3, 4*: 561–572.
Breedlove, B. 2002. "The Continuing Education of a Policy Salesman." *Journal of Policy Analysis and Management 21, 1*: 131–136.
Dunn, W.N. 1983. *Values, Ethics, and the Practice of Policy Analysis*. Lexington, MA: Lexington Books.
Fischer, F., and Forester, J. (eds.). 1993. *The Argumentative Turn in Policy Analysis and Planning*. Durham, NC: Duke University Press.
Gerber, Alan S., Donald P. Green, and Christopher W. Larimer. 2008. "Social Pressure and Voter Turnout: Evidence from a Large-Scale Field Experiment." *American political Science Review 102, 1*: 33–48.
Gidron, B., R.M. Kramer, and L.M. Salamon. 1992. *Government and the Third Sector: Emerging Relationships in Welfare States*. San Francisco, CA: Jossey-Bass Inc Pub.
Hammond, J.S., R.L. Keeney, and H. Raiffa. 2015. *Smart Choices: A Practical Guide to Making Better Decisions*. Cambridge, MA: Harvard Business Review Press.
Henderson, M., and C. Chetkovich. 2014. "Sectors and Skills: Career Trajectories and Training Needs of MPP Students." *Journal of Public Affairs Education* 193–216.
Hill, E.G. 2003. "Non-Partisan Analysis in a Partisan World." *Journal of Policy Analysis and Management 22, 2*: 307–310.
Jenkins-Smith, H.C. 1982. "Professional Roles for Policy Analysts: A Critical Assessment." *Journal of Policy Analysis and Management, 2, 1*: 88–100.
Kenny, N., and M. Giacomini. 2005. "Wanted: A New Ethics Field for Health Policy Analysis." *Health Care Analysis 13, 4*: 247–260.
Light, P.C. 2001. *The New Public Service*. Washington, DC: Brookings Institution Press.
Majone, G. 1989. *Evidence, Argument, and Persuasion in the Policy Process*. New Haven: Yale University Press.
Mann, Christopher B. 2010. "Is There Backlash to Social Pressure? A Large-Scale Field Experiment on Voter Mobilization." *Political Behavior 32, 3*: 387–407.
Nelson, R.H. 2002. "Many Ways of Educating the Client." *Journal of Policy Analysis and Management 21, 1*: 126–131.
Orr, L.L. 2002. "Educating the Client." *Journal of Policy Analysis and Management 21, 1*: 117–121.
Patton, Carl V., David S. Sawicki, and Jennifer J. Clark. 1993. *Basic Methods of Policy Analysis and Planning* (2nd Edition). Upper Saddle River, NJ: Prentice Hall.
Patton, Carl V., David S. Sawicki, and Jennifer J. Clark. 2013. *Basic Methods of Policy Analysis and Planning* (3rd Edition). Boston, MA: Pearson.
Pennock, Andrew S. 2023. *The CQ Press Writing Guide for Public Policy* (2nd Edition). Thousand Oaks, CA: Sage Publications.
Radin, Beryl. 2003. "Reflections on Careers in Policy Analysis." *Journal of Policy Analysis and Management 22, 2*: 299–300.
Salamon, L.M. 1987. "Of Market Failure, Voluntary Failure, and Third-Party Government: Toward a Theory of Government-Nonprofit Relations in the Modern Welfare State." *Journal of Voluntary Action Research 16, 1–2*: 29–49.
Salamon, L.M. 1995. *Partners in Public Service: Government-Nonprofit Relations in the Modern Welfare State*. Baltimore, MD: Johns Hopkins University Press.

Salamon, L.M. 2014. *New Frontiers of Philanthropy: A Guide to the New Tools and New Actors that Are Reshaping Global Philanthropy and Social Investing.* New York: Oxford University Press.

Salamon, L.M., and A.J. Abramson. 1981. *The Federal Government and the Nonprofit Sector: Implications of the Reagan Budget Proposals: A Study for Independent Sector, the 501 (c)(3) Group, and the National Society of Fund Raising Executives.* Washington, DC: Urban Institute.

Schick, A. 1976. "The Supply and Demand for Analysis on Capitol Hill." *Policy Analysis* 215–234.

Schultz, D. 2015. "The Distinctiveness of Nonprofits and Their Role in Public Affairs Education." *Journal of Public Affairs Education 21*, *3*: 305–310.

Sinclair, Betsy. 2012. *The Social Citizen: Peer Networks and Political Behavior.* Chicago: University of Chicago Press.

Stone, Deborah. 2012. *Policy Paradox: The Art of Political Decision Making* (3rd Edition). New York: W. W. Norton.

Tong, R. 1986. *Ethics in Policy Analysis.* Englewood Cliffs, NJ: Prentice Hall.

Turetsky, Vicki. 2018. Interview conducted in October 2017 June 2018.

Warwick, D.P., and T.F. Pettigrew. 1983. "Toward Ethical Guidelines for Social Science Research in Public Policy." In *Ethics, The Social Sciences, and Policy Analysis* (pp. 335–368). Boston, MA: Springer.

9
Epilogue

This book was based on two central premises. First, policy analysis involves the harnessing and management of a multitude of information for very complex issues. The analyst is well served by a framework that helps them organize and interrogate that information and then make coherent and evidence-based recommendations. Policy analysis should be logical and transparent, and should marshal data, broadly defined, to bolster a well-formed argument. We present a framework that provides such structure but also leaves space for flexibility in the face of political, institutional, and resource realities, as well as the values and priorities of the analyst and client. The framework is not wed to one particular ideological or disciplinary lens and can therefore be applied pragmatically and across many contexts.

Second, policy analysis can benefit from multiple scholarly perspectives. We incorporate a range of disciplines into the analytical approach presented in this book, including economics, political science, planning, and design. The complexity of public problems means we need a multifaceted framework for addressing them. It is unreasonable to think that we would find such an approach in a single discipline; indeed, multiple lenses provide opportunities to view problems in different ways and to address them holistically and inclusively.

There are several ways that we implement these guiding principles throughout the book.

- Situate the central problem.
- Construct multi-modal and inclusive criteria. We promote a both a methodologically sound and ethical approach.
- Design alternatives that are innovative and realistic.
- Accept that there might not be a singular, ideal recommendation. Marginal changes are also acceptable and can generate meaningful impacts, especially over time.

What's Next?

Executing a logical, evidence-based policy analysis takes more than reading about it—practice makes perfect. Policy analysis is like any other skill: it must be learned, it must be practiced, and it must be honed.

Practice, Practice, Practice

We use the word "practice" to mean two things.

1. Apply the theory to practice: we have presented a method for organizing information and assessing trade-offs across options; now it needs to be applied to actual, timely policy problems. The hands-on experience of policy analysis is necessary for mastering the skill.
2. Practice the method as many times as possible and in a range of settings:
   - Use it for different policy issues.
   - Use it in individual and team situations.
   - Use it in simulated and "live" experiences.
   - Use it for low- and high-stakes scenarios.

Using the Supplemental Cases to Practice the Analytical Framework

At the end of the book, we include additional cases for practicing the analytical framework presented in the previous chapters. They are written with enough information for the student to lay out a complete analysis and even conduct additional research and data collection if you choose to. However, they are also open-ended enough to leave room for a range of problem framings, policy alternatives and analytical criteria. We also include various prompts that help the student change their perspective or potential client for the analysis. Therefore, the cases can be re-used to conduct simulated client-based analytic experiences, either in team or individual settings. We encourage the students to use the analysis of the cases to then also practice presenting their work in memos, reports, and briefings to a panel of experts and faculty (ideally, someone even plays the role of the client).

Even though the simulated analytic exercises using the cases are different than the "live" experiences analysts may have in the field, they are still very useful in one important way. The cases contain limited information on the topic, and sometimes these information gaps cannot even be filled with additional research. These information constraints force the student to confront the realities of scarcity. They need to make assumptions and work with the limited information they have in front of them—this will serve them well when they come across similar challenges in actual analytical projects.

Other Ways to Practice the Framework

In addition to the curated cases we provide, there are many other opportunities for practicing and applying the framework presented in this book:

- Apply the model to issues presented in newspaper articles and other current media.
- Set up mock debates (where students have to take on *both* sides of an issue).
- Arrange an actual project with a real client.
- Generate a matrix for your everyday decisions, like weekend activities and job opportunities.

Over time and across multiple applications, the analyst will discover that each project and scenario requires a slightly different tweaking of the framework. These adjustments become easier and more refined with experience. However, if the analyst is true to the core tenets of the framework—well-articulated problems, evidence-based logic, and evaluative standards that reflect a comprehensive set of interests and use consistent metrics—flexibility should not compromise integrity.

APPENDIX I
CASE FOR ANALYSIS
WATER SHORTAGES IN THE LOWER AND UPPER BASINS OF THE COLORADO RIVER[1]

How Water Connects the Upper and Lower Basins of the U.S.

On June 1, 2023, Governor Katie Hobbs reassured the worried people of Arizona. "My message to Arizonans is this: we are not out of water and we will not be running out of water" (*Governor Hobbs Unveils 100-Year Study to Protect Valley Groundwater Supplies and Announces $40 Million Investment in Arizona Water Resiliency Fund* 2023). But despite this sunny conclusion, there was dismaying news, particularly for residents in the Phoenix metropolitan area and, perhaps most of all, for the home developers looking to take advantage of the surging demand for new houses in Phoenix. At this press conference, Governor Hobbs announced that there would be a restriction on new homes in the major cities of Arizona unless they could meet 100 years of demand for water without relying on the scarce groundwater. The Phoenix metropolitan area was one of the fastest growing in the United States (US Census Bureau 2023), and this demand for new homes was coupled with a massive housing shortage in the city (Arizona Department of Housing 2022). The news that this restriction would be necessary to prevent severe water shortages in the future came as an alarming signal that policies and behavior would need to shift to make life sustainable in the southwest.

But Phoenix and Arizona's water problems did not exist in isolation. While Arizona relies on groundwater as a backup, its main source of water is the Colorado River, which runs through the seven states that make up the upper and lower basins of the river's watershed. The upper basin states consist of Colorado, New Mexico, Utah, and Wyoming, while the lower basin is California, Arizona, and Nevada (see Appendix A). This division between the upper and the lower basin was established in 1922 by the Colorado River Compact, which allocated the shares of water from the Colorado River (Gelt 1997). Crucially, however, this water sharing agreement greatly overestimated the amount of water that would actually be available in the years to come. The abundance of water promised at the time led to consequential agricultural decisions, such as farmers relying on "thirsty crops" like alfalfa and hay to feed livestock, a practice which persists to this day.

By 2007 it had become obvious that there would have to be new policies to manage the water supply from the Colorado River. The states along the river had experienced eight years of drought, the worst period since record keeping began, and the United States Department of the Interior found it necessary to issue new guidelines to conserve water, such as standardizing drought severity based on the water level of Lake Mead and reducing water deliveries during droughts (Bureau of Reclamation 2007). Even at this stage, the federal government recognized that the current water sharing agreements and increasing shortages would be a source of tension and conflict, stating in their report that "Under these conditions, conflict over water is unsurprising and anticipated. Declining reservoir levels in the Basin led to interstate and inter-basin tensions" (Bureau of Reclamation 2007). These new "Interim Guidelines for the Operation of Lake Powell and Lake Mead" had the objectives of improving the government's management of the water supply by considering the trade-offs between the frequency and magnitude of water delivery and the effects of water shortages, and by enhancing the predictability of shortages and creating new mechanisms for storage and delivery of water.

Despite these guidelines, in August of 2021, Secretary of the Interior Deb Haaland announced the first-ever Tier 1 shortage for the Colorado River (see Appendix B). The level of water shortage for the Colorado River is based on the surface level of Lake Mead, located in Nevada and Arizona. A Tier 1 shortage occurs when the level of Lake Mead falls below 1,075 feet (Bureau of Reclamation 2007). By the following August the situation had become even more drastic. A year after the Department of the Interior announced the first Tier 1 shortage they announced that the water levels of Lake Mead had dropped below the Tier 2a threshold of 1,050 feet.

The Downstream Effects of Drought

Effects on Food Production

At this rate of decline the effects could be catastrophic, and not just for the states along the river but for the entire United States and possibly even beyond. While its dry climate does not immediately suggest that this would be the case, Yuma County, Arizona, is known as the winter lettuce capital of the world, supplying 90 percent of the nation's leafy greens between November and March. But even beyond threatening salads across the country, half of that water is being used to grow feed for cattle and livestock. Water shortages, whether imposed by nature or by governments, could have the downstream effect of causing nationwide shortages of many staple foods.

Effects on Electricity Production

Electricity is another major concern associated with water shortages from the Colorado River. In Nevada, Arizona, and California, about 1.3 million people get their electricity from the Hoover Powerplan, a hydroelectric plant that relies on the flow of water through the (Hoover Dam Frequently Asked Questions and Answers 2017). The water level of Lake Mead had already dropped 25 feet between 2022 and 2023, from 1,075, to 1,050 feet. If the water level ever got below 950 feet, the "minimum power pool," the Hoover Dam would no longer be able to generate electricity. At the "deadpool" level of 895 feet, water wouldn't be able to flow through the dam at all (Hager 2023).

Strategies to Resolve the Crisis

Within the Department of the Interior, the Bureau of Reclamation is the federal agency that manages the water supply in the western half of the United States. The agency has constructed more than 600 dams and reservoirs across the west, most famously the Hoover Dam, which holds back Lake Mead.

The Federal Bureau of Reclamation Plan

In October 2022, the Bureau of Reclamation began work on emergency interim guidelines for the water supply to the seven states (US Department of the Interior 2023a). These guidelines, known as the Supplemental Environmental Impact Statement (SEIS), considered a variety of policy alternatives that would revise the 2007 guidelines, such as requiring the lower basin states to provide a plan to the Bureau for keeping Lake Mead above 1,000 feet any time the level was projected to fall below 1,025 feet (Revised Draft Supplemental Environmental Impact Statement 2023). Some other alternatives that the Bureau rejected were to decommission the Glen Canyon Dam or to import water from other places like the Pacific Ocean. Most importantly, as the federal agency that controls the operation of the Hoover Dam and the Glen Canyon Dam, the tool most readily available to the Bureau is to reduce the supply of water to the states by decreasing the amount of flow through these dams.

Two Competing State Plans

Additionally, six of the states, all but California, managed to agree on a plan to reduce their allotment and consumption of water from the river and leave more of it in Lake Mead. California made its own plan, preferring instead to rely on previously agreed-upon allocations of water to the states. It would not be fair, however, to call this mere stubbornness on the part of California. The six-state plan proposed to reduce water allocations in five "reaches," making larger cuts to the supply further downstream. As the lowest state in the lower basin, California would stand to lose the largest share of their current supply. There are good reasons California would be extremely reluctant to accept such large cuts to its water supply. The state is the largest agricultural producer in the country by far, producing more than 10% of the nation's agricultural commodities (Cash Receipts by Commodity State Ranking n.d.), and possesses more surface irrigated land than any other state (Dieter et al. 2017). Fifty-eight percent of the hydroelectric power created by water running through the Hoover Dam goes to California, compared to just

23 percent and 19 percent going to Nevada and Arizona, respectively (Energy Kids n.d.).

California had been experiencing severe drought conditions for years. Their groundwater, which accounts for 60 percent of the state's water usage, had already been depleted to its lowest point ever recorded. More than 2,000 household wells had gone dry in just three years, and the state had to bring in emergency water supplies, particularly for the poorest residents of the state (Sommer 2023). Now the state was being asked to make drastic cuts to its supply from the Colorado River.

The two plans were irreconcilable. Seemingly at an impasse, the federal government once again threatened to step in and impose their plan on the seven states, an outcome that nobody wanted. So in May of 2023, the lower basin states, California, Arizona, and Nevada, agreed to cut 3 million acre-feet of water usage. One acre-foot is considered the planned annual usage for one single family home. In a letter to the Bureau of Reclamation, the lower basin states emphasized that their plan eliminated the need for federal intervention. To further prevent the imposition of the plan laid out in the SEIS, all seven states also jointly sent a letter to the Bureau asking them to delay implementation of the SEIS and review the lower basin plan. However, they stated in the letter that "nothing in this letter should be construed as an Upper Basin endorsement of the Lower Basin Plan (Buschatzke et al. 2023)."

Concerned that the federal government might soon impose water restrictions on them, the states all moved to form their own plans to deal with the crisis. The Colorado state legislature voted, nearly unanimously, to form the Colorado River Drought Task Force. The task force moved with a sense of urgency, meeting ten times between July and December 2023, and in the end they made eight recommendations to the Colorado legislature to improve the state's water infrastructure and drought resiliency (Wallace and Beall 2024).

These different levels of government, federal, states, coalitions of states, and local governments were all scrambling to devise plans to deal with the crisis that were often in conflict with one another. Their competing interests and different powers made developing an equitable strategy a monumental task.

Arizona v. Navajo Nation

While the states were arguing over the proper allocation of their water rights, another party was advocating that the federal government had an obligation to help fulfill their rights and access to the water of the Colorado River. Long before the 1922 Interstate Compact that allocated water from the river to the seven states, an 1868 peace treaty with the Navajo Nation had created a reservation roughly the size of West Virginia, establishing a "permanent home" for the tribe (*Arizona v. Navajo Nation* 2022). While numerous later court cases and agreements, including the 1922 compact and infrastructure projects such as the Hoover Dam, affected the water available to the tribe, nobody had ever actually assessed the rights of the Nation.

Just as the states themselves were experiencing alarming water shortages, the Navajo reservation was also in a dire situation. On some parts of the reservation 91 percent of people lacked access to water, and the average Navajo household used less than one-tenth of the water that was typical for an American household (*Arizona v. Navajo Nation* 2022). Despite the federal government's guarantees of a permanent home, the rapidly declining availability of usable water was a clear and present threat.

In June of 2023, the Supreme Court ruled in a 5–4 decision that the 1868 treaty "did not require the United States to take affirmative steps to secure water for the Tribe" (*Arizona v. Navajo Nation* 2022). Justice Brett Kavanaugh, writing for the majority, argued that if the court granted the relief sought by the Navajo Nation, the federal government might have to build infrastructure to secure water or that such a decision would even require the government to farm the land, mine the minerals, or harvest the timber.

However, Justice Neil Gorsuch, writing in dissent of the opinion, said that "the court rejects a request the Navajo Nation never made . . . [the Navajo Nation wants] the United States to identify the water rights it holds for them. And if the United States has misappropriated the Navajo's water rights, the Tribe asks them to formulate a plan to stop doing so prospectively" (*Arizona v. Navajo Nation* 2022).

The citizens of the Navajo Nation rely on the water from the Colorado River for their livelihoods and have done so since long before settlers from Europe first stepped foot in the region. Many people who live on the reservation have less than 10 gallons of water on hand at any given time, while the average American uses 88 gallons per day. They must carefully balance hygiene and consumption to avoid running out or having to make long trips to fill jugs and barrels (US Water Alliance 2017). It is not clear at this time how the plans created by the seven states, or the SEIS created by the Bureau of Reclamation, propose to address the needs of the 170,000 people who live on Navajo land.

Reducing the Water Consumption of Agriculture
On December 14, 2022, the Upper Colorado River Commission, made up of representatives from Colorado, New Mexico, Utah, and Wyoming, issued a request for proposals (RFP) to invite users of the Colorado River system to submit plans to voluntarily reduce consumption of water from the river (Upper Colorado River Commission 2022). The pilot program offered $150 per acre-foot of reduced water usage as the "fixed price" option or allowed participants to propose plans with a different amount of compensation with justification for that amount.

The funding for this program came from federal money allocated through the Inflation Reduction Act of 2022, which reserved $4 billion for water infrastructure and conservation efforts in the Colorado River Basin. Of this $4 billion, $125 million was allocated for this new program (Biden-Harris Administration Announces New Steps for Drought Mitigation Funding from Inflation Reduction Act 2022). By the deadline for submissions, 22 proposals had met the preliminary criteria for consideration by the Commission, though very little information about these potential projects was made available to the public, and it is not publicly known how much water these projects collectively propose to conserve (Sackett 2023).

Many farmers interpreted the program to be essentially paying them not to grow crops on parts of their fields, leaving them fallow (Dodd 2023); $150 per acre-foot of water conserved translates to about $400 per acre of field that farmers choose to leave fallow, but some farmers were reluctant to take the government up on this offer, saying that the amount offered was less than what they would bring in by growing on the land. The difference between what the federal government was offering and what farmers said they would need is immense. Save the River, a coalition of farmers and agribusiness leaders, was calling for $1,500 per acre-foot of conservation (Jean-Charles 2023).

Efforts to conserve water from the Colorado River are likely to be stymied if farmers are not part of the solution. Seventy-nine percent of the water taken from the river is used by the agriculture industry, with over half of that amount used to grow feed for livestock (Shao 2023). Reducing the production of these water-intensive crops would mean that meat and dairy producers could not support as many of the animals that consume them. The United States is the world's second-largest meat producer, and Americans consume more meat per capita than the people of any other country on Earth (Ritchie et al. 2023).

Conclusion

The problems caused by the unsustainable use of water from the Colorado River are being felt at every level, from the people of cities like Phoenix who cannot address a severe housing shortage to people all across the country whose supply of meat, dairy, and leafy greens are threatened. The solutions, too, are being negotiated at every level of government. State governments are working to respond to the crisis while trying to establish an equitable distribution for an already-scarce resource. The people of the Navajo Nation are ignored by the US government, which refuses to even tell them how much of their water it is holding. The seven states along the river struggle to reach an agreement, and the federal Department of the Interior threatens to impose one.

The winter of 2022–2023 was particularly wet in the region, with snowpack reaching 130 percent above average (Hufham 2024). This piece of good fortune temporarily alleviated some of the drought conditions and the urgency of developing an immediate policy response for political leaders. Nevertheless, the situation is far from resolved. As the seven states put it in their May 22, 2023, letter to the Bureau of Reclamation, "[we] recognize that having one good winter does not solve the systemic challenges facing the Colorado River" (Buschatzke et al. 2023). The current agreement between the states is set to expire in 2026, and a new one will need to be finalized before that to prevent a crisis. Whatever strategies are pursued among the upper and lower basin states, the implications of their actions will extend miles beyond the banks of the Colorado.

Appendix A Map of the Lower and Upper Basins

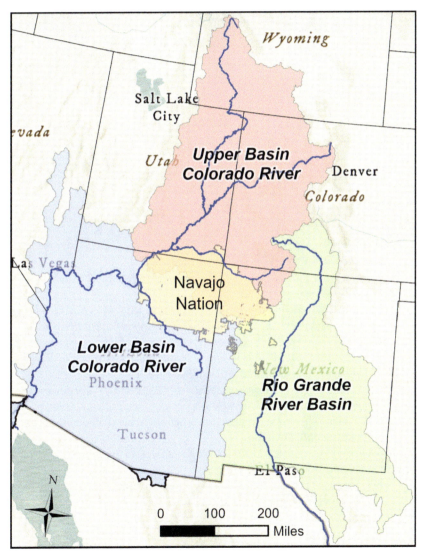

Source: Navajo Water Rights Commission: https://nnwrc.navajo-nsn.gov/. Reprinted with permission.

Appendix B Tier 1 Shortage Guidelines

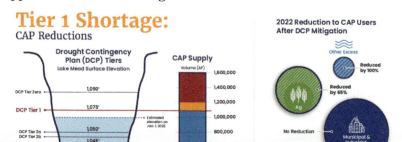

Source: Know Your Water News, Central Arizona Project: https://knowyourwaternews.com/tier-1-shortage-cap-reductions/. Reprinted with permission.

Appendix C

Useful Links:

Colorado River Shortage 2022 Fact Sheet:
www.azwater.gov/sites/default/files/media/ADWR-CAP-FactSheet-CoRiverShortage-081321.pdf

Department of the Interior press release on SEIS:
www.doi.gov/pressreleases/interior-department-announces-next-steps-protect-stability-and-sustainability-colorado

KUNC—"Six States Agree on a Proposal for Colorado River Cutbacks, California has a Counter"
www.kunc.org/environment/2023-01-31/six-states-agree-on-a-proposal-for-colorado-river-cutbacks-california-has-a-counter

NY Times—"Arizona Limits Construction Around Phoenix as Its Water Supply Dwindles"
www.nytimes.com/2023/06/01/climate/arizona-phoenix-permits-housing-water.html

NY Times—"The Colorado River Is Shrinking. See What's Using All the Water."
www.nytimes.com/interactive/2023/05/22/climate/colorado-river-water.html

Discussion Questions and Prompts for Analysis

1. You are advising the governor of Arizona on how to address the state's water shortage and bring balance to the competing interests desperate for a stable and secure water supply, including agribusiness, real estate developers, and local residents. Any policy recommendation will have tradeoffs, helping some groups more than others. What options should the governor consider? What criteria should be employed to evaluate them? What would you recommend? Why?
2. You are the chief lobbyist for Arizona's largest agricultural producers. What arguments should you make to convince the governor and state legislature that the supply of water for lettuce and other major crops should not be reduced? What alternative strategies would you propose, and why?
3. You are an advisor to the US Secretary of the Interior, tasked to advise her on how the federal government should balance the competing claims of the lower and upper basins. What criteria should drive any decision? What options should be considered?

Note

1. This case was written by Aaron Bierstein.

Bibliography

Arizona Department of Housing. 2022. *Fiscal Year 2022 Annual Report*.
Arizona Department of Water Resources. n.d. *Phoenix AMA Groundwater Supply Updates*. www.azwater.gov/phoenix-ama-groundwater-supply-updates
Arizona v. Navajo Nation, Citation Pending, US Supreme Court. 2022. www.supremecourt.gov/opinions/22pdf/21-1484_aplc.pdf
Biden-Harris Administration Announces New Steps for Drought Mitigation Funding from Inflation Reduction Act. 2022. U.S. Department of the Interior (October 12). www.doi.gov/pressreleases/biden-harris-administration-announces-new-steps-drought-mitigation-funding-inflation
Bland, A. 2023. "Colorado River Deal: What Does It Mean for California?" *CalMatters* (May 22). https://calmatters.org/environment/water/2023/05/colorado-river-states-agreement/
Bureau of Reclamation. 2007. *Record of Decision—Colorado River Interim Guidelines for Lower Basin Shortages and the Coordinated Operations for Lake Powell*

and Lake Mead. Bureau of Reclamation (December). www.usbr.gov/lc/region/programs/strategies/RecordofDecision.pdf#page=9

Buschatzke, T., J.B. Hamby, E. Lopez, B. Gebhart, R. Mitchell, J.J. Entsminger, and G. Shawcroft. 2023. *Seven States Letter*. Colorado River Basin States Representatives of Arizona, California, Colorado, Nevada, New Mexico, Utah, and Wyoming (May 22). www.doi.gov/sites/doi.gov/files/seven-states-letter-5-22-2023.pdf

Cash Receipts by Commodity State Ranking. n.d. US Department of Agriculture Economic Research Service. https://data.ers.usda.gov/reports.aspx?ID=17844#P2fa97c4879eb4635af642e8db3515163_3_251iT0R0x0

City of Phoenix Water Services Department. 2011. *2011 Water Resource Plan*. City of Phoenix. www.phoenix.gov/waterservicessite/Documents/d_046975.pdf#search=Water%20Resource%20Plan

Colorado General Assembly. 2023. *Colorado River Drought Task Force | Colorado General Assembly*. https://leg.colorado.gov/bills/sb23-295

Colorado River Shortage 2022 Fact Sheet. 2017. Central Arizona Project (November 9). www.azwater.gov/sites/default/files/media/ADWR-CAP-FactSheet-CoRiverShortage-081321.pdf

Dieter, C.A., M.A. Maupin, R.R. Caldwell, M.A. Harris, T.I. Ivanhnenko, J.K. Lovelace, N.L. Barber, and K.S. Linsey. 2017. *Estimated Use of Water in the United States in 2015*. U.S. Geological Survey. https://doi.org/10.3133/cir1441

Dodd, E. 2023. "Water Shortage has Farmers Afraid of Biden Conservation Funding." *Business Insider* (March 19). www.businessinsider.com/water-california-colorado-farmers-fear-drought-climate-change-biden-funding-2023-3

Energy Kids. n.d. *Hoover Dam Hydroelectric Plant: A Report from Energy Ant — My Trip to the Hoover Dam Near Boulder City, Nevada*. US Energy Information Administration. https://www.eia.gov/kids/for-teachers/field-trips/hoover-dam-hydroelectric-plant.php#:~:text=Nineteen%20percent%20of%20the%20electricity,that%20is%20270%20miles%20away

Fitchette, T. 2022. *Saving the Colorado River*. Agribusiness & Water Council of Arizona (September 14). https://agribusinessarizona.org/saving-the-colorado-river

Gelt, J. 1997. *Sharing Colorado River Water: History, Public Policy and the Colorado River Compact | Water Resources Research Center | The University of Arizona*. Water Resources Research Center (August 1). https://wrrc.arizona.edu/publication/sharing-colorado-river-water-history-public-policy-and-colorado-river-compact

Governor Hobbs Unveils 100-Year Study to Protect Valley Groundwater Supplies and Announces $40 Million Investment in Arizona Water Resiliency Fund. 2023. Office of the Governor Katie Hobbs (June 2). https://azgovernor.gov/office-arizona-governor/news/2023/06/governor-hobbs-unveils-100-year-study-protect-valley

Hager, A. 2023. *Six States Agree on a Proposal for Colorado River Cutbacks, California has a Counter*. KUNC (January 31). www.kunc.org/environment/2023-01-31/six-states-agree-on-a-proposal-for-colorado-river-cutbacks-california-has-a-counter

Healy, J. 2023. "Arizona Limits Construction Around Phoenix as Its Water Supply Dwindles." *The New York Times* (June 1). www.nytimes.com/2023/06/01/climate/arizona-phoenix-permits-housing-water.html

Hoover Dam Frequently Asked Questions and Answers. 2017. Bureau of Reclamation (November 9). www.usbr.gov/lc/hooverdam/faqs/powerfaq.html

Hufham, A. 2024. *Colorado River Basin has Last Year to Thank for Stability Despite Drought*. The Salt Lake Tribune (January 4). www.sltrib.com/news/environment/2024/01/04/how-last-years-winter-continues/

Interior Department Announces Next Steps to Protect the Stability and Sustainability of Colorado River Basin | U.S. Department of the Interior. 2023. US Department of the Interior (April 11). www.doi.gov/pressreleases/interior-department-announces-next-steps-protect-stability-and-sustainability-colorado

James, I. 2023. "Water Concerns Prompt New Limits on Growth in Arizona." *Los Angeles Times* (June 1). www.latimes.com/environment/story/2023-06-01/phoenix-arizona-water-crisis

Jean-Charles, P. 2023. *To Save the Colorado River, Farmers will be Paid not to Farm. Some are Looking to Cash in*. Agriculture Dive (October 6). www.agriculturedive.com/news/colorado-river-farm-agriculture-drought-conservation/695862/

Luedke, T., and M. DiPaolo. 2020. *Arizona Water Rights—The Copper State's Water Rights System*. aquaoso (December 1). https://aquaoso.com/water-rights/arizona-water-rights/

Magill, B. 2023. *US Sets New Colorado River Drought Plan to Take Effect in 2027*. Bloomberg Law (October 19). https://news.bloomberglaw.com/environment-and-energy/us-sets-new-colorado-river-drought-plan-to-take-effect-in-2027

Metropolitan and Micropolitan Statistical Areas Totals: 2020–2023. 2024. Census Bureau (March 11). www.census.gov/data/tables/time-series/demo/popest/2020s-total-metro-and-micro-statistical-areas.html#v2022

Navajo Nation Water Rights Commission. n.d. *Supporting Navajo Water Rights Through Public Advocacy*. https://nnwrc.navajo-nsn.gov/

Notice of Intent to Prepare a Supplemental Environmental Impact Statement. 2023. Southern Nevada Water Authority (January 31). www.snwa.com/assets/pdf/seis-letter.pdf

Popat, M., and T. Davis. 2023. "Arizona Panel Urges Big Overhaul of Rural Groundwater Rules." *Arizona Daily Star* (December 1). https://tucson.com/news/local/environment/arizona-panel-groundwater-governor-rural-pumping-regulation-legislature/article_39e1d0f6-8ee9-11ee-9cfa-971a31b1a398.html

Record of Decision. 2007. Bureau of Reclamation (December 1). www.usbr.gov/lc/region/programs/strategies/RecordofDecision.pdf

Revised Draft Supplemental Environmental Impact Statement. 2023. Bureau of Reclamation (October). www.usbr.gov/ColoradoRiverBasin/documents/NearTermColoradoRiverOperations/20231019-Near-termColoradoRiverOperations-RevisedDraftEIS-508.pdf

Ritchie, H., P. Rosado, and M. Roser. 2023. *Meat and Dairy Production*. Our World in Data (December). https://ourworldindata.org/meat-production#which-countries-eat-the-most-meat

Sackett, H. 2023. "Little Information Released on Conservation-Program Proposals." *Sky-Hi News* (April 9). www.skyhinews.com/news/little-information-released-on-conservation-program-proposals/

Selin, S. 2023. *FY 2024 Strategic Plan—ADWR*. Arizona Department of Water Resources (July 15). www.azwater.gov/sites/default/files/media/FY_2024_Strategic_Plan_-_ADWR.pdf

Shao, E. 2023. "See How the Colorado River Water Gets Used Up." *The New York Times* (May 22). www.nytimes.com/interactive/2023/05/22/climate/colorado-river-water.html

Sommer, L. 2023. "Why California's Drought Won't Really End, Even Though It's Raining." *NPR* (March 23). www.npr.org/2023/03/23/1165378214/3-reasons-why-californias-drought-isnt-really-over-despite-all-the-rain

Tinetti, J. 2022. *Department of Interior Announces Tier 2 Shortage on the Colorado River*. CSG West (August 18). https://csgwest.org/2022/08/18/department-of-interior-announces-tier-2-shortage-on-the-colorado-river/

Upper Colorado River Commission. 2022. *Pre-Solicitation Notice of Request for Proposals Regarding a Potential Funding Opportunity for Voluntary Participation in a System Conservation Pilot Program for 2023* (December 14). www.ucrcommission.com/wp-content/uploads/2022/12/SCPP-for-2023-Notice-of-Pre-Solicitation-Request-for-Proposals-Dec-13-2022.pdf

US Census Bureau. 2023. *Metropolitan and Micropolitan Statistical Areas Population Totals: 2020-2023*. www.census.gov/data/tables/time-series/demo/popest/2020s-total-metro-and-micro-statistical-areas.html#v2022

US Department of the Interior. 2023a. *Interior Department Announces Next Steps to Protect the Stability and Sustainability of Colorado River Basin | U.S. Department of the Interior*. DOI.gov (April 11). www.doi.gov/pressreleases/interior-department-announces-next-steps-protect-stability-and-sustainability-colorado

US Department of the Interior. 2023b. *Lower Basin Plan Letter* (May 22). www.doi.gov/sites/doi.gov/files/lower-basin-plan-letter-5-22-2023.pdf

US Water Alliance. 2017. *Closing the Water Access Gap in the United States—A National Action Plan*. US Water Alliance (November 9). https://static1.squarespace.com/static/5e80f1a64ed7dc3408525fb9/t/6092ddcc499e1b6a6a07ba3a/1620237782228/Dig-Deep_Closing-the-Water-Access-Gap-in-the-United-States_DIGITAL_compressed.pdf

Wallace, C., and J. Beall. 2024. "Colorado River Drought Task Force Releases Final Report." *Western Livestock Journal* (January 5). www.wlj.net/top_headlines/colorado-river-drought-task-force-releases-final-report/article_e6883276-abdd-11ee-bbe8-ffb1822bc324.html

APPENDIX II
CASE FOR ANALYSIS
REGULATING SHORT-TERM RENTALS[1]

Much Ado About Short-Term Rentals

The mayor turned over the matter in her mind. On her desk lay a memo from a representative of the United Hotel Owners Association[2] asking that the city consider a ban on short-term rental units. These units, which had been popping up across the city in rapidly increasing numbers over the past few years, were houses or apartments owned privately but available to rent through a popular online app. Owners could list their home, or even just a bedroom for people to stay in, for costs that were often much lower than a hotel. Tourists and guests often found more personalized or roomier accommodations than a standard hotel room. Vacation rentals had existed since the 1950s but took off in force in the late 90s and early 2000s with the proliferation of the internet. The biggest name in short-term rentals, Airbnb, began in 2008 as the first internet platform that allowed users to book a single room in a host's house and gave them the ability to pay using a credit card over the internet (The History of Short-Term Rentals n.d.).

The problem was that, according to some, particularly hotel owners, these rental units were little more than illegal hotels that did not operate with the same standard of safety or health regulations that a hotel would be expected to maintain. Unregistered units could have fire code violations that could possibly endanger guests, such as missing smoke detectors or a lack of emergency escape exits (Verzoni 2022). Bug infestations and unsanitary conditions had been reported with alarming regularity (Bloom 2021). These issues did not only impact the guests of these properties, but fires could spread to neighboring buildings; loud parties could disrupt others in the area; and some people expressed concerns that their quiet, residential neighborhood might increasingly cater to the needs of out-of-town guests rather than the people who actually lived there.

There was also the issue of housing in the city. Critics of the rentals claimed that they drove up housing prices by reducing the amount of available affordable housing for residents (Zaveri 2023). They argued that the units being listed as short-term rentals would otherwise be leased as long-term residences, therefore trimming an already scarce supply of housing and pushing overall prices up. The mayor had to consider that housing prices were rapidly becoming completely unaffordable for a lot of people and that the rise of these rentals could be contributing to the problem.

Finally, the hotel owners complained that short-term rentals harmed workers who relied on their jobs in the legal hotel industry and even went so far as to suggest that police, fire departments, and schools might not be as well funded without the tax revenue from their businesses (Zaveri 2023). There was some validity to this: hotels paid over $41 billion in state and local taxes in the United States in 2021 (American Hotel & Lodging Association 2023). The mayor had repeatedly had calls and meetings with frantic hotel owners already struggling to survive after years of a global pandemic that brought business to a standstill, and now their bookings were increasingly being encroached upon by the short-term rental market. If the mayor didn't act quickly to alleviate these concerns, the city might face a more catastrophic backlash from its well-organized hospitality industry, which could impact the precarious rebound of the tourism industry since COVID.

Not All Short-Term Rentals Are the Same

Rhetoric about short-term rentals typically conflated two different types of owners with very different interests and operations. On the one hand were individual owners, usually people who owned one or two homes and wanted to make a little extra money on the side to supplement their incomes or retirement funds. These "mom and pop" owners made up 94% of all short-term rentals (New York State Office of the Attorney

General Eric T. Schneiderman 2014). They were more dispersed and typically lacked the significant political influence of corporate owners who were able to spend lavishly on lobbyists and campaign donations.

The other group were commercial owners. These owners operated short-term rental units more like a chain of boutique hotels. Typically, these were owners who possessed three or more properties and were operating them as a business and not simply utilizing the service of the app to help make ends meet at home. While these owners only made up 6 percent of the total, they accepted 36 percent of the bookings in 2022 (New York State Office of the Attorney General Eric T. Schneiderman 2014).[3]

Conflicting Interests

Several cities had already passed laws that effectively banned short-term rental units. These laws did not distinguish between individual and commercial property owners, which some people have thought to be unfair.

An organization known as Protecting Homeowner Rights and Independence (PHORI) was formed to fight back against the new law in their city (Restore Homeowner Autonomy & Rights n.d.) and its effect on individual owners. They claimed that the law takes away homeowners' autonomy and was intended to force them out of the short-term rental market in order to make more room for luxury hotels. They primarily saw the regulation as serving the interests of hotel owners facing competition from this smaller budget option. Larger corporate owners had more ability and resources to be able to adapt their units to the new regulations and stay in business. Some rental owners questioned whether the law was really about safety and sanitation at all.

The new laws also seemed to some to disregard the benefits of short-term rentals. While the hotels in the center of the city were unhappy about the added competition, the mayor heard from some small business owners in the less busy areas that these units had brought new people to the area. Some of these were visitors from other states and countries who might otherwise have never found these businesses if they had been staying in a traditional hotel closer to the center of the city (World Travel & Tourism Council 2022).

Others protested that the new regulations threatened large supplements to their fixed incomes in their retirement years. Hosts operating short-term rental units could make tens of thousands of dollars per year (Lenzen 2023). The average host income in the United States in 2021 was $44,235 (Airbnb Calculator—Estimate Your Short-Term Rental Revenue n.d.) (see Appendix A), so in many cases the impact to these owners could be enormous.

And tourists appreciated having alternative options to traditional hotels, which could feel impersonal and monotonous. In some places, 70 percent of tourists were renting out entire houses instead of rooms (Guttentag et al. 2018), which was something most hotels simply could not accommodate. Guests frequently found it to be a more affordable option. A student on a very limited budget was able to visit Milan, the most expensive city in Italy, spending only €99 for three nights, and didn't particularly mind sharing the apartment with a woman and her cat.

The Law

The mayor considered some of the legislation from other cities that were also navigating how to manage the growing presence of these short-term rentals. While local variations existed, restrictions on short-term rentals in different cities and jurisdictions mostly involved some very similar rules. In a typical case, these new regulations applied to rentals of fewer than 30 days, which included nearly all vacation or business bookings.

Owners were required to register their units with the city government, paying a registration fee on the order of $150. While this requirement might not seem to present much of an encumbrance, the office in charge of processing these applications often moves very slowly. One law, passed in January 2022, had received 4,624 registration applications by September 2023 and had only processed 405 of them, leaving the rest in a legally ambiguous position (Brand and Jeffry-Wilensky 2023). Owners had to wait an average of 50 days for approval from the city to continue operating their units for rent, while if more information was needed or corrections were required, the process might take an average of 87 days (Brand and Jeffry-Wilensky 2023). Until permitting went through, their rental units would sit vacant.

Other restrictions aimed to prevent the operation of short-term rentals as hotels. Only two guests were allowed on a reservation, regardless of the size of the property. The owner of the unit was required to physically occupy the unit. A common practice had been to rent out a particular part of a home, keeping it separate from the rest of the residence by means of locked doors. The new law required that all interior doors must be unlocked, with guests having access to the entire property (City of New York 2021).

Other cities introduced less direct measures to combat the spread of "illegal letting." The city council of Paris, France, voted on a proposal to ban small key boxes that had popped up everywhere to facilitate guests being able to enter units without having to meet the owners face to face (O'Sullivan 2024). Ostensibly, this regulation was proposed on aesthetic grounds; the boxes were considered by many an eyesore and a form of "pollution." It did not escape the notice of the media, however, that the ban on key boxes amounted to a restriction of the rentals they were meant to facilitate.

Some cities chose to regulate short-term rentals by limiting them to certain geographic areas or capping the number of them allowed within the city. The city of New Orleans banned short-term rentals in most of the French Quarter (Local Housing Solutions 2022), and Portland, Maine, limited the number of non-owner-occupied rentals to just 300 (Billings 2017). Other cities have opted to allow the rentals to continue virtually unrestricted but with additional taxes for "internet-based" short-term rentals (Local Housing Solutions 2022).

Doubts

The mayor also knew that not everybody accepted the reasoning behind the new laws, and some speculated that ulterior motives might be at play. Some of the more intuitive claims did not seem to be strongly backed by evidence. Most suspect was the assertion that short-term rentals were substantially contributing to housing shortages. While some evidence existed that short-term rental units might have a modest effect on increasing housing costs, the percentage of total housing units being used as short-term rentals in one city, where this issue was most at the fore, was only 0.39 percent (Zaveri 2023). Of these, a significant number were people renting out their own homes, which might not otherwise be on the regular housing market even if they weren't being used in this way.

Opponents of short-term rental companies argued that landlords were evicting tenants in order to convert their properties into the more profitable "illegal hotel" business (Bhuiyan 2015). In an attempt to enforce their regulation, New York City began issuing dozens of fines to real estate companies found to have violated the law by converting apartments into short-term rental units (Jones 2024). It was unclear how widespread or impactful these conversions had been, but they had gotten a lot of attention.

Others noticed that much of the criticism of these companies came from hotel owners and associations representing them. Both hotel associations and short-term rental companies engaged in heavy lobbying efforts to convince legislators to support their cause. Money flowed into political campaigns from both sides of the issue. A state attorney general whose office authored a critical report on short-term rentals was found to have accepted over $100,000 in campaign donations from hotel executives and unions that represent hospitality workers (O'Brien 2015).

The mayor recognized that the concerns raised about short-term rentals were real and serious. The fact that they were not subject to the same safety or health regulations as hotels and were exempt from the occupancy taxes that hotels were required to pay could lead to consequential social and fiscal problems. But there were also other interests at play, with less of an eye to the public good. The challenge would be sorting out which arguments were being advanced in good faith and which might be more self-interested.

The Future of Short-Term Rentals

Few, if any, jurisdictions have banned short-term rentals outright, even if local laws force them to radically change the way that they operate. Some have accused short-term rental companies of attempting to get around these laws or not encouraging owners to register with municipalities, as required, believing that they can get the law overturned in court (Brand and Jeffrey-Wilensky 2023). Without strong encouragement from rental companies to register, and a slow-moving approval process on the part of city governments, few properties have been able to register and operate legally.

In this legal limbo, a rash of "black market" short-term rental options have appeared, particularly on social media (Hoover 2023). Owners typically list their properties on social media platforms for people to see and handle the bookings on their own, skirting the companies entirely. This practice has the consequence of perhaps being even less safe and aggravating the concerns that ostensibly have led to these regulations in the first place.

And while it is one thing to regulate short-term rentals, it is another to actually enforce these regulations. Even after these laws have been passed, owners continue to list their properties, in violation of the law, and guests continue to book them (Shaban et al. 2016). In most cases they are not caught, and few people have actually faced penalties for operating illegally. Lawmakers have sought ways to make the implementation and enforcement of these policies more effective, but there has not yet been a silver-bullet solution.

Conclusion

The mayor's path forward was not clear. Could she manage to balance the concerns of the hotel and tourism industries with those of owners supplementing their retirement income by renting out a spare bedroom? Were there ways of making sure that visitors to the city were safe in their accommodations while also allowing them to have a range of options to meet their needs and preferences? Did any laws in other places seem to strike the right balance? With the economic troubles from the pandemic still mounting and an election year rapidly approaching, these questions needed to be answered quickly and decisively.

The rise of the internet had facilitated an attendant informal "sharing" economy that allowed individuals to make money on their own terms without the need to start businesses of their own. In cities across the world, taxi drivers faced threats from ridesharing apps. Traditional offices had, in some places, given way to shared workspaces.

These spaces and practices were inherently more difficult to regulate, control, and make safe for users, especially while maintaining their trademark flexibility. Yet fighting against them may be about as useful as trying to hold back the tide. As in the case of short-term rental units, individual owners, commercial operators, and the renters themselves may have such varying concerns and priorities that a single policy cannot effectively address them all. How can one threat, like health and safety or severe housing shortages, be mitigated without propagating an even more problematic response, such as shadow networks for renting that are without any oversight? And would overly restrictive regulation drive these short-term rental platforms out of the city, possibly undermining tourism and a crucial source of revenue? The mayor's next move would need to take all these factors into account.

Discussion Questions and Prompts for Analysis

1 You are advising the mayor on how to respond to the concerns raised about the growth of short-term rentals. Is public intervention warranted? What options should the mayor consider? What criteria should be employed to evaluate them? What would you recommend? Why?
2 You have been hired as a consultant for a group of organizations that advocate for and develop affordable housing in the city. What kind of arguments would you develop to convince the mayor that affordable housing is at risk in the context of expanding short-term rentals? What alternative strategies would you propose to clamp down on the short-term rentals, and why?
3 You are a policy analyst for a local council member who represents a neighborhood outside of the central district and that has one of the highest concentrations of short-term rental units (but no hotels). How would you propose responding to the concerns about short-term rentals so that you balance both your neighborhood constituents' interests and those of the city more broadly? What criteria should drive any decision? What options should be considered?

Notes
1 This case was written by Aaron Bierstein.
2 Organizations cited are fictionalized and loosely based on real-life examples.
3 Information from this source has been adapted to apply to the current case.

References

Airbnb Calculator—Estimate Your Short-Term Rental Revenue. n.d. AllTheRooms. www.alltherooms.com/resources/articles/airbnb-calculator/

American Hotel & Lodging Association. 2023. *Report: Hotel-Generated State and Local Tax Revenue to Reach New Highs in 2023* (February 21). www.ahla.com/news/report-hotel-generated-state-and-local-tax-revenue-reach-new-highs-2023

Bhuiyan, J. 2015. *NYC Council Members Take Airbnb to Task at Oversight Hearing.* Buzzfeed News (January 20). www.buzzfeednews.com/article/johanabhuiyan/nyc-council-members-take-airbnb-to-task-at-oversight-hearing

Billings, R. 2017. "Portland's New Rules Limit Short-Term Rentals, Add Fees for Hosts." *Portland Press Herald* (March 27). www.pressherald.com/2017/03/27/portland-enacts-rules-for-short-term-rentals/

Bloom, L.B. 2021. "Is Airbnb Safe? New Report Exposes Scams, Bug Infestations, Discrimination." *Forbes* (October 11). www.forbes.com/sites/laurabegleybloom/2021/10/11/is-airbnb-safe-new-report-exposes-scams-bug-infestations-and-more/?sh=6c9d0ded493b

Brand, D., and J. Jeffrey-Wilensky. 2023. "NYC Only has 405 Legal Airbnb and Other Short-Term Rentals Available After Crackdown." *Gothamist* (September 28). https://gothamist.com/news/after-crackdown-nyc-only-has-405-legal-airbnb-and-other-short-term-rentals-available

City of New York. 2021. *Local Law 18 of 2022* (November 13). www.nyc.gov/assets/specialenforcement/downloads/pdfs/LL18-of-2022.pdf

Guttentag, D., S. Smith, and M. Havitz. 2018. "Why Tourists Choose Airbnb: A Motivation-Based Segmentation Study." *Journal of Travel Research* 57, 3: 342–359.

The History of Short-Term Rentals. n.d. Keycafe Blog. https://blog.keycafe.com/the-history-of-short-term-rentals/

Hoover, A. 2023. "New York's Airbnb Ban is Descending into Pure Chaos." *WIRED* (October 9). www.wired.com/story/airbnb-ban-new-york-illegal-listings/

Jones, S. 2024. "NYC has Issued $16.3M in Fines as It Cracks Down on Short-Term Rentals." *Bisnow* (May 14). www.bisnow.com/new-york/news/hotel/new-york-city-to-reach-155m-in-settlements-from-illegal-short-term-rentals-124244

Lenzen, C. 2023. "East Dallas Short-Term Rental Operators Sue City Over New Regulations." *Community Impact* (October 30). https://communityimpact.com/dallas-fort-worth/lake-highlands-lakewood/government/2023/10/30/east-dallas-short-term-rental-operators-sue-city-over-new-regulations/

Local Housing Solutions. 2022. *Regulating Short Term Rentals* (September 9). Retrieved May 19, 2024, from https://localhousingsolutions.org/housing-policy-library/regulating-short-term-rentals/

New York State Office of the Attorney General Eric T. Schneiderman. 2014. *Airbnb in the City* (October). https://ag.ny.gov/sites/default/files/reports/AIRBNB_REPORT.pdf#page=11

O'Brien, R. 2015. *Hotel Industry Targets Upstart Airbnb in Statehouse Battles* (July 15). The Center for Public Integrity. https://publicintegrity.org/politics/state-politics/hotel-industry-targets-upstart-airbnb-in-statehouse-battles/

O'Sullivan, F. 2024. "Paris May Ban Key Boxes in Battle Against Short-Term Stays." *Bloomberg.com* (January 17). www.bloomberg.com/news/articles/2024-01-17/airbnb-vrbo-paris-may-ban-key-boxes-in-battle-against-short-term-lets

Restore Homeowner Autonomy & Rights. n.d. www.rhoar.org/

Shaban, B., J. Carroll, and K. Nious. 2016. "Thousands Violate SF Housing Laws Using Airbnb, Few Face Penalties." *NBC* (December 7). www.nbcbayarea.com/news/local/bay-legal-thousands-violate-sf-housing-laws-few-face-penalties/73239/

Verzoni, A. 2022. *Short-Term Rental Safety.* National Fire Protection Association (June 28). www.nfpa.org/news-blogs-and-articles/blogs/2022/06/28/short-term-rental-safety

WorldTravel & Tourism Council. 2022. *Best Practices—Short-Term Rentals* (July). https://wttc.org/Portals/0/Documents/Reports/2022/Best%20Practices-%20Short%20Term%20Rentals.pdf

Zaveri, M. 2023. "What to Know About New Airbnb Regulations in NYC." *The New York Times* (September 5). www.nytimes.com/2023/09/05/nyregion/airbnb-regulations-nyc-housing.html

INDEX

Note: Page numbers in *italics* indicate figures and page numbers in **bold** indicate tables on the corresponding page, and references following "n" refer notes.

Ackerman, Frank 180, 185, 188–189
administrative costs 161
administrative data 261–262
administrative feasibility 17, 120, 188
adverse selection 44
Advocacy Coalition Framework (ACF) 19
advocacy coalitions 19
advocacy organizations as source of information 243
affordability restrictions in zoning 75
Affordable Care Act 53, 77–79
agencies, research and statistical 244, **245**; *see also specific name*
Agendas, Alternatives, and Public Policies (Kingdon) 18
aggregate ratings 211
Aid for Families with Dependent Children 58
allocative efficiency 186, 187
alternative models of policy analysis: defining the problem and 39–40; design approaches 26–28; economic efficiency and 23; incrementalist model 28–33; overview 26; rational model and 21, **22**
alternative policy options: analogous policies 72, 96; background information 249; behavioral economics and, insights from 81–93, 96; best practices, cautionary note on 72–73; brainstorming 80–81, 96; child support debt case study and 97–105; client suggestions 71; constraints and, imagining policies without 81; criteria and, confusing with 137; design thinking and, insights from 93–96; futures thinking 81; government intervention, standard modes of 76–80, 96; ideal solution, building of 81; impacts of 23; incremental changes to status quo 70–71; juxtaposition of 68; multiple variations 73–75; names given to 68; overview 5, 69–70, 96; past policies addressing similar issues 71–72; policies in other places addressing similar issues 71; prediction and 195; recommendations for policy and 67; sources for, overview of 69–70, 96; status quo 70
American Bar Association 288
American Civil Liberties Union (ACLU) 143n2
American Community Survey (ACS) 258, 260, **260–261**

Amy, Douglas J. 289, 292
analogous policies 72, 96
analytical matrix 138–139
anchoring 83
applied research, policy analysis as 235, 268
architecture of problem 45
The Argumentative Turn in Policy Analysis and Planning (Fischer and Forester) 296
Arizona v. Navajo Nation 312–313
Attract framework 89–90, 198
audience, understanding/knowing 49–51, 284–285
Automatic Collection System **147**, 151, **151–152**, 152, **169–171**, **174**, **175**, **188**
Automatic Forgiveness of Arrears Due to Incarceration Alternative (AFAI) 103, 140, 219, 225–226, 229–230
Automatic systems 82
availability 83–84
avoided cost method 165

backloading costs 170
backward mapping 124
Baltimore's Responsible Fatherhood Project 101
Bardach, Eugene 21, **22**, 25, 26, 45, 73, 204, 246
Baumgartner, Frank 19, 32
behavioral economics, insights from: alternative policy options and 81–93, 96; anchoring 83; availability 83–84; confirmation bias 84; framing choices 83; loss aversion 82–83; nudge concept and 84–93; optimism 84; overconfidence 84; overview 81–82, 96; representativeness 84; status quo bias 82
Behavioral Insights Team (United Kingdom) 86, 198
benefit-cost ratio (BCR) 176
benefits: explicit 163; external 161; frontloading 170; identifying which to include 160–163, 181; implicit 163; internal 161; monetary values to, assigning 163–168; primary 161–162; secondary 161–162; up-front **172**
best practices 72–73, 266–269
bias 82–84, 86, 139, 293
binary criteria 209
Bipartisan Policy Center 45
Bloomberg, Michael 87
Boardman, Anthony E. 159, 182
bounded rationality 24, 30, 38
bounding 137, 173, 184
brainstorming 80–81, 96
Brennan Center 241
budgets 187, 259
building off ideal solution 81
Bureau of Reclamation 309–311, 314
Bush (George H.) 78

"cap and trade" allowances 78
capital costs 201
carbon tax 78
Caro, Robert 19
case for analysis: short-term rentals 321–328; water shortages in lower and upper basins (Colorado River) 307–317, *315*
case studies 266–268; *see also* child support debt case study; voter participation case study
categorical measures 130, 132–136, 195–196
causation of problem, mapping 49
Center for Policy Research 99
central problem, identifying 37, 47–49, *48*, 56
child support: financial institution 79–80; function of 58; increased funding for genetic testing 80; share information and with-held for 58
child support debt case study 10, 231n3; Aid for Families with Dependent Children and 58; alternative policy options and 97–105; Automatic Collection System and **147**, 151, **151–152**, 152, **169–171**; automatic forgiveness of arrears due to incarceration 102–104; causation of problem and 49; causes of, common

59–61; child support enforcement policies and 41–42; Child Support Recovery Act and 41; Clean Slate option and 220; cost-benefit analysis and 168–169, **169–170**; cost-effectiveness analysis and 186–187, **188**; criteria and 110, 131, 133, 140–143; custodial parents/children 62–63, 229; data sources for 269–270, **270–271**; "deadbeat dads" and 4, 9, 41, 79; Deadbeat Parents Punishment Act and 41; debt leveraging and 98; defining the problem and 37–38, 40–43, 57–63; description of 4; discounting and 146–147, **147**; effectiveness assessment standard and 121; ethics and 297–299; Families Forward and 99–100; feasibility assessment standard and 123–125; Flexibility, Efficiency, and Modernization in Child Support Programs Final Rule and 10; function of child support and 58; government intervention and 79; impact of debt and 61; market failure and 43–45; Match Plus Outreach and 99–100, 104–105, 221–223, **223**; Medicaid and 58; noncustodial parents and 8–9, 41, 62; objectives and 109–110; Office of Child Support Enforcement and 58, 298; outcomes, comparison of 227–231, **228**; Participation Incentive Program and 98–99, 104, 219–220, **220**; Personal Responsibility and Work Opportunity Reconciliation Act and 8; prevalence of child support and 57–58; recap 97, 139–140, 218–219; recommendations for policy and 219–231; research and 237, **238–239**, 269–270, **270–271**; researching nature of the problem and 43–47; research plan and 237, **238–239**; Responsible Employed Active Loving program and 101; Responsible Fatherhood Project and 101; Scott case and 7, 37–38, 48; Social Security and 57; summary of 4, 7–10; Targeted Workforce Development Program and 147, **147**, 151, **151**, **152**, **169–170**; Temporary Assistance for Needy Families and 57, 58; trade-offs, weighing 227–231, **228**; unpaid child support debt and 8, 59, 63; Workforce Development alternative and 101–102, 105, 223–225, **224**

child support enforcement (CSE) policies 38, 41–42, 111, 146, 169

Child Support Recovery Act (1992) 41

civic duty 11–12; *see also* voter participation case study

Civil Rights Acts (1964) 33

civil rights movement 33

Clark, Jennifer J. 81

Clean Slate option 220

clearance points 17

client: alternative policy options and 71; criteria and, input on 112–116, *114*, *115*, 139; policy analysts as advocates of 15–16, 277; voter participation case study and 128

client advocates 15–16, 277

Clinton, Bill 41

Cobb, Roger W. 49, 53

co-creation 94–95

Code of Medical Ethics 288

Colorado River, water shortages in lower/upper basins 307–317, *315*

communication skills 296–297; audience and, knowing 284–285; brevity and 285–286; importance of 284; impression and, making good 287; organization and 285–286; outlines and 285; resources for oral and written 287; visual presentations and 286

comprehensiveness and criteria 117, 129–130, 139, 141

conditional cash transfer program *(Oportunidades)* (Mexico) 194–195

confirmation bias 84

Congressional Budget Office (CBO) 150

consequences, unintended 8–9, 205–206

Conservative–Liberal Democratic Coalition Government 86

INDEX

Consumer Price Index 202
contestable concept 242
contingent valuation 166–168
cost assessment standard 120, 125–127, 139, 201–202, 209
cost-benefit analysis (CBA): allocative efficiency and 59, 186; applying time value of money methods (Step 4) 168–175; assigning monetary values to costs and benefits (Step 3) 163–168; assumptions and, justifying 177–178; benefit-cost ratio and 176; bounded projection 190; bounding outcomes of 184; child support debt case study and 168–169, **169–170**; conducting 157; cost-effectiveness analysis as alternative to 186; critiques of 182, 185; defining 155, 157–160; determining who or what has standing (Step 1) 160; discounting in context of 172; distributive effects and, testing for 185–186; distributive justice and, omission of 185; dollar amount on priceless items, possibility of 178–181; efficiency assessment standard and 127; flexible use of 183–186; formula 157; forward-looking, uncertainty of 181–183; hedonic price models and 166; historical perspective of 155–156; human life and, valuing 179–180; identifying costs and benefits to include (Step 2) 160–163, 181; innovation of 157–158; internal rate of return and 173–174; intuition of 157; Kaldor Hicks criterion and 159; marginal valuation and 164; model of, fundamental 157; neoclassical economics and 158; overview 145–146, 155–157, 189–190; Pareto efficiency and 159; Pareto improvement and 159; practicing, challenges of 177–181; pragmatic use of 183–184; rationale behind 159; sensitivity analyses and 173–175; steps in 159–177; trade-offs and, weighing 214; using decision criterion for moving forward (Step 5) 175–177

cost-effectiveness analysis (CEA): as alternative to cost-benefit analysis 186; approaches to 187; child support debt case study and 186–187, **188**; environmental impact statement and 145; fixed budget approach to 187; fixed effectiveness approach to 187; measures of success and effectiveness and 186; multi-faceted approach to 188–189; overview 145–146, 189–190; supplementing, with other criteria 188–189; technical efficiency and 186; trade-offs and, weighing 214–215

costs: administrative 161; backloading 170; bearers of, considering 202; capital 201; delayed **172**; explicit 163; external 161; housing, US 260, **260–262**; identifying which to include 160–163, 181; implicit 163; internal 161; marginal 164; monetary value to, assigning 163–168; nominal 201; opportunity 163; per diem 165; primary 161–162; secondary 161–162; spillover 162; tragic 179

Cozzolino, Elizabeth 259
criminalization 76
criteria: alternatives and, confusing with 137; analytical matrix 138–139; background information 109; bias in analysis and 139; binary 208; bounding analysis and 137; categorical measures and 130, 132–136, 195–196; child support debt case study and 110, 131, 133, 140–143; client input on 112–113, *114*; combining several 119; comprehensiveness and 117, 129–130, 141; context and 112; cost assessment standard and 120, 125–127, 139; deciding on a set of 118–119; decision 175–177; defining 109–111; design thinking and 112–113; effectiveness assessment standard and 120–122, 131, 139; efficiency assessment standard and 120, 127–131, 139; eliminating from final analysis 119–120; equity assessment standard

and 120, 122–123, 139; evaluative 110; feasibility assessment standard and 120, 123–125, 139; formulating 112–116; function of 118; generic, as guideline 120–127; grading across 211; implementation of policy and 124–125; invariant, omitting 211–212; labels for, creating 131–133; measures 127, *132*, 132–137, 139; mutual exclusiveness and 117, 118, 129–130, 141; non-redundant 118, 139; objectives and 109–110, *110*, 131, *132*, 139–140; outcomes and, projected 133; overview 5–6, 137; for pedestrian safety 118; pitfalls of 138; proxy and 120; quantitative measures and 126, 132–134, 195–196, 209; reconciling measures across sub-criteria and 136; voter participation case study and 128–130; weighting 130, 138, 209

Dark Money (Mayer) 19–20
databases 257–263, **260**, **261**, 269
data sets 257–258, 269
"deadbeat dads" *see* child support debt case study
Deadbeat Parents Punishment Act (1998) 41
debt leveraging 98
decision criterion, using to move forward 175–177
decision trees 199
decriminalization 76
defining the problem: alternative models and 39–40; audience and, understanding 49–51; background information 37; causation of problem and, mapping 49; central problem and, identifying 37, 47–49, *48*, 56; child support debt case study and 37–38, 40–43, 57–63; context and 40–42; framing nature of the problem and, evidence for 53–55, 57–63; iterative and reflective process 56; Kingdon and 40; narratives and 39–40; norm-setting and 39; overview 5, 37–38, 56; policy analysis and, importance

of 56; probing nature of the problem 47; public attention and, dimensions for gaining 53–54; rational model and 38–39; related problems and, identifying 47, 48, 56; researching nature of the problem and 43–47; Stone and 39, 43; underlying problems and, identifying 47–48, *48*, 56; voter participation case study and 55; *see also* problem statement
delayed costs **172**
Department of Social Service 37, 57, 298
Dery, David 39
Design for Policy (Bason) 28
design thinking: as alternative model 26–28; alternative policy options and, insights from 93–96; criteria and 112–113; description of 26–28
discount factor 147
discounting: child support debt case study and 146–147, **147**; in cost-benefit analysis context 172; discount factor and 147; discount rate and 148–152, **151**, **152**, 169, 170, 172–174, **174**, 178; government agencies that most commonly use 150; importance of 146; intuition behind 146; long-term impacts and 178; net present value and 151; overview 145, 189–190; present value and 146–151, *149*, **151**, **152**; voter participation case study and 153–155, **155**
discount rate 148–152, **151**, **152**, 169, 170, 172–174, **174**, 178
distributive effects, testing for 185–186
distributive justice and cost-benefit analysis, omission of 185
documents: accuracy of, varied 241; advocacy organizations and 243; documents leading to 246; federal 244; finding relevant 243–247; non-peer-reviewed 242; peer-reviewed 244; people leading to 246–247; policy analysts' use of 240–243; qualitative context and 53; types of 240–241
dollar amount on priceless items, possibility of 178–181

dominated alternatives, eliminating **207**, 210–211, 217
double counting 162
Dunn, William N. 45, 283, 295

Earned Income Tax Credit 32
EAST (Easy, Attract, Social, Timely) framework 86–91, 198
Easy framework 86–89
economic efficiency 25
economics and rational model 24–26
effectiveness assessment standard 120–122, 196–201, 212
efficiency assessment standard 120, 127–131, 139
Emory, Allison D. 259
empathy 94, 113
employment of policy analysts: with client 16; as consultant 15–16; in new public service 276; in nonprofit sector 279–280; in private sector 280–282; in public sector 277–279; settings of, varied 276–279; themes of 276
environmental impact statement (EIS) 145
Environmental Protection Agency 33, 162
equitable outcome 122
equitable process 122
equity assessment standard 120, 122–123, 139, 202–203
equity, concept of 122–123
estimation *see* prediction
ethics: of American Bar Association 288; analyses *versus* practices and 289–291; challenges to incorporating into policy analysis 291–293; child support debt case study and 297–299; code for policy analysts and 288–289; fiduciary model of 291; personal model of 291; perspectives in considering 290; in policy analysis, implementing 293–296; principles of lifting up issues in policy analysis and 294–295; values and 288; voter participation case study and 293
evaluation of program 17

evidence-based policy analysis 1–3, 33, 304
evidence for framing nature of the problem 53–55
experimentation 95
explicit costs and benefits 163
exploratory inquiry 45
external costs and benefits 161
externalities 43, 161

fairness assessment standard 120, 122–123, 131, 139
Families Forward 99–100
FDsys (Federal Digital System) 244
feasibility assessment standard 120, 123–125, 139, 203–205; *see also* specific type
Federal Bureau of Reclamation Plan 310
fiduciary model of ethics 291
final policy analysis 216–217
financial assessment standard 120, 125–127
financial feasibility 120, 126–127, 143
Fischer, Frank 25, 288, 296
fixed budget approach 187
fixed effectiveness approach 187
Flexibility, Efficiency, and Modernization in Child Support Programs Final Rule (2016) 10
focus groups 247, 255–256, 269
food stamps *see* Supplemental Nutrition Assistance Program (SNAP)
forecasting error 182
Forester, John 288, 296
Fragile Families and Child Wellbeing Study 258–259
framework for policy analysis 3–4, 33; *see also* rational model
framing choices 83
framing the issue 53–55, 57–63
free riders 206
frontloading benefits 170
futures thinking 81

Garbage Can Model 40
gasoline taxes 78
Google Scholar 243

Gordon, Eric 95
Gorsuch, Neil 312
Government Accountability Office (GAO) 242, 244
government failure 45
government intervention, standard modes of 76–80, 96; *see also specific type*
grants 76
Greater Avenues for Independence (GAIN) (California) 73
greenhouse gas emissions, government intervention and 77–78
group interviews 247, 255–256

Haaland, Deb 308
Halpern, David 86–87, 89–92
Hambleton, Robin 92
Hammond, John S. **22**, 137
Hanf, Ruth 262
health care and insurance 77–79; insure health coverage directly 79; mandate and Medicaid expansion 78; stiffer penalties against parents 79; subsidies and regulations 78–79
hedonic price models 166
Heinzerling, Lisa 180, 185, 188–189
Heritage Foundation 241
Hobbs, Katie 307
Hobson's choice 68
homelessness problem 45–47; reducing 196, 199, *200*
horizontal equity 122
Housing and Community Development Representative 278
housing costs in United States 260, **260–262**
Huffington Post 242
human life, valuing 179–180
hybrid recommendations for policy 216

ideal solution, building off 81
IDEO (design firm) 80
impact categories *see* criteria
implementation of policy: criteria and 124–125; feasibility and 204; prediction and 205; program evaluation and studies of 17; robustness and ease of 204–205
implementation of program 16
implicit costs and benefits 163
imputed income 59–60
incarceration 102–104
inclusionary zoning 73–75
incremental changes to status quo 70–71
incremental policy analysis 24, 28–33
Independent Budge Office (New York City) 242
Inflation Reduction Act (2022) 313
information, imperfect 44
information sources: administrative data 261–262; agencies, research and statistical 244, **245**; budgets 259; databases 257–263, **260**, **261**, 269; data sets 257–258; focus groups 247, 255–256, 269; group interviews 247, 255–256; Internet searches 244, 246; public events 256–257; site visits 257, 269; social science data 262; surveys 263–266; think tanks 241, 242, **245**; *see also* documents; interviews
inheritance tax 68
in-person interviews 251–252
in-person surveys 266
inquiry, exploratory 45
Inside the Nudge Unit (Halpern) 86
inspections for cars 77
instinct, trusting 296
intergenerational equity 122–123
internal costs and benefits 161
internal rate of return (IRR) 173–174
Internet searches 244, 246
Inter-University Consortium for Political and Social Research (University of Michigan) 258
interviews: conducting 252–253; group 247, 255–256, 269; in-person 251–252; interviewees and 247–250; interviewers and, multiple 254–255; method of 251–252; phone 251–252; policy analysis and 247–250; preparing for 250–251; recording 253–254; writing up 254
invariant criteria, omitting 211–212

Jenkins-Smith, Hank 276
Johnson, Lyndon 19
Jones, Bryan 19, 32

Kahneman, Danny 81, 82, 84
Kaldor Hicks criterion 159
Kavanaugh, Brett 312
Kingdon, John 18, 40

legal feasibility 204
libertarian paternalism 85, 92
Library of Congress 244
Light, Paul 276
Lindblom, Charles 24, 26, 28–32, 70
Lipsky, Michael 124
literature reviews 53, 267, 269
Livermore, Michael A. 158, 178, 183
loss aversion 82–83
lower bound 184

MacRae, Duncan 160
mainstream perspectives of policy analysis 5; *see also* rational model
Majone, Giandomenico 39, 111, 283–284, 291
mandates 8, 78
marginal costs 164
marginal dollar 164
marginal valuation 164
market failures 43–45, 165
market prices 164–165
markets: for emissions 78; nonexistent or unpredictable 44
Match Plus Outreach 99–100, 104–105, 140, 218, 221–223, **223**, 229–230
Mayer, Jane 19
Mayor's Management Report (New York City) 261, 271n4
measurement error 182–183
measures: applying 139; bounding analysis and 137; categorical 132–136, 195–196; costs and benefits 160–163; quantitative 126, 132–134, 195–196, 209; reconciling across sub-criteria 136
Medicaid 58, 78–79
Medicare 79

microeconomics 23, 25
Microsoft Excel 148–149, *149*
Microsoft PowerPoint 216, 285–286
monetary values to costs and benefits, assigning 163–168
monopolies 44–45
moral hazards 44, 206
Mugar, Gabriel 95
multi-attribute trade-off approach 188–189
multiple advocacy 284
multiple criterion analysis 188–189
multiple streams 18
multiple variations of alternative policy options 73–75
mutual exclusiveness and criteria 117, 118, 129–130, 139, 141

nature of problem: framing 53–55; probing 47; researching 43–47
neoclassical economics 25, 33, 158
Nepomnyaschy, Lenna 259
net benefits 170, **171**, 172
net present value (NPV) 150, 151, 168–170, 173–178, **174**, 184
new public service 276
nominal costs 201
nonprofit sector, employment of policy analysts in 279–280
non-redundant criteria 118, 139
nonuse value 180
norm-setting 39
Nudge (Thaler and Sunstein) 85
nudge concept and limitations 84–85, 92–93
Nudge Unit (United Kingdom): EAST framework of 86–91, 198; establishment of 86; Halpern and 86; prototyping and 94; purpose of 86
Nussbaum, Martha 179

Obama Administration 10, 86, 103, 150, 156
objectives: child support debt case study and 109–110; client input on 112–113, *114*; context and 111; criteria and 109–110, *110*, 131, *132*,

139–140; defining 109; equity-oriented 112; maximizing 131; minimizing 131; overview 5, 139–140
objective technicians 276
Office of Child Support Enforcement (OCSE) 42, 58, 135, 269, 298
Office of Management and Budget (OMB) 150
oligopolies 45
omission error 182
online resources for job searches **283**
online survey platforms 264–265
online voter registration system 153, **155**
open data platforms 259
opportunity costs 163
optimism 84
Osborn, Alex 70
outcomes: child support debt case study 227–231, **228**; comparison of 193, 206–215, **207**, 217; criteria and projected 133; dominated alternatives and, eliminating **207**, 210–211, 217; equitable 122; grading across criteria and 211; invariant criteria and, omitting 211–212; prediction and most likely 194; trade-offs and, weighing 212–214, 217; *see also* prediction
outlines in communication 285
overconfidence 84

paradox in distributive problems 123
Pareto efficiency 159
Pareto improvements 159
Participation Incentive Program (PIP) 98–99, 104, 140, 219–220, **220**, 229–230
past policies addressing similar issues 71–72
Patashnik, Eric M. 21, **22**, 25–26, 45, 73, 204, 246
Patton, Carl V. **22**, 70, 71, 81, 290, 291, 295
per diem costs 165
personal model of responsibility 291
Personal Responsibility and Work Opportunity Reconciliation Act (1996) 8

phone interviews 251–252
policies in other places addressing similar issues 71
policies without constraints, imagining 81
policy adoption 19
policy advocates 276, 282–284
policy analysis: as applied research 235, 268; critiques of 3; defining 15–16; defining the problem and, importance of 56; design thinking and 26–28; ethical challenges 291–293, 297; ethical practices *versus* ethical 289–291; ethics and, implementing into 293–296; evidence-based 1–3, 33, 304; final 216–217; flexible 34; framework for 3–4, 33; framing problem and 3; incremental 24, 28–33; interviews and 247–250; iterative 34, 218; logic and 1, 303; mainstream perspectives of 5; multidisciplinary perspective of 2, 289; overview 5, 33–34; persuasive 34; policy making and 17–20; in policy process 16–20; practicing 304–306; preliminary 216–217; premises behind 1–2, 303; as problem solving 1; program evaluation *versus* 16–17; program implementation *versus* 17; stages of 21, 33; subjectivity of 111; supplemental cases 304–305; texts on 2–3; workshopping 217; *see also* implementation of policy; recommendations for policy; research in policy analysis; technical methods of policy analysis; specific model
policy analysts: in all sectors 276–282; challenges of incorporating ethics into policy analysis and 291–293; as client's advocates 15–16, 277; communication skills and 284–287, 296–297; conducting ethical policy analysis and 293–295; as consultants 15–16; documents used by 240–243; dominated and practically dominated alternatives 217; ethical analyses

versus ethical practices and 289–291; ethical code for 288–289; instinct and, trusting 296; latitude in decision-making 23; moral obligation 297; in new public service 276; in nonprofit sector 279–280; as objective technicians 276; online resources for job searches and **283**; overview 6–7, 275, 296–297; as policy advocates 276, 282–284; in private sector 280–282; professional positioning of 288–289; in public sector 277–279; recommendations for policy and 68, 193, 215–217; resources for building skills 7; roles of 276–277; satisfying minimum requirement and 209; standing in current analysis and 116; *see also* employment of policy analysts
policy change 18–19
policy entrepreneurs 18
policy implementation *see* implementation of policy
policy making 17–20; *see also* alternative policy options
policy monopolies 19
Policy Paradox (Stone) 39
policy process 16–20; *see also* policy analysis
policy recommendations *see* recommendations for policy
policy windows 18, 125
political campaigns 11, 326
political feasibility 81, 130, 143, 203–205, **207**, 213, 214, **226**, 229, 230, 237
political power 19
positivism 24–26
Posner, Richard A. 167
Practical Guide for Policy Analysis (Bardach and Patashnik) 25–26
practicing policy analysis 304–306
prediction: alternative policy options and 195; categorical measures and 195–196; challenges with 194–196; comparison of outcomes and 206–215, **207**, 217; cost assessment standard and 201–202, 209; decision trees and 199; effectiveness assessment standards and 196–201; equity assessment standard and 202–203; and estimation 194–205; feasibility assessment standard and 203–205; free riders and 206; implementation of policy and 205; limited information and 194–196; moral hazards and 206; outcomes and, most likely 194; probabilities and 200; quantitative measures and 195–196; recommendations for policy and 193–205; rent seeking and 206; sensitivity analyses and 205; uncertainty and 199; unintended consequences and 205–206
preliminary policy analysis 216–217
present value (PV) 146–151, *149*, **151**, **152**, 168, 201
Pressman, Jeffrey 17, 124
Priceless (Ackerman and Heinzerling) 180
priceless items, possibility of putting dollar amount on 178–181
prices: contingent 166; hedonic price models and 166; market 164–165; shadow 165
primary costs and benefits 161–162
private sector, employment of policy analysts in 280–282
probabilities 200
probing the nature of the problem 47
problem definition *see* defining the problem
problem sensing 45
problem solving: framing problem and 3–4; government recognition of problem and 18; multiple streams and 18; policy analysis as 1; *see also* defining the problem
problem statement: analytically manageable 51–52; articulating 51–52, 56; concise and digestible 51; establishing 37, 40–52; meticulously

worded 51; non-prescriptive 52; open-ended 52; pitfalls 52; *see also* defining the problem
program evaluation 16–17
program implementation 16–17
projected outcomes and criteria 133; *see also* prediction
projection *see* prediction
Protecting Homeowner Rights and Independence (PHORI) 323
prototyping 95–96
proxy 120
public attention to problem, gaining 53–54
public events 256–257, 269
public goods 43–44
public sector, employment of policy analysts in 277–279
Punctuated Equilibrium Theory (PET) 19, 32

qualitative data 53
quantitative criteria 195–196, 209
quantitative data 53
quantitative measures 126, 132–134, 195–196, 209
questionnaires 264

rationality 21, 23
rational model: alternative models and 21, **22**; cognitive limits of 24; critiques of 23–26; defining the problem and 38–39; design thinking and 23–26; economics and 27; flexible use of 33–34; framework of 20–21; incrementalist model and 28–33; open-ended 34; overview 16; positivism and 24–26; rationality and 23; texts on policy analysis and 2–3
recommendations for policy: alternative policy options and 67; child support debt case study and 219–231; choices of 216; final policy analysis and 216–217; hybrid 216; making formal 20, 216; outcomes and, comparing 206–215, **207**; overview 6, 193, 217–218; policy analysis and 20; policy analysts and 68, 193, 215–217; prediction and 193–205; preliminary policy analysis and 216–217; ranking 218; uncertainty and 194
Reflective systems 82
regression analysis 166
regulation 77–79
related problems, identifying 47, 48, 56
rent seeking 206
representativeness 84
research agencies 244, **245**, 259
researching nature of the problem 43–47
research in policy analysis: agencies and, statistical and research 244, **245**; best practices and 266–269; budgets 259; case studies and 266–269; child support debt case study and 237, **238–239**, 269–270, **270–271**; databases 257–263, **260**, **261**, 269; data sets and 257–258, 269; documents and 240–243; focus groups and 247, 255–256, 269; interviews and 247–256, 268; literature reviews and 268; overview 6, 268–269; people and 246–247; public events and 256–257, 269; purpose of 235–236; research in other fields *versus* 236; research plan and 236–240, **237–238**; role of 235–236; site visits and 257, 269; surveys and 263–266, 269
research plan 236–240, **238–239**, 268
Responsible Employed Active Loving (R.E.A.L.) program (Westchester, NY) 101
Responsible Fatherhood Project program (Baltimore) 101–102
return on investment (ROI) 176
Revesz, Richard L. 158, 178, 183
robustness 204
Rochefort, David A. 49, 53
Roth, Bernard 27–28

Sabatier, Paul 19
same-sex marriage issue 33

satisfying minimum requirement 209
Sawicki, David S. 81
Schick, Allen 283, 294
"Science of Muddling Through, The" (Lindblom) 28, 70
Scott, Walter 7, 37–38, 48, **270**
secondary costs and benefits 161–162
Sen, Amartya 160, 167
sensitivity analyses 168, 173–174, 205
service provision 261
shadow prices 165
short-term rentals 321–328
Simon, Herbert A. 24, 30, 38
site visits 257, 269
Smith, Hank Jenkins 19, 276
Social framework 90, 198
social movements 33
social networks 12
social return on investment (SROI) 156
social science data 262
Social Security Act 58
Sorensen, Elaine 61
spillover costs 162
staff time, converting into dollars 202
stagist methodology 23
stakeholders *see* client
standing, determining who or what has 159, 160
State Elections Legislative Database 263
State's Child Support Program 104
statistical agencies 244, **245**
status quo 70; incremental changes to 70–71
status quo bias 82
Stiglitz, Joseph 159
Stokey, Edith **22**, 150, 177
Stone, Deborah 25, 31, 39, 43, 68, 111, 123, 178
subsidies 76, 78, 79, 85, 87
Sunstein, Cass 82, 83, 85, 92, 93, 180, 183–185
supplemental cases 304–305
Supplemental Environmental Impact Statement (SEIS) 310, 311, 313
Supplemental Nutrition Assistance Program (SNAP) 32, 50

surveys 263–266, 269
System 1 82
System 2 82

Targeted Workforce Development Program **147**, **151**, **152**, **169–172**, **174**, **188**
taxation 68, 76
tax credits 32, 78
technical efficiency 186
technical feasibility 123–125
technical methods of policy analysis: background information 145; cost-benefit analysis 145, 155–186; cost-effectiveness analysis 145, 186–189; discounting 145–155; overview 6, 145–146; *see also* specific method
Temporary Assistance for Needy Families (TANF) 58, 231n4
Thaler, Richard 82, 83, 85, 92
think tanks 20, 241, 242, 245
time inconsistent preferences 91
Timely framework 90–91, 198
time value of money methods, applying 168–175; *see also* discounting
Tong, Rosemarie 275, 291
trade-offs, weighing 212–214, 217, 227–231, **228**
traditional model 16, 28
tragic costs 179
transaction costs, high 44
Turetsky, Vicki 103
Tversky, Amos 81, 84

Um, Hyunjoon 259
uncertainty 181–183, 190, 194, 199, 217
underlying problems, identifying 47–48, *48*, 56
unintended consequences 4, 8, 205–206
United Hotel Owners Association 321
unpaid child support debt *see* child support debt case study
up-front benefits **172**
upper bound 184
Urban Policy Lab (New School) 257

US Census Bureau 258, 262
US Election Assistance Commission 263

valuation error 182
Vera Institute for Justice 150
vertical equity 122
Vining, Aidan R. **22**
visual presentations 286–287
voter ID laws 4
voter participation case study: barriers to voting and, legal and institutional 12; civic duty and 11; client and 128; criteria and 128–130; databases on 263; defining the problem and 55; description of 4–5; discounting and 153–155, **155**; EAST framework and 86–91; ethics and 293; online registration system and 153, **155**; outcomes and, comparing 206, **207**, 210; political campaigns and 11; social networks and 12; summary of 3–4, 10–12; trade-offs and, weighing 212–214, 217; voter ID laws and 4; Voter Rights Act and 4
Voter Rights Act (2013) 4
voting policy, dueling views on 241

Waller, Maureen R. 103
water shortages, lower and upper basins (Colorado River) 307–317, *315*
weighing trade-offs 212–214, 217, 227–231, **228**
weighting criteria 130, 138, 209
Weimer, David L. **22**
welfare reform act 8, 58
welfare-to-work programs 73
Whittington, Dale 160
Wikipedia 242
Wildavsky, Aaron 17, 124
willingness-to-accept (WTA) 167
willingness-to-pay (WTP) 26, 166–167
willingness-to-sell (WTS) 167
Workforce Development alternative 101–102, 105, 140, 152, 218, 223–225, **224**, 229–230
workshopping policy analysis 217

Zeckhauser, Richard **22**, 150, 177
Zerbe, Richard O., Jr. 160
zoning, inclusionary 73–75
Zoom (videoconferencing) 247, 252, 255